Health and Human Development Series

ALCOHOL-RELATED COGNITIVE DISORDERS: RESEARCH AND CLINICAL PERSPECTIVES

HEALTH AND HUMAN DEVELOPMENT SERIES

JOAV MERRICK, EDITOR

Adolescent Behavior Research: International Perspectives
Joav Merrick and Hatim A. Omar
2007. ISBN: 1-60021-649-8

Complementary Medicine Systems: Comparison and Integration
Karl W. Kratky
2008 ISBN 978-1-60456-475-4

Pain in Children and Youth
Patricia Schofield and Joav Merrick
2008 ISBN 978-1-60456-951-3

Obesity and Adolescence: A Public Health Concern
Hatim A. Omar, Donald E. Greydanus, Dilip R. Patel and Joav Merrick
2009 ISBN 978-1-60456-821-9

Health and Happiness from Meaningful Work: Research in Quality of Working Life
Søren Ventegodt and Joav Merrick
2009 ISBN 978-1-60692-820-2

Behavioral Pediatrics 3rd Edition
Donald E. Greydanus, Dilip R. Patel, Helen D. Pratt and Joseph L. Calles, Jr.
2009. ISBN: 978-1-60692-702-1

Poverty and Children: A Public Health Concern
Alexis Lieberman and Joav Merrick
2009 ISBN 978-1-60741-140-6

Living on the Edge: The Mythical, Spiritual, and Philosophical Roots of Social Marginality
Joseph Goodbread
2009. ISBN 978-1-60741-162-8

Alcohol-Related Cognitive Disorders: Research and Clinical Perspectives
Leo Sher, Isack Kandel and Joav Merrick (Editors)
2009. ISBN 978-1-60741-730-9

Health and Human Development Series

ALCOHOL-RELATED COGNITIVE DISORDERS: RESEARCH AND CLINICAL PERSPECTIVES

LEO SHER, ISACK KANDEL
AND JOAV MERRICK
EDITORS

Nova Science Publishers, Inc.
New York

NOTICE TO THE READER

The Publisher has taken reasonable care in the preparation of this book, but makes no expressed or implied warranty of any kind and assumes no responsibility for any errors or omissions. No liability is assumed for incidental or consequential damages in connection with or arising out of information contained in this book. The Publisher shall not be liable for any special, consequential, or exemplary damages resulting, in whole or in part, from the readers' use of, or reliance upon, this material.

Independent verification should be sought for any data, advice or recommendations contained in this book. In addition, no responsibility is assumed by the publisher for any injury and/or damage to persons or property arising from any methods, products, instructions, ideas or otherwise contained in this publication.

This publication is designed to provide accurate and authoritative information with regard to the subject matter covered herein. It is sold with the clear understanding that the Publisher is not engaged in rendering legal or any other professional services. If legal or any other expert assistance is required, the services of a competent person should be sought. FROM A DECLARATION OF PARTICIPANTS JOINTLY ADOPTED BY A COMMITTEE OF THE AMERICAN BAR ASSOCIATION AND A COMMITTEE OF PUBLISHERS.

LIBRARY OF CONGRESS CATALOGING-IN-PUBLICATION DATA

Alcohol-related cognitive disorders : research and clinical perspectives / [edited by] Leo Sher, Isack Kandel, Joav Merrick.
    p. ; cm.
  Includes bibliographical references and index.
  ISBN 978-1-60741-730-9 (hardcover : alk. paper)
 1. Alcoholism--Complications. 2. Fetal alcohol syndrome. 3. Cognition disorders. I. Sher, Leo. II. Kandel, Isack, 1960- III. Merrick, Joav, 1950-
  [DNLM: 1. Alcohol-Related Disorders--complications. 2. Alcohol-Induced Disorders, Nervous System. 3. Cognition Disorders--etiology. 4. Fetal Alcohol Syndrome. WM 274 A352595 2009]
  RC565.A44425 2009
  362.292--dc22   2009015101

Published by Nova Science Publishers, Inc. ✢ New York

CONTENTS

PREFACE

This book discusses the different mental and physical aspects of alcohol abuse, including prenatal fetal intoxication. It explores the many types of social behavior affected by the excessive use of alcohol and the physical repercussions of this syndrome. It covers a vast variety of alcohol related conditions by many select consultants in this field. Alcohol addiction is one of the major disorders encompassing society world round. Its devastating effect on social stability and inter-personal relationships requires aggressive treatment and new ways to evoke the eventual success of sobriety.

A book of this magnitude should prove helpful to students, laymen, and professionals in the medical and mental health field.

Chapter 1 - Fetal Alcohol Spectrum Disorders (FASDs) represent a continuum of development disabilities associated with maternal consumption of alcohol during pregnancy. This spectrum of disorders, which includes the Fetal Alcohol Syndrome (FAS), is characterized by a wide range of physical, cognitive, and behavioral impairments. Estimates of the number of live births in the United States meeting criteria for a diagnosis of FAS range from .5 to 2 infants per 1,000, with the prevalence of the entire continuum of FASDs estimated to be 1 in 100. This chapter discusses some of the complexities involved in diagnosing individuals affected by prenatal alcohol exposure, provides a review of the neurocognitive and neurobehavioral deficits commonly seen in this population, and examines how such deficits may manifest during different developmental periods across the life span. Additionally, strategies for assessing these deficits are described, and specific measures that are appropriate for alcohol-exposed individuals are presented. The challenges of working with this under-identified and underserved population are highlighted, as well as the importance of early diagnosis and intervention.

Chapter 2 - While structural information regarding anatomical abnormalities found in the brains of individuals with fetal alcohol syndrome (FAS) and fetal alcohol spectrum disorders (FASD) has been thoroughly investigated, few functional neuroimaging studies have been performed. The major structural anomalies are outlined and the results of the functional neuroimaging studies are described in detail. Links between the anatomical region of impairment, functional impairment, and the cognitive dysfunction found in FASD are proposed. A literature search revealed only five studies of functional neuroimaging in individuals with FASD. One study used positron emission tomography (PET), three used single photon emission computed tomography (SPECT), and one used functional magnetic resonance imaging (fMRI) to evaluate brain metabolism and function. Of these, only fMRI actually examined task-related functional changes in the brain related to cognition. Although there is significant variability in the results, due to the heterogeneity of the syndrome and the few studies performed to date, clear regions of impairment related to cognitive dysfunction are described. The most consistent results involve the impairment of the frontal cortex, specifically the prefrontal cortex and medial frontal lobe, which is related to executive function, working memory, response inhibition, and attention. Consistent impairment was also noted in the temporal brain region, implicated in problems with emotions, memory, learning, and language functions.

Chapter 3 - Studies examining maternal alcohol consumption during pregnancy have mainly examined the effects on the individual after birth. The observation of the fetus during pregnancy, the time period of exposure, can enable a better understanding of the effects of alcohol on the fetus. Because the behavior of the fetus is directly reflective of the functioning of its central nervous system, the effect of alcohol on neural system functioning and integrity may be assessed. This chapter reviews the few studies that have examined the effects of alcohol on the behavior of the human fetus. Studies reveal that chronic and acute alcohol exposure influences behavior and, significantly, at lower doses than are considered important when evaluating effects after birth. There appears to be a dose-dependent effect, and the influence of alcohol on the behavior of the fetus persists after alcohol has been cleared from the mother's blood stream. Possible mechanisms of action include a direct effect of alcohol on the developing nervous system; and, an indirect effect of alcohol induced disruption of normal behavioral patterns central to the development of the brain and CNS. Observing the fetus's behavior may thus enable the mechanisms underlying alcohol-induced effects on the individual to be better understood.

Chapter 4 - Fetal Alcohol Spectrum Disorder (FASD) is a prevalent preventable disorder with a significant societal burden related to the cognitive and behavioral disabilities associated with this disorder. This chapter reviews published work on FASD diagnosis, surveillance and screening programs. Challenges inherent to FASD diagnosis remain, and complicate attempts to estimate FAS prevalence. In addition, the drive toward diagnostic accuracy has led to formulation of screening protocols for children at school ages after many disabilities associated with FASD are established.

The authors present the design and selected findings from a regional multi-stage screening project piloted in Wisconsin. Small for gestational age (SGA) newborns with birth head circumference less than 10th percentile were selected in the first screening stages. Those meeting these criteria were evaluated for growth, development and FAS facial features at about two years of age. Of newborns meeting the initial screening criteria, 30% demonstrated growth deficits and developmental delays at about 2 years of age. Children with any FAS facial feature (of 177 children assessed, n=13 with 2 or 3 facial findings, n=77 with one facial finding) showed greater deficits in growth and a greater proportion were developmentally delayed. These findings demonstrate the potential value of embedding screening for FAS within a multistage screening method to identify infants at risk for developmental delay. Because this model would be a part of larger population screening for developmental delay, cost efficiencies could be achieved. Problems relating to protection and confidentiality that inevitably accompany screening to identify FASD would also be reduced in a screening model that focuses on identification of children at risk for developmental delay rather than confirmation of the etiologic source of the delays.

Chapter 5 - Prenatal exposure to alcohol can lead to long-term impairments in cognition and behavior and represents a major public health concern. This chapter reviews studies examining the social and behavioral functioning of individuals with prenatal alcohol exposure. Social and behavioral functioning are important domains for study because deficits in these areas can lead to problems in everyday functioning and to maladjustment in later life. Most research with individuals with prenatal alcohol exposure has used caregiver or self-report questionnaires or semi-structured interviews to sample behavior. The vast majority of studies indicate significant difficulties with interpersonal functioning, internalizing and externalizing behavior problems, and high rates of psychopathology. Recent intervention studies conducted with individuals with prenatal alcohol exposure have shown promising results in improving the social skills and behavioral functioning in this population. Finally, this chapter concludes with recommendations for future studies in this area.

Chapter 6 - This chapter will discuss relevant issues in the diagnosis of mental disorders comorbid with fetal alcohol spectrum disorders (FASD). The authors present a theoretical model of the effect of prenatal alcohol exposure on neurobehavioral development and a systematic review of published data on the mental disorders in subjects with an FASD. They have found that prenatal alcohol exposure is associated with high rates of mental disorders, 48 papers reporting on 3,343 subjects. The most common mental disorder comorbid with FASD is attention deficit - hyperactivity disorder occurring in 48% of subjects with FASD. Cognitive impairment is also very common. It appears that prenatal alcohol exposure have differential effects on outcomes leading to large increases in rates of some, but apparently not most mental disorders. The authors discuss strategies to improve the diagnosis of mental disorders in FASD and the multiplicity of uses for this important data.

Chapter 7 - Prenatal alcohol exposure can result in life-long primary and secondary disabilities in affected individuals. Adolescents with Fetal Alcohol Spectrum Disorder (FASD) and/or prenatal alcohol exposure display high rates of many risky behaviors. In this chapter, the authors review the risky behaviors common in adolescents with FASD, including trouble with the law, delinquency, substance abuse, disrupted school experience and dropping out of school, inappropriate sexual behavior, suicidality, psychopathology, and maladaptive behavior. Next, they review factors that are related to high risk behaviors in individuals with FASD, which include executive functioning deficits, impaired decision making, and abnormalities of the prefrontal cortex. Finally, we discuss why adolescence is a period of increased risk taking and poor decision making, and how individuals with FASD are particularly vulnerable during adolescence.

Chapter 8 - Fetal Alcohol Spectrum Disorders (FASDs) currently represent the leading cause of mental retardation in North America, ahead of Downs syndrome and cerebral palsy. The damaging effects of alcohol on the developing brain have a cascading impact on the social and neurocognitive profiles of affected individuals. Researchers investigating the profiles of children with FASD have found impairments in learning and memory, executive functioning, and language, as well as hyperactivity, impulsivity, poor communication skills, difficulties with social and moral reasoning, and psychopathology. The primary goal of this chapter is to examine current issues pertaining to the identification of a behavioural phenotype in FASD, as well as addressing related screening and diagnostic concerns. The authors conclude that future research initiatives comparing children with FASD to non-alcohol exposed children with similar cognitive and socioemotional profiles should aid in uncovering the unique behavioural phenotype for FASD.

Chapter 9 - Alcohol is arguably the most widely used and studied drug in human history. The acute effects of alcohol in humans have been studied in laboratories for over a century.

Much of the interest in alcohol concerns its debilitating effects on human performance. Originally this interest was fueled by well-founded concerns that alcohol could impair the drinker's ability to operate an automobile. Before the advent of breath analysis devices, "road-side" behavioral tests of motor coordination and mental ability were the only means of detecting "impaired drivers". Thus there was much interest in discerning which aspects of human behavior were most disrupted by a given dose of alcohol. This chapter concerns the acute impairing effects of alcohol on cognitive functions in healthy, non-alcohol dependent adults. The chapter begins by describing how different aspects of human performance are not equally sensitive to the impairing effects of alcohol and that the wealth of research on these differences poses unique challenges for summarizing and communicating this large body of evidence. The chapter then discusses speeded and divided attention tasks as methods commonly used to assess the acute cognitive impairing effects of alcohol and the cognitive theories that have been offered to account for the findings based on these tasks. This is followed by a review of more contemporary methods and techniques that focus on how the drug impairs specific cognitive mechanisms that underlie the control and regulation of behavior. The chapter concludes by explaining how acute impairments of such mechanisms might actually contribute to the abuse potential of alcohol for some individuals.

Chapter 10 - In this chapter the authors examine the influence of acute alcohol on attentional lapses whilst performing a sustained attention task (SART). The sample consisted of 17 male and seven females. A dose of alcohol achieving 80mg/100ml was administered to subjects before completion of the task. Alcohol led participants to make more errors as the session progressed and report a greater incidence of mind wandering. Importantly, alcohol reduced individuals' ability to recover from a lapse in attention. Although the sample size is small, the study did enable the authors to gain insight into the detrimental effects of acute alcohol ingestion on mind wandering. The authors anticipate that through the use of thought probes in the context of the SART and a larger sample size, they hope to shed further light on this phenomenon.

Chapter 11 - This chapter is a secondary analysis of acute alcohol effects on intrusion errors in social drinkers in immediate free recall and delayed free recall tasks. The authors' aim was to examine further the mechanism through which intrusion errors occur in delayed recall. Intrusion errors occur when individuals produce information that is not relevant to the task. Previous research suggests that alcoholics are less able than controls to inhibit intrusions (a reflective cognitive function) under both no-intoxication and acute benzodiazepine Halcion intoxication conditions. They hypothesized that acute alcohol intoxication in social drinkers would cause more intrusion errors reflecting impaired reflective cognitive function in the delayed, compared to the immediate, free recall task. Twenty-two (11 male) volunteers participated in two counterbalanced sessions (alcohol, no-alcohol). In the alcohol session, free recall tasks were completed at blood alcohol concentrations between 80-84 mg/dl. Results showed that participants committed significantly more intrusion errors in a delayed recall task during acute alcohol intoxication compared to their no alcohol performance level. In contrast, in the immediate free recall task, participants' number of intrusion errors did not differ between alcohol and no-alcohol conditions. The authors suggest that by increasing the susceptibility to interference, acute alcohol intoxication caused more intrusion errors in the delayed, than in the immediate free recall task. Finally, the implications of these results in terms of alcohol prevention and intervention are suggested.

Chapter 12 - This chapter describes an experiment designed to examine the effects of caffeine expectancy on intentional control of behavior under alcohol. A process dissociation paradigm was used to measure the separate influence of automatic and intentional controlled processes on performance of a word-stem completion task. Forty social drinkers studied a list of words, received either alcohol or a placebo, and then performed a word-stem completion task designed to measure intentional control of behavior. Before performing the task, two groups (i.e., one alcohol and one placebo group) also received decaffeinated coffee, which has been shown effectively to establish caffeine expectancy. The results indicated that the expectation of receiving caffeine was sufficient to counteract the impairment of intentional control seen under alcohol. Those individuals who received both alcohol and decaffeinated coffee demonstrated better intentional control than those who received alcohol alone. Moreover, the performance of the alcohol-decaffeinated coffee group did not differ from placebo. No treatment significantly affected automatic processes. The expectation of receiving caffeine under alcohol was sufficient to counteract the impairing effects of the drug.

Chapter 13 - With the widespread use of alcohol in our society, research on the effects of alcohol on memory has clinical importance. In addition, an investigation of the amnesia produced by alcohol can be a powerful tool for elucidating normal and abnormal memory mechanisms. The purpose of this chapter was to provide a review of placebo-controlled laboratory studies of the acute effects of alcohol administration on memory in healthy adult social drinkers. Acute alcohol administration impairs working memory, episodic memory, and semantic memory, but does not appear to impair implicit memory or automatic, non-conscious memory processes. Alcohol produces relatively greater impairment of episodic memory encoding than retrieval processes. Whereas episodic memory is impaired following acute alcohol administration (anterograde amnesia), episodic memory for information presented prior to alcohol administration is enhanced under certain conditions (retrograde facilitation). Although extensive research has been conducted on the acute effects of alcohol on memory, many interesting questions surrounding the effects of alcohol on memory (e.g., the selectivity of alcohol's effects on different working memory processes; the conditions under which episodic memory retrieval is impaired; the mechanisms underlying retrograde facilitation; the effects of ascending versus descending blood levels on different memory processes), as well as the relationship between memory effects and emotion/mood, remain to be explored. Further hypothesis-driven memory research with alcohol using behavioral and neuroimaging techniques has the potential both to enhance the understanding of the clinical implications of alcohol use and to elucidate basic cognitive and brain mechanisms.

Chapter 14 - Driving and flying are common ways of transportation. The impairing effects of alcohol intoxication on driving and flying skills have been extensively studied. It has been shown that driving and flying skills are impaired in a dose-dependent manner. Public health campaigns have drawn attention to the dangers of drunk driving and strict flying rules regarding alcohol use have been established. In contrast, driving and flying during alcohol hangover (ie, when blood alcohol concentrations are zero) received relatively little scientific attention. A literature review was performed to identify all clinical trials that examined the impact of alcohol hangover on driving and flying. The few studies that have been published (N=11) showed that driving performance and flying during alcohol hangover were significantly impaired. Public health campaigns should therefore point at the risks of driving the day after a heavy drinking session and flying regulations should adopt a strict zero alcohol policy.

Chapter 15 - Studies on cognitive functions in alcoholism have reported a range of deficits affecting, among other domains, executive functions, and social cognition. The impairment pattern is consistent with the so-called frontal lobe hypothesis, which asserts a specific vulnerability of the prefrontal cortex to the neurotoxic effects of alcohol. This chapter aims to give an overview of the neuropsychological profile relating to executive functions and social cognition in alcoholism by reviewing both patient and functional neuroimaging studies. The implications of such impairments for the therapy of alcoholism will also be addressed.

Chapter 16 - Etiological models for alcohol use disorders have traditionally proposed trait and cognitive explanations for initiation, maintenance, and dependence. Numerous studies have shown that heavy drinkers and subjects suffering from alcohol dependence have reduced performance on neurocognitive tests compared with controls. Alcohol dependence is an important risk factor for suicidal behavior. The large population of individuals with alcohol dependence, the relative frequency of suicides and suicide-related behaviors in this population, and the devastating effects of attempted and completed suicides on individuals, families, and society make this an important area for research. Data suggest that neuropsychological dysfunction may play a role in determining risk for suicidal acts. Suicide attempters have been characterized as "cognitively rigid" based on self-ratings and performance on mental flexibility tasks. Depressed subjects with a history of high-lethality suicide attempts exhibited deficits in executive functioning that were independent of deficits associated with depression alone. Alcohol use disorders are associated with both cognitive impairment and suicidal behavior. It is possible that cognitive abnormalities contribute to increased suicidality in individuals with alcohol use disorders. Future studies of the role of cognitive abnormalities in the pathophysiology of suicidal behavior are merited.

Chapter 17 - Long lasting or excessive alcohol consumption can result in alcoholic Korsakoff syndrome, characterized by severe anterograde and also retrograde memory deficits, as well as impairments in temporal orientation. In addition, further neuropsychological reductions can accompany the syndrome. Executive dysfunctions and emotional abnormalities are commonly reported in patients with Korsakoff's pathology but also seen in non-amnesic subjects with alcohol dependency. In patients with Korsakoff syndrome, the additional deficits mentioned are most commonly less severely pronounced than are amnesic symptoms. For the cognitive decline in patients suffering from this disease, damage to diencephalic and prefrontal brain regions are the most prominent neural correlates. Most likely, lesions within the mammillary bodies and parts of the thalamus are responsible for memory deterioration, whereas prefrontal damage primarily contributes to executive dysfunctions. Still a topic of debate is whether the direct alcoholic neurotoxic effects cause the brain changes in patients with Korsakoff's pathology or whether malnutrition and thiamine deficiency, potentially influenced by a genetic predisposition, are more strongly related to the diencephalic lesions that might be specific for Korsakoff syndrome. In the course of the disease, evidence suggests that cognitive impairments remain more or less stable over time. Therefore, the syndrome can be viewed as a single entity and it does not necessarily result in alcohol-related dementia.

Chapter 18 - Alcoholism may result in impaired cognition and dementia. The increased risk of dementia in older individuals interferes with the differential diagnosis, especially when an elderly patient with a long history of alcohol abuse is the case. The aim of the chapter is to evaluate the diagnostic value of the putative cerebrospinal fluid (CSF) biomarkers tau (τ), β-

amyloid 1–42 (Aβ42) and their ratio in differentiating alcohol related dementia (ARD) from others of vascular or degenerative aetiology. Double-sandwich ELISAs (Innotest htau antigen and β-Amyloid (1–42), Innogenetics) were used to quantify the above markers in a total of 151 patients and 82 controls. Patient groups comprised: 24 ARD, 17 vascular dementia, 11 dementia with Lewy bodies, 23 frontotemporal dementia and 76 Alzheimer's disease (AD) patients. Tau protein succeessfully differentiated ARD from AD with 88% specificity and 86% sensitivity. Aβ42 alone had a specificity of 86% and a sensitivity of 70%, while tau/Aβ42 ratio was better than τ alone with corresponding values 100% and 91% respectively. For the discrimination of ARD from other dementias the diagnostic value of the above markers is substantially lower. In conclusion, the combined use of CSF τ and Aβ42 seems to be a useful tool in the differential diagnosis of ARD from AD, while in other primary dementias only a positive result may be useful.

Chapter 19 – The authors examined the relationships between alcohol use, cognitive and affective variables, and the potential differential benefits of training for older adults drinkers and non-drinkers who participated in a randomized trial implemented between 2001-2006. Participants, who were living independently in the community, were randomly assigned to either twelve hours of memory training or health promotion classes. Outcomes included depression, health, cognition, verbal, visual, memory, and performance-based IADLs. The sample was 79% female, 17% Hispanic and 12% African-American. The typical participant had an average age of 75 years with 13 years of education. In the memory intervention group, there were 135 individuals (63 drinkers, 72 non-drinkers). In the health promotion condition, there were 129 individuals (58 drinkers and 71 non-drinkers). At baseline, drinkers scored higher on cognition, verbal memory, and lower on depression than non-drinkers. Alcohol use was positively related to physical health at baseline as measured by the Physical Component Summary Score of the Medical Outcomes Health Scale (SF-36).

The authors found significant effects for the time*drinking*treatment group interaction in the repeated measures ANCOVA for the Mini Mental Status Examination, the Hopkins Verbal Learning Test, and the SF-36 Mental Health sub-scale. The time*drinking*group interactions were not statistically significant for any of the other outcomes. This study demonstrated that older adults benefited from targeted psychosocial interventions on affective, cognitive and functional outcomes.

In addition, the SeniorWISE study provides empirical support to the research evidence emphasizing the health benefits of moderate alcohol consumption in older adults.

Chapter 20 - The aim of this chapter is to discuss how acute and chronic alcohol consumption affects on cognitive functions. In general, greater deficits in executive functions compared with other cognitive functions have been reported in patients suffering from alcohol addiction with deficits in problem solving, abstraction, planning, organizing and working memory. The acute effects of alcohol cause a decline in explicit memory processes. Alcohol impairs memory formation, at least in part, by disrupting activity in the hippocampus. Persisting neuropsychological deficits after cessation of alcohol consumption may lead to alcohol amnestic disorder and dementia associated with alcoholism. Considerable inconsistencies in neuropsychological study results will be discussed referring to variations in methodological designs such as amount of alcohol assumed or length of alcohol abuse. Despite advances in human neuroimaging techniques, detecting clear relations between brain structures and specific cognitive functions has so far been difficult.

Chapter 21 - Both human immunodeficiency virus (HIV) and alcohol use contribute to neuropsychological (NP) impairment, and a relatively large proportion of HIV seropositive individuals have histories of heavy alcohol use. Evidence from neuropathological, and both structural and functional neuroimaging studies have supported the direct central nervous system effects of both HIV and alcohol. HIV preferentially affects frontal regions of the brain as well as subcortical structures including the basal ganglia, while alcohol has been shown to result in cortical atrophy and cerebellar and frontal damage. These central nervous system changes are clinically manifested through psychomotor slowing, memory impairments, slowed reaction time, and executive dysfunction in persons with HIV. Alcohol use and abuse are associated with similar deficits as well as dysfunction in domains including visuoperception. While some studies have observed a synergistic effect between alcohol and HIV on NP performance, particularly reaction time, this has not been consistent. Whether HIV and alcohol exert purely independent, additive or interactive NP effects remains unresolved, and this may in part be due to methodological issues inherent in the measurement of alcohol use, comorbidities such as substance use, and other co-factors, such as socioeconomic status and neurologic history. The picture of NP decline due to HIV continues to evolve in the era of highly active antiretroviral therapy (HAART), and it is still unclear whether such changes will mitigate the impact of alcohol on NP functioning in persons with HIV.

Chapter 22 - Ancient scripture and paintings together with several medical reports on the effect of alcohol on the newborn over the past three hundred years finally led to the description of the fetal alcohol syndrome in the 1970s by French and American research groups. Maternal alcohol abuse during pregnancy can result in the specific pattern of malformations and neurocognitive deficits characteric of this syndrome. Diagnostic criteria and classifications have been developed and in the 1990s reports showed the long term consequences for these children. In recent years several studies from different countries have shown that prenatal alcohol exposure will lead to life long consequences on physical development, intellectual development, behavior, social development, occupation, independence, sexuality or sexual behavior and increased risk of suicidality. In this review of long-term observation studies we found that the prenatal exposure to alcohol have permanent and life long damage, which impair both the social and occupational future of the person exposed with a need for life long assistance in order for that person to function at an optimal level. Primary prevention and early intervention with general public health educational efforts seems to be the best way forward.

In: Alcohol-Related Cognitive Disorders
Editors: L. Sher, I. Kandel, J. Merrick pp. 1-2

ISBN: 978-1-60741-730-9
© 2009 Nova Science Publishers, Inc.

INTRODUCTION

ALCOHOL USE AND THE BRAIN

Leo Sher, Isack Kandel and Joav Merrick

Alcohol related problems are a major public health concern in the western world. Alcohol use disorders (AUD) are also an important social and medical problem [1-3], as well as less severe alcohol-related problems, associated with significant social costs [4] For example, in 1998 the social costs of AUD in the United States (US) were estimated at $184.6 billion. Although alcohol-abusing drinkers and their families bear some of these costs (e.g., medical and legal costs), the non-abusing population also bears costs related to the adverse social consequences of problems, such as alcohol-related motor vehicle crashes, crime, violence, and increased health care costs. Because of the enormous social costs they impose, AUD as well as other alcohol-related problems are of major concern to clinicians, researchers, and policymakers. For example, as of 2004 in the US, 45 states, the District of Columbia, and Puerto Rico had enacted laws making it illegal to drive with a blood alcohol concentration of .08 grams per deciliter or higher.

Alcohol use disorders are associated with well-known neurological and psychiatric signs and symptoms, including seizures (unrelated to active drinking or with-drawal), withdrawal syndromes (seizures, hallucinations, delusions, delirium), psychotic syndromes (paranoia, hallucinations, and delusions in a clear sensorium), peripheral neuropathy (usually in the lower extremities, bi-lateral, symmetrical, and sensorimotor in type) and cognitive deficits (ranging from minor memory problems to dementia and the anmestic syndrome) [2,5]. AUD are associated with suicidal behavior [6]. In the US, about half of the nearly 20 million individuals with alcoholism seem to be free of cognitive impairments [7]. In the remaining half, however, neuropsychological difficulties can range from mild to severe. For example, up to two million individuals with alcoholism develop permanent, and debilitating conditions requiring lifetime custodial care. Examples include alcohol-induced persisting amnesic disorder (also called Wernicke-Korsakoff syndrome) and dementia, which seriously affects many mental functions in addition to memory (e.g., language, reasoning, and problem-solving abilities).

Multiple studies of the neurobiological effects of alcohol have been performed [1,6,8,9]. According to one hypothesis, atrophy of the cerebral cortex and white matter, as well as possible atrophy of basal forebrain regions, can result from the neurotoxic effects of alcohol

[8]. Furthermore, thiamine deficiency can result in damage to portions of the hypothalamus. Brain imaging, using magnetic resonance imaging, has revealed that several brain structures in persons with a history of chronic alcohol dependence are smaller in volume than the same brain structures in non-alcoholic control subjects. The areas that are particularly affected are the frontal lobes, which are involved in reasoning, judgment, and problem solving. Older people are especially vulnerable to the damaging effects of alcohol. The effects of alcohol on neurotransmitter systems in the brain have also been extensively studied [10-12]. Further studies of the effects of alcohol on the brain are merited to bring better knowledge and ways to prevent and treat.

REFERENCES

[1]   Kandel I, Merrick J, Sher L, eds. *Adolescence and alcohol: An international perspective*. London-Tel Aviv: Freund, 2006.

[2]   Winokur G, Clayton PJ, eds. *Medical basis of psychiatry*, 2nd ed. Philadelphia: WB Saunders, 1994.

[3]   Nikelly AG. Alcoholism: Social as well as psycho-medical problem—The missing "big picture." *J. Alcohol Drug Educ.* 1994:1-12.

[4]   Bray JW, Zarkin GA. Economic evaluation of alcoholism treatment. *Alcohol. Res. Health* 2006; 29(1):27-33.

[5]   Oscar-Berman M, Marinkovic K. Alcoholism and the brain: An overview. *Alcohol. Res. Health* 2003;27(2):125-33.

[6]   Sher L, Kandel I, Merrick J, eds. *Alcohol and suicide: Research and clinical perspectives*. Victoria, BC: Int Acad Press, 2007.

[7]   Rourke SB, Löberg T. The neurobehavioral correlates of alcoholism. In: Nixon, SJ, ed. Neuropsychological assessment of neuropsychiatric disorders, 2nd ed. New York, NY, USA: Oxford Univ Press, 1996:423–85.

[8]   Lishman WA. Alcohol and the brain. *Br. J. Psychiatry* 1990; 156:635–44.

[9]   Crews FT, Nixon K. Alcohol, neural stem cells, and adult neurogenesis. *Alcohol. Res. Health* 2003; 27(2):197-204.

[10]   Sher L, Oquendo MA, Li S., Huang Y, Grune-baum MF, Burke AK, et al. Lower CSF homo-vanillic acid levels in depressed patients with a history of alcoholism. *Neuropsychopharmacology* 2003;28(9):1712-9.

[11]   Valenzuela CF. Alcohol and neurotransmitter interactions. *Alcohol. Health Res. World* 1997;21: 144–8.

[12]   Chastain G. Alcohol, neurotransmitter systems, and behavior. *J. Gen. Psychol.* 2006;133(4):329-35.

PART ONE: FETAL ALCOHOL SPECTRUM DISORDERS

In: Alcohol-Related Cognitive Disorders
Editors: L. Sher, I. Kandel, J. Merrick pp. 5-28

ISBN: 978-1-60741-730-9
© 2009 Nova Science Publishers, Inc.

Chapter 1

FETAL ALCOHOL SPECTRUM DISORDERS: NEUROCOGNITIVE AND NEUROBEHAVIORAL IMPAIRMENT

Blair Paley and Mary J. O'Connor

ABSTRACT

Fetal Alcohol Spectrum Disorders (FASDs) represent a continuum of development disabilities associated with maternal consumption of alcohol during pregnancy. This spectrum of disorders, which includes the Fetal Alcohol Syndrome (FAS), is characterized by a wide range of physical, cognitive, and behavioral impairments. Estimates of the number of live births in the United States meeting criteria for a diagnosis of FAS range from .5 to 2 infants per 1,000, with the prevalence of the entire continuum of FASDs estimated to be 1 in 100. This chapter discusses some of the complexities involved in diagnosing individuals affected by prenatal alcohol exposure, provides a review of the neurocognitive and neurobehavioral deficits commonly seen in this population, and examines how such deficits may manifest during different developmental periods across the life span. Additionally, strategies for assessing these deficits are described, and specific measures that are appropriate for alcohol-exposed individuals are presented. The challenges of working with this under-identified and underserved population are highlighted, as well as the importance of early diagnosis and intervention.

INTRODUCTION

Prenatal alcohol exposure is considered the leading cause of developmental disabilities of known etiology [1]. Fetal Alcohol Syndrome (FAS), the most severe consequence of such exposure, is defined by a characteristic pattern of facial anomalies, growth retardation, and central nervous system dysfunction [1]. Significant cognitive, behavioral, and emotional difficulties have been documented among individuals with FAS [2-7], as well as in individuals with prenatal alcohol exposure but without all the features of FAS [4,8,9]. The term Fetal Alcohol Spectrum Disorders (FASDs) [10] has been proposed to represent individuals experiencing significant impairments associated with prenatal alcohol exposure, including not only those with FAS but also those who might be diagnosed with other related conditions, such as Partial FAS, Alcohol Related Neurodevelopmental Disorder (ARND), or Alcohol Related Birth Defects (ARBD).

The number of live births in the United States meeting the criteria for a diagnosis of FAS is estimated to range from .5 to 2 infants per 1,000, with the prevalence of the entire continuum of FASDs estimated to be 1 in 100 [11]. The cost of FAS alone in the United States is estimated to be over 2 billion dollars per year [12]. This chapter will briefly review the diagnostic criteria for FAS and some of the challenges in diagnosing FAS and other alcohol-related conditions, provide an overview of the neurocognitive and neurobehavioral deficits found among individuals with FASDs, and describe some of the methods for assessing such deficits.

DIAGNOSIS

In 2004, the United States Centers for Disease Control and Prevention (CDC) National Center on Birth Defects and Developmental Disabilities in coordination with the National Task Force on Fetal Alcohol Syndrome and Fetal Alcohol Effects published guidelines on diagnosing FAS [13]. According to these guidelines, a diagnosis of FAS is based on the following: (a) evidence of three essential facial abnormalities: short palpebral fissures, a smooth philtrum, and a thin vermillion border or upper lip; (b) evidence of either prenatal or postnatal growth deficiency; and (c) evidence of central nervous system (CNS) dysfunction, which may include: structural abnormalities (e.g., microcephaly), neurological problems (e.g., seizures that are not due to some type of postnatal insult), or functional impairments (e.g., global cognitive delay). Although confirmation of prenatal alcohol exposure can provide increased evidence for the diagnosis of FAS, it is not required. In many cases, prenatal alcohol exposure may be reasonably suspected, but cannot be confirmed (e.g., child was adopted and the biological mother was an alcoholic). In cases in which prenatal alcohol exposure cannot be confirmed, ruling out other disorders that might present similarly to FAS is especially important. Exposure to other teratogens, such as phenytoin, can cause presentations similar to FAS. Certain genetic disorders, such as Williams syndrome or Noonan syndrome, also can present similarly to FAS.

Fetal Alcohol Spectrum Disorders is a relatively new term that has come into usage to convey that although some individuals with prenatal alcohol exposure will meet the full criteria for a diagnosis of FAS, in reality, the majority of individuals with prenatal alcohol exposure exhibit some but not all of the criteria of FAS. The term FASDs is meant to convey the presence of a continuum of effects, and that some individuals can be mildly affected in one area but moderately or severely affected in another area. For example, an individual might not exhibit the characteristic facial dysmorphology, but still experience profound cognitive and behavioral impairments. The term FASDs is not a clinical diagnosis in and of itself but rather is an umbrella term intended to include several alcohol-related diagnoses, including FAS, Partial FAS (also referred to as Atypical Fetal Alcohol Syndrome in some diagnostic systems), ARND, and ARBD. The latter three diagnostic terms (Partial FAS, ARND, and ARBD) were proposed in the Institute of Medicine's report, Fetal Alcohol

Syndrome: Diagnosis, Epidemiology, Prevention, and Treatment [14], for individuals who do not meet all the criteria for FAS. Currently, however, some debate remains regarding the precise criteria that distinguish among these other diagnostic categories. The term Fetal Alcohol Effects (FAE), which has been used in prior research to describe individuals who do not exhibit all the sequelae of FAS but still have experienced significant impairments associated with prenatal alcohol exposure, is used less commonly now in the current literature.

Several diagnostic approaches have been proposed to evaluate individuals for FAS and related conditions [13,15-19]. Although there is general agreement among these various approaches regarding the basic criteria for FAS, several important differences exist regarding the specific thresholds that must be met for the various criteria. For example, these approaches can differ regarding what specific criteria to use as thresholds for growth deficiency or facial dysmorphology. Furthermore, a clear agreement has not yet been reached regarding how to distinguish FAS diagnostically from other related conditions, such as Partial FAS or ARND. Despite such challenges, these approaches offer both clinicians and researchers better methods for evaluating individuals with prenatal alcohol exposure that will lead to increased validity and reliability in their diagnostic decisions.

NEUROLOGICAL IMPAIRMENTS

Facial anomalies and growth retardation may be the most easily recognized sequelae of prenatal alcohol exposure, but the CNS abnormalities affecting neurocognitive and neurobehavioral functioning are clearly the most debilitating. Numerous studies have provided evidence of differences in brain size, shape, and symmetry among individuals with prenatal alcohol exposure [20], as well as abnormalities in specific brain structures, including the corpus callosum, cerebellum, and basal ganglia [20-25].

Specifically, alcohol-exposed individuals have a smaller overall brain volume. In addition to reductions in brain volume, white matter density appears to be reduced, but gray matter density is increased in certain regions [25]. The cerebellum, which plays a role in movement, especially balance and coordination, as well as attentional abilities, has been found to be smaller and characterized by abnormalities, particularly in the anterior regions of the vermis [21,22,24]. The basal ganglia, which governs voluntary movement, and certain cognitive functions, such as the ability to shift from one task to another, the inhibition of inappropriate behavior, and spatial memory, is smaller, primarily due to the reduced size of the caudate [26]. The corpus callosum, which plays a role in attention, reading, learning, verbal memory, and executive functioning, has been found to be smaller, thinning or completely absent (agenesis) [27]. Agenesis is present in about 6.8% of the FAS population, compared with about 2.3% in developmentally disabled populations, and 0.3% in the general population [20]. Among alcohol-exposed individuals, the reduction in the size of the corpus callosum appears specific to the splenium [28]. In addition to the decreased size of the corpus callosum, abnormalities in shape and location have been documented [25]. In light of the significant impact that in utero alcohol exposure can have on fetal brain development, not surprisingly alcohol-affected individuals show a vast range of cognitive and behavioral impairments.

Among alcohol-exposed individuals, cognitive functioning, as reflected by standardized scores on IQ tests, can vary widely, with studies documenting scores that can range from profoundly retarded to above average [4]. Indeed, most alcohol-exposed individuals are not mentally retarded but they typically fall below the average range of intellectual functioning [29-31]. For example, researchers found in a sample of 415 adolescents and adults a mean IQ of 80 for patients diagnosed with FAS and a mean IQ of 88 for those diagnosed with FAE [7]. In a sample of children with prenatal alcohol exposure, the mean IQ was 74.4 among those who met full criteria for FAS, and 83.6 for those who did not exhibit the physical features of FAS [29].

In addition to deficits in general intellectual functioning, a wide range of neurocognitive deficits among individuals with prenatal alcohol exposure is well-documented. Attentional problems are among the most common deficits observed in this population [32-34] Individuals with FASDs frequently present with clinical symptoms consistent with a diagnosis of ADHD and are most often diagnosed as the inattentive subtype of ADHD as defined by the DSM-IV [35]. The prevalence rates of ADHD appear to increase significantly with increasing levels of prenatal alcohol exposure (36). Notably, there may be differences in the types of attentional problems exhibited by individuals with FASDs as compared with non-alcohol exposed individuals with ADHD. In a study examining different aspects of attention, children with FAS or FAE performed most poorly on measures of encoding (the ability to learn and manipulate new information and shifting attention); in contrast, non-exposed children with ADHD performed most poorly on measures of focused and sustained attention [37]. Noteworthy, however, are the findings that children with FASDs also show deficits in focused and sustained attention when compared with non-exposed, non-psychiatric controls [33,38,39].

Learning and memory problems have also been frequently observed in this population. Difficulties learning from experience are considered one of the hallmark impairments associated with prenatal alcohol exposure. In a classic animal study [40,41], alcohol-exposed chicks (alcohol was injected into the airspace of the chicks' eggs) had much greater difficulty learning how to circumvent a barrier to reach a reward (food) compared with non-exposed chicks. Indeed, some of the exposed chicks were never able to learn how to avoid the barrier even after being shown the correct route for 4 days in a row. In comparison, none of the non-exposed chicks had this much difficulty learning the correct route. Among humans, clinical reports frequently describe alcohol-exposed individuals as having great difficulty learning from previous experiences. Many parents report that their alcohol-exposed children are unable to predict that the same behavior will produce the same result no matter how many learning trials they have. Other parents lament that their children seem unable to learn from negative consequences. For many of these individuals, unfortunately, their difficulty in avoidance learning might be interpreted as demonstrating a lack of remorse or as a moral failing rather than as a function of their cognitive deficits. Some studies suggest that individuals with prenatal alcohol exposure also have difficulties acquiring new verbal information, although their ability to retain verbal information appears to be less affected [42,43].

Problems in executive functioning, including difficulties in planning, organizing, and sequencing behavior, and problems in abstract and practical reasoning, also appear to be quite prominent in individuals with prenatal alcohol exposure [6,44,45]. Such individuals show deficits in working memory [46-48], verbal and nonverbal fluency [49,50], verbal reasoning and concept formation [51], and nonverbal reasoning and concept formation [30,43]. Impairments in planning [47,51], cognitive flexibility [47,50-52], and response inhibition [50,51] have also been reported. Such deficits have been found to be greater in exposed individuals than what would be predicted from their IQ scores [53] and are still apparent even when controlling for IQ [50,54]. Notably, such deficits are evident in alcohol-exposed individuals, regardless of whether they meet or do not meet the full criteria for FAS [43,51,53,54], and continue into adulthood [3,31,53,55].

Individuals with FASDs can often be quite talkative, and some may appear to have good language skills at a superficial level. Because of their talkativeness, deficits in speech and language can often be overlooked. Indeed, when their communication skills are examined at a more meaningful level, impairments in several areas emerge. Speech disorders, including articulation problems, are not uncommon [56]. Additionally, a myriad of language impairments have also been reported, including receptive [4,30] and expressive [56] language deficits, difficulties with naming and word comprehension [43], and poor semantics, syntax, and pragmatics [57].

Strong evidence has been presented for a host of other neurocognitive impairments among individuals with prenatal alcohol exposure. Impairments in both spatial and auditory memory are well documented in this population [52,58]. A number of studies have found such individuals to have poor arithmetic skills [7,48,59], including deficits in calculation [60] and number comparison [61]. Clinical reports suggest that alcohol-exposed individuals often have difficulties with the concepts of time and money. Visual-spatial problems have also been noted, including problems processing hierarchical stimuli [62], visual motor integration problems [43], and delays in the development of visual perception [59]. Motor problems are also commonly observed in this population. Infants and young children exposed to alcohol in utero have been found to exhibit delays in motor development [63]. Numerous other studies of individuals with prenatal alcohol exposure have found fine motor deficits [43,64,65], poor balance [64,66], and poor coordination [67].

Several studies have also examined the relation between prenatal alcohol exposure and adaptive functioning. Researchers have documented significant impairments across all three domains of the Vineland Adaptive Behavior Scales among children, adolescents, and adults with FAS or FAE [7]. In a study of clinic-referred alcohol exposed and non-exposed children, deficits were documented in both groups across the communication, daily living, and socialization domains of the Vineland Adaptive Behavior Scales; among the alcohol-exposed group, however, deficits in socialization became increasingly significant with age even after controlling for IQ differences between groups [68]. Other studies also found evidence for deficits in socialization in particular. Both parents [69] and teachers [70] rate children with prenatal alcohol exposure as having greater deficits in social skills than unexposed children. Such impairments include difficulty in interpreting social cues, in anticipating the consequences of one's actions, and in understanding social cues, and having problems with communicating in social contexts [55,71-73]. Moreover, such deficits do not appear to be merely a function of general cognitive delays because prenatally exposed children have shown greater impairments socially when compared with non-exposed children having similar levels of developmental delay [74]. Rather, such interpersonal deficits may be related to the impairments in executive functioning commonly seen in this population [75]. Furthermore, findings suggest that social skills deficits are evident well past childhood into adolescence and adulthood [55,76].

Finally, individuals with FASDs present with high rates of secondary disabilities. Children and adults with FAS or other alcohol related conditions are at increased risk for a myriad of comorbid psychiatric disorders [2,31,36,77-80] and are overrepresented in psychiatric samples [81]. School problems are extremely common among children and adolescents with FASDs, including lagging academic skills and a greater likelihood of dropping out of school [7,43,59]. Adults with FASDs are highly likely to experience employment problems, and are much less likely to be able live independently [31]. Among the most troubling of these secondary disabilities, however, is the increased risk for delinquent and criminal behavior [7,9]. Furthermore, recent studies suggest that in juvenile detention and correctional settings, individuals with FASDs are over-represented [82] but frequently unidentified [83].

FASDS ACROSS THE LIFE SPAN

FASDs are not disorders that are 'outgrown' [73], but rather are associated with deficits throughout the life span. The impairments associated with prenatal alcohol exposure, however, are likely to manifest differently during different developmental periods. Both animal [84] and human [85,86] studies demonstrate that the effects of prenatal alcohol exposure are evident as early as infancy. Among infants with prenatal alcohol exposure, studies have revealed higher rates of negative affect and disturbances in attachment relationships [5,87], and poorer habituation [86] and orientation (85). Problems with state [86] and autonomic [85] regulation, increased post-stress cortisol levels (88), and less mature motor behavior and increased level of activity (89,90) have also been shown. Prenatally exposed infants may also frequently present with feeding difficulties and failure to thrive [73]. Delays in cognitive development, including language and visual-motor deficits, also have been documented among 2-year olds who were exposed to alcohol throughout pregnancy [91,92].

Although cognitive deficits may be evident very early on, learning and academic problems may become especially salient during early and middle childhood. Children with FASDs are at increased risk for learning disorders [2] and more likely to be in need of special education services [59]. Such children also commonly present with externalizing behavior, including attentional problems and impulsivity [36,80,93,94]. Continuing problems in attachment relationships and the emergence of internalizing problems and mood disorders have also been observed in children with prenatal alcohol exposure during this period (95,96). Such behavioral and emotional difficulties are likely to interfere further with school functioning and academic performance. Social skills deficits may also become quite salient during this period, and such deficits should represent an important focus of assessment and intervention. Poor peer relationships in latency aged children are associated with a significantly increased risk for delinquency and early withdrawal from school [97-99], outcomes to which individuals with FASDs are already vulnerable.

Adolescents with FASDs are more likely to engage in high-risk behaviors, placing them at increased risk for both victimization and delinquency [7,9,100]. Among adolescents with FASDs, difficulties with peer interactions continue, and problems in romantic relationships are likely to come to the fore. In a longitudinal study of alcohol-exposed individuals, almost

60% of adolescents with FAS or FAE had problems with peer interactions, and almost half had engaged in some type of inappropriate sexual behavior [7]. Adolescents with prenatal alcohol exposure are also at high risk for drug and alcohol abuse [101]. Academic problems are likely to persist, with a recent study finding that approximately 53% of adolescents with FAS or FAE had received suspensions, 29% had been expelled, and 25% had dropped out of school [7]. Academic failures can be extremely demoralizing to individuals with FASDs. When not detected early, such failures persist and often become worse, and may set alcohol-exposed individuals on a course of quitting school, socializing with peers who exert negative influences on them, and becoming increasingly marginalized from the rest of society. Parents of children with FASDs have noted significant challenges in obtaining adequate and consistent school-based services [102]. Unfortunately, research results suggest that individuals who do not meet full criteria for FAS are those who fare more poorly in school and in the legal system, most probably because they are never identified and not provided with early intervention [31].

During adulthood, such basic responsibilities as maintaining a steady job and handling one's finances can overwhelm individuals who had prenatal alcohol exposure [73,101]. Furthermore, adults diagnosed with FAS or FAE have been found to be at increased risk for serious psychopathology, including alcohol or drug abuse or dependence, depression, psychotic disorders, and various personality disorders [77,103]. High rates of legal problems persist into adulthood, and prenatally exposed adults are at increased risk for being incarcerated or confined to a psychiatric hospital [7]. Clearly, the long-term course for individuals affected by prenatal alcohol exposure raises significant concerns. A number of variables have been identified that can serve as protective factors for such individuals, including an early diagnosis [7]. Such findings further highlight the importance of evaluating alcohol-exposed individuals, particularly with regard to the multitude of cognitive and behavioral impairments that may place them at increased risk for developing secondary disabilities.

ASSESSMENT

A multidisciplinary approach is essential when medical and mental health professionals are presented with the challenge of conducting an evaluation of an individual with prenatal alcohol exposure [17,100,104]. Alcohol-exposed individuals frequently present with impairments across multiple domains of functioning and thus are most likely to benefit from an evaluation by a team of professionals who possess expertise across those domains. The broad range of expertise and skills of the team's members will likely lead to the most integrative and comprehensive evaluation of an alcohol-exposed individual's deficits and strengths, and to the recom-mendation of interventions that best serve the needs of the individual and their family.

The components of a multidisciplinary evaluation typically include a clinical interview with parents or with other caregivers, as well as the patient or client when appropriate; a thorough record review; information obtained from teachers, therapists, or other relevant informants either through interviews or questionnaires (e.g., rating scales); behavioral observations; and standardized testing. In addition, a physical examination should be conducted to both assess for dysmorphology and for any medical problems, especially those that are frequently associated with prenatal alcohol exposure. For the purposes of this chapter, we will focus our discussion of assessment on the methods most commonly used for evaluating the neurocognitive and neurobehavioral deficits usually seen in individuals with prenatal alcohol exposure—namely, behavioral obser-vations and standardized testing.

Behavioral Observations

In an individual with suspected or known prenatal alcohol exposure, observations should focus on multiple aspects of their behavior and ideally in multiple settings. Thus, the information obtained by observing such an individual in a clinical setting (e.g., during testing at a psychologist's office or during a pediatric visit) can be quite valuable, but it is also likely to be extremely helpful to observe an alcohol-exposed child in the school setting as well, for example. Observations in settings like school can provide information regarding how the individual functions with varying degrees of structure (e.g., classroom vs. the playground). Observing the individual in different settings can also reveal deficits or strengths that are evident in one environment but not in another.

For example, it is not uncommon for parents of children with FASDs to not recognize their children's significant social impairments, perhaps not only because these children can appear quite friendly (overly friendly actually) but also because parents may compensate, perhaps without even realizing it, for some of the child's difficulties in ways that mask the degree of their child's impairment in this domain. Thus, the opportunity to observe the alcohol-exposed child interacting with his/her peers on the playground may (a) better inform a clinician's understanding of how the child fares when having to function more independently, and (b) ultimately identify an important focus of intervention.

Another benefit of observing the alcohol-exposed individual in multiple settings is that it can provide important information about aspects of the individual's environment that may serve to enhance or, alternatively, further compromise the individual's functioning. For example, as noted earlier, individuals with FASDs commonly experience significant problems in school. Undoubtedly, some of these problems can be attributed to the child's primary cognitive and behavioral deficits. Nevertheless, a classroom that does not provide enough structure or consistency for that particular child, or perhaps teachers who are unaware of or do not fully understand the extent and nature of the child's impairments—particularly if the child has never been properly diagnosed—may have a further impact on the child's functioning.

Conversely, school observations can reveal that the child's classroom environment is functioning in such a way that enhances the child's potential. For example, a teacher might have developed very effective strategies for teaching an alcohol-exposed child and for managing behavior problems, strategies that the parents would benefit from incorporating at home. Obviously such observations can greatly inform the evaluation process, but collecting such data is not always feasible (e.g., observing an alcohol-exposed adult at work would be difficult). In such cases, efforts should be made at least to interview and/or to collect rating scales from other informants (with the appropriate consents), such as school counselors, employers, or spouses, regarding the individual's behavior in other settings. The behavioral domains noted in table 1 would be relevant for any individual presenting in a psychiatric setting, but many are especially important to note in an alcohol-exposed child or adult.

Table 1. Behavioral observations of individuals with prenatal alcohol exposure

Physical appearance
- Does the individual exhibit any apparent facial dysmorphology or other physical anomalies that might be associated with prenatal alcohol exposure?
- Is the individual's appearance consistent with his/her chronological age, or does he appear smaller or younger than would be expected, possibly suggesting growth delay?
- Does he/she have any obvious injuries due to falls or accidents, which might be suggestive of poor balance or coordination?

Activity level
- Does the individual exhibit an excessive level of motor activity? For younger individuals, this may manifest as running around the room or climbing on furniture; for older individuals, this may be evident in frequent fidgeting or constantly moving about in one's chair.

Attention
- Can the individual focus on a particular task for a sustained period of time in a manner that is consistent with his/her developmental level?
- Is the individual easily distractible by meaningless stimuli?
- Does he/she move rapidly from one activity or stimulus (e.g., toys, games) to another, without ever really demonstrating any meaningful interest in any one activity or stimulus?

Impulsive behavior
- Is the individual's level of impulsivity appropriate to his/her developmental level?
- Does he/she seem to think before acting?
- Does he/she engage in high-risk behavior (e.g., trying to climb up to or jump from high places) with little recognition of possible danger?

Social interaction/relatedness
- What is the individual's behavior like upon first meeting or encountering new people? Does he/she seem to differentiate between friends and strangers, or is he/she socially indiscriminant, immediately interacting with strangers or new acquaintances in an overly friendly manner?
- What is the nature and quality of the individual's interactions with adults?
- Does the individual make social bids or initiate interactions with parents/caregivers, and with examiners? Does he/she show a preference for parents/caregivers over a less familiar adult?
- How does the individual respond when others try to engage him/her?
- Is the individual able to maintain meaningful interactions with others or does he/she lose interest quickly?
- What is the nature and quality of the individual's interactions with peers?

Table 1. (Continued)

- Is he/she overly friendly to the point of intrusiveness?
- Does he/she have difficulty respecting physical boundaries (e.g., personal space)?
- Does the individual have difficulty reading social cues (e.g., doesn't recognize when other children don't wish to play)

Affect and mood
- What kind(s) of affect does the individual display? Does he/she display a range of affect across different situations?
- Does the individual's affect appear to change predictably or does his/her affect change without warning?
- How does the individual describe his/her mood state? Is the individual able to articulate his/her internal mood states in an accurate and coherent way?

Emotional regulation skills
- What is the individual's capacity to regulate his/her own emotional arousal?
- What types of strategies does the individual use to soothe him/herself when distressed?
- Does the individual seek comfort out from others when distressed?
- How does the individual respond to the emotional expressions of his/her parents or caregivers? Does he/she appear to notice when others are distressed and can he/she respond appropriately?

Motivation and response to frustration
- Does he/she appear to appraise or be aware of his/her own successes or failures?
- How does the individual handle frustration?
- Does he/she persist when faced with difficult tasks or give up easily?
- Does he/she become angry or throw a tantrum if he/she cannot successfully complete a task?
- Is he/she able to ask others for help?
- Is the individual receptive if others offer unsolicited help?

Response to reinforcement and limits
- Does the individual respond to limits set by the parents/caregivers and/or examiners fairly easily or is he/she largely noncompliant?
- Does the individual respond well to positive reinforcement, such as praise or some type of tangible reinforcer (e.g., a sticker)?
- Does the individual seem to have difficulty understanding contingencies?
- Does the individual appear to have difficulty learning from negative consequences?
- Does the individual repeat the same behavior over and over again with little ability to predict the same outcome?

Structure, routines, transitions
- How does the individual function with varying degrees of structure? Does he/she tend to have more difficulty in unstructured situations?

- Does the individual appear to function better if consistent routines are followed?
- How does the individual respond to transitions? Is the individual likely to become upset or throw tantrums when having to transition from one environment or activity to another?

Play
- Is the individual's play appropriate to his/her development level (e.g., functional vs. imaginative)?
- Does the individual perseverate on one object or theme when playing, or is play more elaborative and varied?
- Does the individual attempt to solicit others to participate in his/her play, or is he/she content to play alone, and perhaps in fact, resists others' attempts to enter into his/her play?
- Is the individual responsive to others' attempts to redirect the play in another direction?

Speech and language
- Is the individual's articulation appropriate to his developmental level? Can he/she be understood by others or does he appear to have some phonological difficulties?
- Does the individual exhibit difficulties in receptive language?
  - Does he/she recognize simple words?
  - Does he/she understand basic questions?
  - Can he/she understand and respond to basic and multi-step instructions?
- Does the individual have difficulties in expressive language?
  - Does he/she use language spontaneously?
  - Is he/she able to use language in a functional/ communicative manner?
  - Can the individual relate a story in a logical, coherent manner or does he/she relate events in a confusing manner?
- What is the quality of the individual's pragmatics?

Motor functioning
- How are the individual's fine motor skills?
  - Can he/she manipulate small objects?
  - Does he/she have difficulty with drawing or writing?
- How are the individual's gross motor skills?
  - Does he/she have difficulty walking, running, jumping, hopping, etc.?
- Does the individual have difficulty with balance or coordination?
  - Does the individual fall or trip easily, frequently stumble?

Behavioral observations of older individuals should also focus on:

Judgment
- Is the individual able to plan out his/her actions and foresee the potential consequences of those actions?
- Does the individual appear able to make decisions in a thoughtful manner and is he/she able to communicate the rationale for his/her decisions?

Table 1. (Continued)

Insight
- Does he/she seem to have an appreciation for the motivations and feelings that underlie his/her behavior?
- Does he/she seem to recognize the impact of his/her behavior on others and can he/she adjust his/her behavior accordingly?

Ability to problem-solve and think abstractly
- Does the individual primarily use trial and error to solve problems or can he/she solve problems hypothetically?
- Does he/she appear to understand metaphors, figures of speech?
- Does he/she appear to understand humor or does he/she respond concretely to sarcasm, jokes or teasing?

Observations should focus on both positive and negative aspects of the individual's presentation and behavior so that areas of both strength and deficit can be identified. Understandably, parents, teachers, and other informants may be more likely to provide information regarding problematic behavior because they are typically seeking help for such behavior. Equally important, however, is that clinicians also note the positive aspects of the individual's presentation or behavior, so that the clinician can not only provide feedback that includes a balanced view of the patient but also make recommendations that both address areas of impairment and capitalize on existing strengths. In addition to the behavioral domains described in table 1, The Fetal Alcohol Behavior Scale [105], a rating scale that parents typically complete, can also be used by the clinician as a guide regarding specific behaviors to look for that commonly present in individuals with prenatal alcohol exposure.

Standardized Measures

A comprehensive testing battery that includes measures of cognitive, neuropsychological, achievement, adaptive, behavioral, social, and emotional functioning is optimal when assessing individuals who have been exposed to alcohol prenatally. Such measures can include tests such as IQ tests that are administered to the patient directly, and rating scales or interviews that are administered to other informants, such as parents or teachers. When conducting such evaluations, one must keep in mind that many alcohol-exposed individuals will have a normal IQ, which may obscure deficits in other areas of cognitive functioning. As noted earlier, prior research has found that executive functioning in individuals with FASDs is often lower than what would be expected based on IQ [53]. In light of such discrepancies, tests of intelligence may not adequately capture the full range of cognitive deficits that may be associated with prenatal alcohol exposure. Consequently, an evaluation of the individual's functioning across multiple domains is necessary to provide useful information to guide treatment planning. Additionally, speech and language testing and occupational and/or physical therapy evaluations might be conducted, or patients may be referred for such assessments if the relevant professionals are not part of the evaluation team.

The assessment battery should include measures that have been standardized and normed on a diverse sample. Testing results should be interpreted in light of relevant cultural factors, language issues, and environmental experiences. Histories of past abuse, neglect, or deprivation, exposure to trauma, and disrupted attachment experiences are not uncommon among individuals with prenatal alcohol exposure, and such experiences may have significant and long-lasting effects on an individual's development even if the individual has since been placed in a more supportive and stable environment. Several studies have shown that many alcohol-affected children experience one or more changes in custody during their lives, either being placed in foster care or being adopted, or being institutionalized [14] Estimates are that two-thirds of affected children are not raised in their biological homes [106], and many experience multiple placements in their lifetime, often of varying quality. Some of the children we see in our clinical practice have been adopted from other countries and may have learned English or begun formal schooling only recently. Thus, an initial evaluation can provide important baseline data regarding the individual's functioning, but once interventions have been consistently implemented and/or the individual has had the benefit of living in a more supportive, stable environment, following the individual for further evaluation is essential.

Provided in table 2 is a list of standardized measures that can be used to evaluate individuals with prenatal alcohol exposure across multiple domains of functioning. These measures have been found to be useful when evaluating individuals for FASDs, based on research or clinical experience or both. Within each domain, different measures are noted for use during different developmental periods. For certain domains (e.g., executive functioning), multiple measures are listed that can be used to assess different aspects of functioning within that particular domain. The particular battery selected for each patient should, however, be based on the referral questions, the goals of the evaluation, and on what data are available from previous evaluations.

Table 2. Standardized measures for individuals with prenatal alcohol exposure

---

Achievement
- The Wechsler Individual Achievement Test – Second Edition [115]

Adaptive
- Vineland Adaptive Behavior Scales, 2nd edition [116]

Attention
- Conners' Rating Scales – Revised [117]
- Conners' Continuous Performance Test-II [118]
- Wechsler Intelligence Scale for Children – Third Edition as a Process Instrument: Digit Span and Spatial Span Subtests [119]

Behavioral/emotional/social
- Antisocial Process Screening Device [120]

Table 2 (Continued)

- Beck Depression Inventory-II [121]
- Brief Symptom Inventory [122]
- Child Behavior Checklist, Caregiver-Teacher Report Form, Teacher Report Form, and Youth Self-Report [123]
- Children's Depression Inventory [124]
- Fetal Alcohol Behavior Scale [105]
- NIMH Diagnostic Interview Schedule for Children Version IV [125]
- Pictorial Depression Scale [126]
- Structured Clinical Interview for DSM-IV™ Axis I Disorders, Clinician Version [127]; Structured Clinical Interview for DSM-IV™ Axis II Disorders [128]
- Cognitive
- Bayley Scales of Infant Development – Third Edition [129]
- Wechsler Preschool and Primary Scale of Intelligence – Third Edition [130]
- Wechsler Intelligence Scale for Children – Fourth Edition [131]
- Wechsler Adult Intelligence Scale – Third Edition [132]

Executive
- Behavior Rating Inventory of Executive Function: Parent and Teacher forms [133]
- Children's Color Trails Test [134]
- Delis-Kaplan Executive Function System [135]
- NEPSY (136)
- Wisconsin Card Sorting Test [137]

Language
- Clinical Evaluation of Language Fundamentals, 4th edition [138]
- Preschool Language Scale, 4th edition [139]
- Test of Language Competence – Expanded Edition [140]

Memory
- California Verbal Learning Test – Children's Version [141]
- Children's Memory Scale [142]
- Wechsler Memory Scale – Third Edition [143]

Visual Spatial/Fine Motor
- Beery-Buktenica Developmental Test of Visual Motor Integration- Fifth Edition [144]
- Finger Tapping Test [145]
- Grooved Pegboard Test [146]

Depending on the needs of the particular patient and their family, administering a particular measure in its entirety may be indicated, or conversely administering only a selected battery of subtests. Other researchers have also provided helpful recommendations regarding measures that may be useful for this population [17,100,107].

CONCLUSIONS

Although awareness and knowledge of the impact of alcohol on fetal development has increased among medical and mental health professionals over the last 30 years since FAS was first identified in the United States, the identification and treatment of FASDs continues to present a number of challenges. Health care professionals may believe that obtaining reliable and accurate information regarding an individual's history of prenatal alcohol exposure is too difficult, and there remains a significant need to improve the training and education of professionals regarding FAS and related conditions [108,109]. Current research suggests, however, that overcoming these obstacles is indeed possible [110, 111]. Given the multitude of primary deficits, as well as the increased risk for secondary disabilities seen in individuals with FASDs, it is essential that professionals working with children, adolescents, and adults who present in medical and/or psychiatric settings remain vigilant for individuals who are affected by prenatal alcohol exposure but remain undiagnosed or even misdiagnosed. Moreover, it is critical that evaluation and interventions focus not only on the alcohol-exposed individual, but on their families as well. Parents of children with FASDs report high levels of stress, and their increased stress seems to be at least partly related to the degree of behavioral and cognitive impairment experienced by their children [93,112]. Early identification and diagnosis can play a profoundly important role in preventing many of the adverse outcomes frequently seen in alcohol-exposed individuals, and support for the efficacy of evidence-based interventions for this population is emerging [113,114]. Such early identification and intervention likely offers the best hope for such individuals and their families.

ACKNOWLEDGMENTS

Support for this paper was provided by research grants U01D000041 and U84/CCU925033 from the Centers for Disease Control and Prevention, Atlanta, GA. The findings and conclusions in this report are those of the authors and do not necessarily represent the views of the Centers for Disease Control and Prevention.

REFERENCES

[1]   Jones KL, Smith DW. Recognition of the fetal alcohol syndrome in early infancy. *Lancet* 1973;2:999-1001.
[2]   Burd L, Klug MG, Martsolf JT, Kerbeshian J. Fetal alcohol syndrome: Neuropsychiatric phenomics. *Neurotoxicol Teratol* 2003;25:697-705.
[3]   Carmichael Olson H, Morse BA, Huffine C. Development and psychopathology: Fetal alcohol syndrome and related conditions. *Semin. Clin. Neuropsychiatry* 1998;3:262-84.

[4]   Mattson SN, Riley EP. A review of the neurobehavioral deficits in children with fetal alcohol syndrome or prenatal exposure to alcohol. *Alcohol. Clin. Exp. Res.* 1998;22:279-94.

[5]   O'Connor MJ. Prenatal alcohol exposure and negative affect as precursors of depressive features in children. *Infant Ment. Health* J. 2001;22:291-9.

[6]   Rasmussen C. Executive functioning and working memory in fetal alcohol spectrum disorder. *Alcohol. Clin. Exp. Res.* 2005;29:1359-67.

[7]   Streissguth AP, Bookstein FL, Barr HM, Sampson PD, O'Malley K, Young JK. Risk factors for adverse life outcomes in fetal alcohol syndrome and fetal alcohol effects. *J. Dev. Behav. Pediatr* 2004;25:228-38.

[8]   Kvigne VL, Leonardson GR, Neff-Smith M, Brock E, Borzelleca J, Welty TK. Characteristics of children who have full or incomplete Fetal Alcohol Syndrome. *J. Pediatr* 2004;145:635-40.

[9]   Schonfeld AM, Mattson SN, Riley EP. Moral maturity and delinquency following prenatal alcohol exposure. *J. Stud. Alcohol.* 2005;66:545-55.

[10]   Warren K, Floyd L, Calhoun F, Stone D, Bertrand J, Streissguth A, et al. Consensus statement on FASD. Washington, DC: *Nat. Org. Fetal. Alcohol Syndr*, 2004.

[11]   May PA, Gossage JP. Estimating the prevalence of fetal alcohol syndrome: A summary. *Alcohol. Res. Health* 2001;25:159-67.

[12]   Harwood H (The Lewin Group for the National Institute on Alcohol Abuse and Alcoholism). Updating estimates of the economic costs of alcohol abuse in the United States: estimates, update methods, and data. Rockville, MD: National Institute on Drug Abuse and the National Institute on Alcohol Abuse and Alcoholism, National Institutes of Health, Department of Health and Human Services; 1998. Report No.: 98-4327. Contract No.: N01-AA-7-1010.

[13]   Centers for Disease Control and Prevention. Fetal alcohol syndrome: *Guidelines for referral and diagnosis*. Atlanta, GA: United States Dept Health Human Serv, 2004.

[14]   Stratton K, Howe C, Battaglia F, editors. *Fetal alcohol syndrome: Diagnosis, epidemiology, prevention, and treatment*. Washington, DC: Inst Med, Nat Acad Press, 1996.

[15]   Astley SJ. Diagnostic guide for fetal alcohol spectrum disorders: The 4-digit diagnostic code. Third ed. Seattle, WA: Univ Washington, 2004.

[16]   Astley SJ, Clarren SK. Diagnosing the full spectrum of fetal alcohol exposed individuals: Introducing the 4-digit diagnostic code. *Alcohol Alcohol* 2000;35:400-10.

[17]   Chudley AE, Conry J, Cook JL, Loock C, Rosales T, LeBlanc N. Fetal alcohol spectrum disorder: Canadian guidelines for diagnosis. *Can. Med. Assoc. J.* 2005;172(5 suppl):S1-21.

[18]   Hoyme HE, May PA, Kalberg WO, Kodituwakku P, Gossage JP, Trujillo PM et al. A practical clinical approach to diagnosis of fetal alcohol spectrum disorders: clarification of the 1996 Institute of Medicine criteria. *Pediatrics* 2005;115: 39-47.

[19]   Manning MA, Hoyme HE. Fetal alchol spectrum disorders: A practical clinical approach to diagnosis. *Neurosci. Biobehav.* Rev. 2007;31,230-8.

[20]   McGee CL, Riley EP. Brain imaging and fetal alcohol spectrum disorders. *Ann. Ist Super Sanita* 2006;42:46-52.

[21] Autti-Rämö I, Autti T, Korkman M, Kettunen S, Salonen O, Valanne L. MRI findings in children with school problems who had been exposed prenatally to alcohol. *Dev. Med. Child Neurol.* 2002; 44:98-106.

[22] O'Hare ED, Kan E, Yoshii J, Mattson SN, Riley EP, Thompson PM et al. Mapping cerebellar vermal morphology and cognitive correlates in prenatal alcohol exposure. *Neuroreport* 2005;16: 1285-90.

[23] Riley EP, McGee CL. Fetal alcohol spectrum disorders: An overview with emphasis on changes in brain and behavior. *Exp. Biol. Med.* 2005; 230:357-65.

[24] Riley EP, McGee CL, Sowell ER. Teratogenic effects of alcohol: A decade of brain imaging. *Am. J. Med. Genet.* 2004;127C:35-41.

[25] Spadoni AD, McGee CL, Fryer SL, Riley EP. Neuroimaging and fetal alcohol spectrum disorders. *Neurosci. Biobehav. Rev.* 2007;31:239-245.

[26] Archibald SL, Fennema-Notestine C, Gamst A, Riley EP, Mattson SN, Jernigan TL. Brain dysmorphology in individuals with severe prenatal alcohol exposure. *Dev. Med. Child Neurol.* 2001; 43:148-154.

[27] Riley EP, Mattson SN, Sowell ER, Jernigan TL, Sobel DF, Jones KL. Abnormalities of the corpus callosum in children prenatally exposed to alcohol. *Alcohol. Clin. Exp. Res.* 1995;19:1198-1202.

[28] Sowell ER, Mattson SN, Thompson PM, Jernigan TL, Riley EP, Toga AW. Mapping callosal morphology and cognitive correlates: Effects of heavy prenatal alcohol exposure. *Neurology* 2001;57: 235-44.

[29] Mattson SN, Riley EP, Gramling L, Delis DC, Jones KL. Heavy prenatal alcohol exposure with or without physical features of fetal alcohol syndrome leads to IQ deficits. *J. Pediatr.* 1997;131:718-21.

[30] May PA, Fiorentino J, Gossage JP, Kalberg WO, Hoyme E, Robinson LK et al. Epidemiology of FASD in a province in Italy: Prevalence of characteristics of children in a random sample of schools. *Alcohol. Clin. Exp. Res.* 2006; 30:1562-75.

[31] Streissguth AP, O'Malley K. Neuropsychiatric implications and long-term consequences of fetal alcohol spectrum disorders. *Semin. Clin. Neuropsychiatry* 2000;5:177-190.

[32] Nanson JL, Hiscock M. Attention deficits in children exposed to alcohol prenatally. *Alcohol Clin. Exp. Res*. 1990;14:656-61.

[33] Lee KT, Mattson SN, Riley EP. Classifying children with heavy prenatal alcohol exposure using measures of attention. *J. Int. Neuropsychol. Soc.* 2004; 10:271-7.

[34] Streissguth AP, Barr HM, Sampson PD, Parrish-Johnson JC, Kirchner GL et al. Attention, distraction, and reaction time at age 7 years and pre-natal alcohol exposure. *Neurobehav Toxicol Teratol* 1986;8:717-25.

[35] Kapp FME, O'Malley KD. Watch for the rainbows. True stories for educators and other caregivers of children with fetal alcohol spectrum disorders. Calgary, Alberta, Canada: Frances Kapp Educ Publ, 2001.

[36] Bhatara V, Loudenberg R, Ellis R. Association of attention deficit hyperactivity disorder and gestational alcohol exposure. *J. Atten. Disord.* 2006;9: 515-22.

[37] Coles CD, Platzman KA, Raskind-Hood CL, Brown RT, Falek A, Smith, IE. A comparison of children affected by prenatal alcohol exposure and attention deficit, hyperactivity disorder. *Alcohol Clin. Exp. Res.* 1997;21:150-61.

[38] Coles CD, Platzman KA, Lynch ME, Freides D. Auditory and visual sustained attention in adolescents prenatally exposed to alcohol. *Alcohol Clin. Exp. Res.* 2002;26:263-71.

[39] Jacobson JL, Jacobson SW. Effects of prenatal alcohol exposure on child development. *Alcohol Res. Health* 2002;26:282-6.

[40] Means LW, Burnette MA, Pennington SN. The effect of embryonic ethanol exposure on detour learning in chicks. *Alcohol* 1988;5:305-8.

[41] Means LW, McDaniel K, Pennington SN. Embryonic ethanol exposure impairs detour learning in chicks. *Alcohol* 1989;6:327-30.

[42] Mattson SN, Riley EP, Delis DC, Stern C, Jones KL. Verbal learning and memory in children with fetal alcohol syndrome. *Alcohol Clin. Exp. Res.* 1996;20:810-16.

[43] Mattson SN, Riley EP, Gramling L, Delis DC, and Jones KL. Neuropsychological comparison of alcohol-exposed children with or without physical features of fetal alcohol syndrome. *Neuropsy-chology* 1998;12:146-53.

[44] Kodituwakku PW. Defining the behavioral phenotype in children with fetal alcohol spectrum disorders: A review. *Neurosci. Biobehav. Rev.* 2007; 31:192-201.

[45] Korkman M, Kettunen S, Autti-Ramo I. Neurocognitive impairment in early adolescence following prenatal alcohol exposure of varying duration. *Child Neuropsychol* 2003;9:117-28.

[46] Burden MJ, Jacobson SW, Sokol RJ, Jacobson JL. Effects of prenatal alcohol exposure on attention and working memory at 7.5 years of age. *Alcohol Clin. Exp. Res.* 2005;29:443-52.

[47] Kodituwakku PW, Handmaker NS, Cutler SK, Weathersby EK, Handmaker SD. Specific impairments in self-regulation in children exposed to alcohol prenatally. *Alcohol Clin. Exp. Res.* 1995; 19:1558-64.

[48] Streissguth AP, Barr HM, Sampson PD. Moderate prenatal alcohol exposure: Effects on child IQ and learning problems at age 7 years. *Alcohol Clin. Exp. Res.* 1990;14:662-9.

[49] Kodituwakku PW, Adnams CM, Hay A, Kitching AE, Burger E, Kalberg WO et al. Letter and category fluency in children with fetal alcohol syndrome from a community in South Africa. *J. Stud. Alcohol.* 2006;67:502-9.

[50] Schonfeld AM, Mattson SN, Lang AR, Delis DC, Riley EP. Verbal and nonverbal fluency in children with heavy prenatal alcohol exposure. *J. Stud. Alcohol* 2001;62:239-46.

[51] Mattson SN, Goodman AM, Caine C, Delis DC, Riley EP. Executive functioning in children with heavy prenatal alcohol exposure. *Alcohol Clin. Exp. Res.* 1999;23:1808-15.

[52] Carmichael Olson H, Feldman JJ, Streissguth AP, Sampson PD, Bookstein FL. Neuropsychological deficits in adolescents with Fetal Alcohol Syn-drome: Clinical findings. *Alcohol Clin. Exp. Res.* 1998;22:1998-2012.

[53] Connor PD, Sampson PD, Bookstein FL, Barr HM, Streissguth AP. Direct and indirect effects of prenatal alcohol damage on executive function. *Dev. Neuropsychol.* 2000;18:331-54.

[54] Kodituwakku PW, Kalberg W, May PA. The effects of prenatal alcohol exposure on executive functioning. *Alcohol Res. Health* 2001;25:192-8.

[55] Streissguth AP, Aase JM, Clarren SK, Randels SP, LaDue RA, Smith DF. Fetal alcohol syndrome in adolescents and adults. *JAMA* 1991;265:1961-7.

[56] Church MW, Eldis F, Blakley BW, Bawle EV. Hearing, language, speech, vestibular, and dentofacial disorders in Fetal Alcohol Syndrome. *Alcohol Clin. Exp. Res.* 1997;21:227-37.

[57] Abkarian GC. Communication effects of prenatal alcohol exposure. *J. Commun. Disord* 1992;25: 221-40.

[58] Streissguth AP, Sampson PD, Carmichael Olson H, Bookstein FL, Barr HM, Scott M et al. Maternal drinking during pregnancy: Attention and short-term memory in 14-year old offspring—A longi-tudinal prospective study. *Alcohol. Clin. Exp. Res.* 1994;18:202-18.

[59] Aronson M, Hagberg B. Neuropsychological disorders in children exposed to alcohol during pregnancy: A follow-up study of 24 children born to alcoholic mothers in Göteborg, Sweden. *Alcohol Clin. Exp. Res.* 1998;22:321-4.

[60] Kopera-Frye K, Dehaene S, Streissguth AP. Impairments of number processing induced by prenatal alcohol exposure. *Neuropsychologia* 1996; 34:1187-96.

[61] Burden MJ, Burden SW, Jacobson JL. Relation of prenatal alcohol exposure to cognitive processing speed and efficiency in childhood. *Alcohol Clin. Exp. Res.* 2005;29:1473-83.

[62] Mattson SN, Gramling L, Delis DC, Jones KL, Riley EP. Global-local processing in children prenatally exposed to alcohol. *Child Neuropsychol.* 1997;2:165-75.

[63] Streissguth AP, Barr HM, Martin DC, Herman CS. Effects of maternal alcohol, nicotine, and caffeine use during pregnancy on infant mental and motor development at eight months. *Alcohol Clin. Exp. Res.* 1980;4:152-64.

[64] Barr HM, Streissguth AP, Darby BL, Sampson PD. Prenatal exposure to alcohol, tobacco, and aspirin: Effects on fine and gross motor performance in 4-year-old children. *Dev. Psychol.* 1990;26:339-48.

[65] Kalberg WO, Provost B, Tollison SJ, Tabachnick BG, Robinson LK, Eugene Hoyme H, et al. Comparison of motor delays in young children with fetal alcohol syndrome to those with prenatal alcohol exposure and with no prenatal alcohol exposure. *Alcohol Clin. Exp. Res.* 2006;30:2037-45.

[66] Roebuck TM, Simmons RW, Mattson SN, Riley EP. Prenatal exposure to alcohol affects the body to maintain postural balance. *Alcohol Clin. Exp. Res.* 1998;22:252-8.

[67] Jones KL, Smith DW, Ulleland CN, Streissguth AP. Pattern of malformation in offspring of chronic alcoholic mothers. *Lancet* 1973;1:1267-71.

[68] Whaley SE, O'Connor MJ, Gunderson B. Comparison of the adaptive functioning of children prenatally exposed to alcohol to a nonexposed clinical sample. *Alcohol Clin. Exp. Res.* 2001; 25:118-24.

[69] Roebuck TM, Mattson SN, Riley EP. Behavioral and psychosocial profiles of alcohol exposed children. *Alcohol Clin. Exp. Res.* 1999;23:1070-6.

[70] Brown RT, Coles CD, Smith IE, Platzman KA, Silverstein J, Erikson S et al. Effects of prenatal alcohol exposure at school age. II: Attention and behavior. *Neurotoxicol Teratol* 1991;13:369-76.

[71] Carmichael Olson H. The effects of prenatal alcohol exposure on child development. *Infants Young Child* 1994; 6:10-25.

[72] Coggins TE, Friet T, Morgan T. Analyzing narrative productions in older school-age children and adolescents with fetal alcohol syndrome: An experimental tool for clinical applications. *Clin. Linguist Phon* 1997;12:221-236.

[73] Streissguth AP. *Fetal alcohol syndrome: A guide for families and communities.* Baltimore, MD: Paul H. Brookes, 1997.

[74] Thomas SE, Kelly SJ, Mattson SN, Riley EP. Comparison of social abilities of children with fetal alcohol syndrome to those of children with similar IQ scores and normal controls. *Alcohol Clin. Exp. Res.* 1998;22:528-33.

[75] Schonfeld AM, Paley B, Frankel F, O'Connor MJ. Executive functioning predicts social skills following prenatal alcohol exposure. *Child Neuro-psychol.* 2006;12:439-52.

[76] Ladue RA, Streissguth AP, Randels SP. Clinical considerations pertaining to adolescents and adults with fetal alcohol syndrome. In Sonderegger TB, ed, *Perinatal substance abuse: Research findings and clinical implications.* Baltimore, MD: Johns Hopkins Univ Press, 1992:104-31.

[77] Famy C, Streissguth AP, Unis AS. Mental illness in adults with fetal alcohol syndrome or fetal alcohol effects. *Am. J. Psychiatry* 1998;155:552-4.

[78] Fryer, SJ, McGee, CL, Matt, GE, Riley, EP, Mattson, SN. Evaluation of psychopathological conditions in children with heavy prenatal alcohol exposure. *Pediatrics* 2007; 119;733-41,

[79] O'Connor MJ, Shah B, Whaley SE, Cronin P, Gunderson B, Graham J. Psychiatric illness in a clinical sample of children with prenatal alcohol exposure. *Am. J. Drug Alcohol Abuse* 2002;28:743-54.

[80] Steinhausen HC, Spohr HL. Long-term outcome of children with fetal alcohol syndrome: Psychopathology, behavior, and intelligence. *Alcohol Clin. Exp. Res.* 1998;22:334-8.

[81] O'Connor, MJ, McCracken J, Best A. Under recognition of prenatal alcohol exposure in a child inpatient psychiatric setting, *Ment. Health Aspects Dev. Disabil* 2006;9,105-8.

[82] Fast DK, Conry J, Loock CA. Identifying fetal alcohol syndrome among youth in the criminal justice system. *J. Dev. Behav. Pediatr.* 1999;20:370-2.

[83] Burd L, Selfridge R, Klug M, Bakko S. Fetal alcohol syndrome in the United States corrections system. *Addict. Biol.* 2004;9:177-8.

[84] Schneider ML, Roughton EC, Lubach GR. Moderate alcohol consumption and psychological stress during pregnancy induce attention and neuromotor impairments in primate infants. *Child Dev.* 1997;68:747-59.

[85] Smith I, Coles C, Lancaster J, Fernhoff P, Falek A. The effect of volume and duration of exposure on neonatal physical and behavioral development. *Neurobehav. Toxicol. Teratol.* 1986;8:375-81.

[86] Streissguth AP, Barr HM, Martin DC. Maternal alcohol use and neonatal habituation assessed with the Brazelton scale. *Child Dev.* 1983;54:1109-18.

[87] O'Connor MJ, Sigman M, Kasari C. Attachment behavior of infants exposed prenatally to alcohol: Mediating effects of infant affect and mother-infant interaction. *Dev. Psychopathol.* 1992;4:243-56.

[88] Jacobson SW, Bihun JT, Chiodo LM. Effects of prenatal alcohol and cocaine exposure on infant cortisol levels. *Dev. Psychopathol.* 1999;11:195-208.

[89] Autti-Rämö I, Granstrom ML. The psychomotor development during the first year of life of infants exposed to intrauterine alcohol of various duration. *Neuropediatrics* 1991;22:59-64.

[90] Coles CD, Smith I, Fernhoff PM, Falek A. Neonatal neurobehavioral characteristics as correlates of maternal alcohol use during gestation. *Alcohol. Clin. Exp. Res.* 1985;9:454-60.

[91] Autti-Rämö I, Korkman M, Hilakivi-Clarke L, Lehtonen M, Halmesmaki E, Granstrom ML. Mental development of 2-year-old children exposed to alcohol in utero. *J. Pediatr* 1992;120: 740-6.

[92] Korkman M, Hilakivi-Clarke LA, Autti-Rämö I, Fellman V, Granstrom ML. Cognitive impairments at two years of age after prenatal alcohol exposure or perinatal asphyxia. *Neuropediatrics* 1994;25: 101-5.

[93] Paley B, O'Connor MJ, Kogan N, Findlay R. Prenatal alcohol exposure, child externalizing behavior, and maternal stress. *Parenting Sci. Pract.* 2005;5:29-56.

[94] Sood B, Delaney-Black V, Covington C, Nordstrom-Klee B, Ager J, Templin T et al. Prenatal alcohol exposure and childhood behavior at age 6 to 7 years: I. dose-response effect. *Pediatrics* 2001; 108(2),1-9.

[95] O'Connor MJ, Kogan N, Findlay R. Prenatal alcohol exposure and attachment behavior in children. *Alcohol. Clin. Exp. Res.* 2002;26:1592-1602.

[96] O'Connor MJ, Paley B. The relationship of prenatal alcohol exposure and the postnatal environment to child depressive symptoms. *J. Pediatr. Psychol.* 2006;31:50-64.

[97] Kupersmidt JB, Coie JD, Dodge KA. The role of poor peer relationships in the development of disorder. Asher SR, Coie JD, editors. *Peer rejection in childhood.* Cambridge, MA, USA: Cambridge Univ Press, 1990:274-305.

[98] Paetsch JJ, Bertrand LD. The relationship between peer, social, and school factors, and delinquency among youth. *J. Sch. Health* 1997;67:27-33.

[99] Patterson GR, Forgatch MS, Yoerger KL, Stool-miller M. Variables that initiate and maintain an early-onset trajectory for juvenile offending. *Dev. Psychopathol* 1998;10:531-47.

[100] Carmichael Olson H, Clarren SG. FAS diagnostic and prevention network. *Manual for psychological assessment and treatment planning for individuals with FAS and related conditions.* Seattle, WA, USA: Univ Washington, 1996.

[101] Streissguth AP, Barr HM, Kogan JA, Bookstein FL. Understanding the occurrence of secondary disabilities in clients with fetal alcohol syndrome and fetal alcohol effects. Final report. Seattle, WA, USA: Univ Washington School of Medicine, *Fetal Alcohol and Drug Unit*; 1996. Report No.: 96-06. Sponsored by the Centers for Disease Control and Prevention.

[102] Ryan S, Ferguson DL. On, yet, under the radar: Students with fetal alcohol syndrome disorder. *Except Child* 2006;3:363-79.

[103] Baer JS, Sampson PD, Barr HM, Connor PD, Streissguth AP. A 21-year longitudinal analysis of the effects of prenatal alcohol exposure on young adult drinking. *Arch. Gen. Psychiatry* 2003;60:377-85.

[104] Bertrand J, Floyd LL, Weber MK; Fetal Alcohol Syndrome Prevention Team, Division of Birth Defects and Developmental Disabilities, National Center on Birth Defects and Developmental Disabilities, Centers for Disease Control and Prevention (CDC). Guidelines for identifying and referring persons with fetal alcohol syndrome. *MMWR Recomm. Rep.* 2005;54,1-15.

[105] Streissguth AP, Bookstein FL, Barr HM, Press S, Sampson PD. A fetal alcohol behavior scale. *Alcohol Clin. Exp. Res.* 1998;22:325-33.

[106] National Organization on Fetal Alcohol Syndrome. Fetal alcohol spectrum disorders: Special focus. Washington, DC, USA: *Nat. Org. Fetal Alcohol Syndr*, 2002.

[107] Canadian Paediatric Society. Fetal alcohol syndrome: Position statement. *Paediatric Child Health* 2002;7:161-74.

[108] Diekman ST, Floyd RL, Decoufle P, Schulkin J, Ebrahim SH, Sokol RJ. A survey of obstetrician-gynecologists on their patients' alcohol use during pregnancy. *Obstet Gynecol* 2000;95:756-63.

[109] Nevin AC, Parshuran V, Nulman I, Koren G, Einarson A. A survey of physician knowledge regarding awareness of maternal alcohol use and the diagnosis of FAS. *BMC Fam. Pract.* 2002;3:2-8.

[110] Floyd RL, O'Connor MJ, Bertrand J, Sokol R. Reducing adverse outcomes from prenatal alcohol exposure: A clinical plan of action. *Alcohol Clin. Exp. Res.* 2006;30:1271-5.

[111] Paley B, O'Connor MJ, Baillie S, Guiton G, Stuber M. Integrating case topics in medical school curriculum to enhance multiple skill learning: Using fetal alcohol spectrum disorders as an exemplary case. *Acad Psychiatry.* In press.

[112] Paley B, O'Connor MJ, Frankel F, Marquardt M. Predictors of stress in parents of children with fetal alcohol spectrum disorders. *J. Dev. Behav. Pediatr.* 2006;27:396-404.

[113] Laugeson E, Paley B, Schonfeld AM, Carpenter EM, Frankel F, O'Connor MJ. Adaptation of children's friendship training for children with fetal alcohol spectrum disorders. *Child and Family Behavior Therapy.* In press.

[114] O'Connor MJ, Frankel F, Paley B, Schonfeld AM, Carpenter E, Laugeson E et al. A controlled social skills training for children with fetal alcohol spectrum disorders. *J. Consult Clin. Psychol.* 2006; 74:639-48.

[115] Wechsler D. *Wechsler Individual Achievement Test*, Second edition. San Antonio, TX, USA: Psychol Corp, 2001.

[116] Sparrow SS, Cicchetti DV, Balla DA. *Vineland Adaptive Behavior Scales*, Second edition (Vineland II), Survey interview form/Caregiver rating form. Livonia, MN, USA: Pearson Assessments, 2005.

[117] Conners CK. *Conners' Rating Scales*, Revised. New York, NY, USA: Multi-Health Systems, Inc, 2000.

[118] Conners CK, MHS Staff. *Conners' Continuous Performance Test II (CPT-II).* New York, NY, USA: Multi-Health Systems Inc, 2000.

[119] Kaplan E, Fein D, Kramer J, Delis D, Morris R. *Wechsler Intelligence Scale for Children, Third edition as a Process Instrument.* San Antonio, TX, USA: Psychol Corp, 1999.

[120] Frick PJ, Hare RD. *Antisocial process screening device.* Toronto, ON, Canada: Multi-Health Systems, 2001.

[121] Beck AT, Steer RA, Brown GK. Manual for the BDI-II. San Antonio, TX, USA: Psychol Corp, 1996.

[122] Derogatis LR. *BSI Brief Symptom Inventory. Administration, scoring, and procedures manual. Fourth edition,* Minneapolis, MN, USA: NCS Pearson, 1993.

[123] Achenbach TM, Rescorla LA. Manual for the ASEBA school-age forms and profiles. Burlington, VT, USA: Univ Vermont, *Res. Center Children Youth Fam.*, 2001.

[124] Kovacs M. The childhood depression inventory. New York, NY, USA: Multi-Health Serv, 1992.

[125] Shaffer D, Fisher P, Lucas CP, Dulcan MK, Schwab-Stone ME. NIMH diagnostic interview schedule for children version IV (NIMH DISC-IV): Description, differences from previous versions, and reliability of some common diagnoses. *J. Am. Acad. Child. Adolesc Psychiatry* 2000;39:28-38.

[126] O'Connor MJ, Kasari C. Prenatal alcohol exposure and depressive features in children. *Alcohol Clin. Exp. Res*. 2000;24:1084-92.

[127] First MB, Spitzer RL, Gibbon M, Williams JBW. Structured clinical interview for DSM-IV™ axis I disorders, Clinician Version. Washington, DC, USA: *Am. Psychiatr* Publ, 1996.

[128] First MB, Spitzer RL, Gibbon M, Williams JBW. *Structured clinical interview for DSM-IV™ axis II disorders*. Washington, DC, USA: Am Psychiatr Publ, 1997.

[129] Bayley N. *Bayley Scales of Infant Development. Third edition*. San Antonio, TX, USA: Harcourt Assessment, 2005.

[130] Wechsler D. *Wechsler preschool and primary scale of intelligence*, Third ed. San Antonio, TX, USA: Psychol Corp, 2002.

[131] Wechsler D. *Wechsler intelligence scale for children*, Fourth edition. San Antonio, TX, USA: Psychol Corp, 2003.

[132] Wechsler D. *Wechsler adult intelligence scale*, Third edition. San Antonio, TX, USA: Psychol Corp, 1997.

[133] Gioia GA, Isquith PK, Guy SC, Kenworthy L. Behavior rating inventory of executive function. Lutz, FL, USA: *Psychol. Assess Resources*, 2000.

[134] Llorente AM, Williams J, Satz P, D'Elia L. Children's color trails test. Lutz, FL, USA: *Psychol. Assess Resources*, 2003.

[135] Delis DC, Kaplan E, Kramer, JH. *Delis-Kaplan Executive Function System*. San Antonio, TX, USA: Psychol. Corp, 2001.

[136] Korkman M, Kirk U, Kemp S. *NEPSY: A developmental neuropsychological instrument*. San Antonio: TX, USA: Psychol Corp, 1998.

[137] Heaton RK, Chelune GJ, Talley JL, Kay GG, Curtiss G. Wisconsin Card Sorting Test. Lutz, FL, USA: Psychol Assess Resources, 1993.

[138] Semel E, Wiig EH, Secord WA. *Clinical evalu-ation of language fundamentals*. 3rd ed. San Antonio, TX: Psychol Corp, 2004.

[139] Zimmerman IL, Steiner VG, Pond RE. *Preschool Language Scale*, Fourth edition. San Antonio, TX: Harcourt Assessment, 2002.

[140] Wiig EH, Secord W. *Test of language competence*, expanded edition. San Antonio, TX: Psychol Corp, 1989.

[141] Delis DC, Kramer JH, Kaplan E, Ober BA. *California verbal learning test, children's version*. San Antonio, TX: Psychol Corp, 1994.

[142] Cohen MJ. *Children's memory scale*. San Antonio, TX: Psychol Corp, 1997.

[143] Wechsler D. *Wechsler memory scale*, Third edition. San Antonio, TX: Psychol Corp, 1997.

[144] Beery KE, Buktenica NA. *Developmental test of visual motor integration*, Fourth edition. Parsipanny, NJ: Modern Curriculum Press, 1997.

[145] Halstead WC. *Brain and intelligence*. Chicago, IL: Univ Chicago Press, 1947.

[146] Reitan RM, Davison LA. *Clinical neuropsychology: Current status and applications.* Washington, DC: VH Winston, 1974.

In: Alcohol-Related Cognitive Disorders
Editors: L. Sher, I. Kandel, J. Merrick pp. 29-56

ISBN: 978-1-60741-730-9
© 2009 Nova Science Publishers, Inc.

Chapter 2

NON-INVASIVE NEUROIMAGING IN FETAL ALCOHOL SPECTRUM DISORDERS

Krisztina L. Malisza

ABSTRACT

While structural information regarding anatomical abnormalities found in the brains of individuals with fetal alcohol syndrome (FAS) and fetal alcohol spectrum disorders (FASD) has been thoroughly investigated, few functional neuroimaging studies have been performed. The major structural anomalies are outlined and the results of the functional neuroimaging studies are described in detail. Links between the anatomical region of impairment, functional impairment, and the cognitive dysfunction found in FASD are proposed. A literature search revealed only five studies of functional neuroimaging in individuals with FASD. One study used positron emission tomography (PET), three used single photon emission computed tomography (SPECT), and one used functional magnetic resonance imaging (fMRI) to evaluate brain metabolism and function. Of these, only fMRI actually examined task-related functional changes in the brain related to cognition. Although there is significant variability in the results, due to the heterogeneity of the syndrome and the few studies performed to date, clear regions of impairment related to cognitive dysfunction are described. The most consistent results involve the impairment of the frontal cortex, specifically the prefrontal cortex and medial frontal lobe, which is related to executive function, working memory, response inhibition, and attention. Consistent impairment was also noted in the temporal brain region, implicated in problems with emotions, memory, learning, and language functions.

INTRODUCTION

Fetal alcohol syndrome (FAS), partial FAS (pFAS) and alcohol related neurodevelopmental disorders (ARND) are collectively referred to as fetal alcohol spectrum disorders (FASD). To design possible interventions, it is necessary to characterize and understand the effects of alcohol on the central nervous system (CNS). Functional neuroimaging methods provide a means to do so. This paper will focus on functional neuroimaging findings in FASD affected individuals. This area will see significant growth as the non-invasive techniques, such as functional magnetic resonance imaging (fMRI), and multimodal experiments using electroencephalography (EEG), combined with fMRI become more prevalent in the clinical realm. Since these techniques do not subject individuals to harmful radiation, it is now possible for children to participate in research studies. This benefits not only the affected populations but also allows for the acquisition of neuroimaging data from healthy children to provide reliable baseline, normative data.

The incidence of FASD is high in Canada and the United States [1,2]. The direct costs of FASD, due to increased health support, social services, and special education requirements, are estimated to be over one million US dollars per affected individual [1]. The use of neuroimaging techniques for the recognition and confirmation of FASD could result in a reduction in secondary disabilities that are preventable after diagnosis and after targeted and adapted interventions and treatment of the affected child [3]. This decrease should translate into substantial benefits for society, the affected individuals and their families.

FETAL ALCOHOL SPECTRUM DISORDERS

The action of ethanol in the body, particularly in the CNS is not well understood. Although, moderate alcohol consumption does not pose significant long-term health risks to adult humans, the effects of ethanol in the developing organism are far more serious. The diagnosis of FASD is currently based on a four-digit diagnostic code that evaluates four criteria: growth deficiency, facial phenotype, CNS damage or dysfunction, and gestational alcohol exposure (4). Multidisciplinary teams are necessary to complete this diagnosis and to provide treatment options [1,5]. The most devastating consequences of FASD are the effects on the CNS. Whereas the other characteristics are easily defined, CNS damage is not. Significant brain dysfunction is found in the majority of individuals with FASD. Deficits are observed in the following areas: attention, communication (receptive and expressive language), cognitive function (IQ), comprehension (reading, mathematical reasoning, abstract thought), memory (visual, verbal, working memory, long and short term), executive function (reasoning, planning, judgment, abstraction, problem solving), adaptive/social skills (behavior), and neurological abnormalities [1].

Children with FAS often have intellectual impairment and on average, are classified as being mildly retarded, whereas those without the full syndrome tend to have higher IQ scores [1]. Although subjects with ARND frequently do not demonstrate many of the facial features characteristic of FAS, such individuals nonetheless show neurological deficits that may include CNS neurodevelopmental and/or cognitive or behavioral abnormalities [5]. The attention problems found in FASD, and more specifically in ARND-affected patients, are similar to those in individuals with Attention Deficit Hyperactivity Disorder (ADHD), resulting in increased difficulties with diagnosis [6,7]. Confounding further is the likelihood that comorbid conditions exist within some individuals. This can lead to FASD not being diagnosed, being misdiagnosed, or medical advice not being sought. Understanding the differences in neurocognitive function between the subgroups of FASD helps to determine and tailor treatment options.

The diagnosis of FASD is particularly difficult as symptoms are often not obvious or not yet present in young children. Accurate diagnosis is important because many secondary disabilities could be prevented with appropriate intervention. Common secondary disabilities include mental health problems, disrupted schooling, delinquency, alcohol/drug problems, inappropriate sexual behavior, dependent living, and unemployment [8]. The critical age at which intervention would no longer be effective is uncertain. The evidence indicates that although the younger brain is more readily amenable to learning and change, older brains have not lost this capacity [9].

The mechanisms governing interactions of ethanol with the developing fetus are not well understood. A popular hypothesis is that ethanol interferes with growth factor signal transduction (10,11), which, in turn, suggests that the timing and duration of ethanol exposure during gestation should critically affect the type and severity of symptoms [12]. This view could explain the wide range of behavioral, sensory-motor, and cognitive deficits associated with FASD. Exposure to ethanol in the first trimester seems to lead to the characteristic facial dysmorphology and midline brain anomalies [13]. Such anomalies as microcephaly can be caused by ethanol exposure any time during pregnancy; yet, cessation of ethanol consumption after the second trimester appears to improve head growth [14]. Exposure to ethanol during second and third trimesters can lead to neuronal loss [15], extensive gliosis (16), and altered neuronal circuitry [17]. Purkinje cells have been shown to be vulnerable to ethanol exposure in the third trimester [16].

The CNS manifestations of FAS are diverse. The effects of alcohol as a teratogen are very well documented [12,18-20]. A variety of anatomical changes have been reported post mortem, such as reduced volume of the basal ganglia and cerebellar vermis and brain overall, neuronal migration anomalies, hydrocephalus, cortical thinning and abnormalities in corpus callosum, cerebellum, and brainstem [21]. The corpus callosum and cerebellar vermis seem to be particularly sensitive to ethanol [21]. Children with obvious anatomical changes often have low IQ scores, whereas children with normal IQ scores tend to have no detectable anatomical abnormalities [1,22]. Common cognitive deficits include delayed language development, visual and auditory attention impairments, memory deficits, and difficulties in mathematical reasoning [23-29]. Sensory-motor deficits are also reported [30-33]. Ophthalmologic and hearing disorders have a high prevalence in FAS patients [1].

Extensive damage of executive function seems to be closely linked with FASD [23-25,34]. The function of the prefrontal cortex in working memory is well established [35-39]. In particular, fMRI studies show neuronal activation of the prefrontal and parietal cortices increases with greater levels of working memory load in healthy individuals [23,24,39]. The dorsolateral prefrontal cortex, posterior parietal cortex and Broca's area have been identified in working memory function [24,36-38,40,41]. Children with prenatal alcohol exposure have deficits in explicit memory with impaired recall, but have intact recognition memory and no deficit in implicit memory, as measured by a priming task [28].

Attention is a major cognitive deficit characteristic of FAS and prenatal alcohol exposure [6,26,42-47]. As mentioned above, FASD and ADHD share common features, often leading to the misdiagnosis of individuals with FASD, and in particular ARND. Despite these similarities, few studies have directly compared FASD and ADHD. Studies using conventional psychiatric measures and measures of neurocognitive function suggest distinct patterns of deficits between FAS and ADHD groups (43). Among the clinical implications is the finding that for children with FASD, ADHD is more likely to be the earlier-onset, inattention subtype, with co-morbid developmental psychiatric and medical conditions (48). Co-morbid psychiatric disorders in FASD include anxiety, mood, conduct, or explosive disorders.

Previous studies involving measures of sustained attention using the continuous performance task (CPT) did not show significant differences between adolescents with FASD without dysmorphology and control subjects [24,42]. Nevertheless, significant errors of omission were observed in the alcohol exposed individuals, which suggested a deficit in visual perception [42]. Streissguth et al [45,47] reported significant differences between prenatal alcohol-exposed individuals and controls on a CPT test, with poorer performance associated with higher alcohol exposure. Also acknowledged is that the resulting poorer performance of FAS individuals may result from impulsivity rather than attention [47].

Functional neuroimaging methods can potentially provide finer, less subjective measures of alcohol-related changes in brain function. These techniques may assist in determining unequivocal diagnosis where it was not previously possible. The accurate diagnosis of individuals with FASD will offer increased potential for early and tailored intervention and access to social and educational programs.

FUNCTIONAL NEUROIMAGING METHODS

Positron Emission Tomography, or PET, is an invasive imaging technique involving radionuclide injection (^{11}C, ^{18}F, ^{15}O or ^{13}N) [49]. The radiopharmaceutical injected emits positrons that collide with electrons to produce two gamma rays, which travel at approximately 180° apart and are detected by scintillation crystals around the patient. Photomultiplier tubes convert the photons to electrical signals that are used to produce the images. Since gamma rays are emitted in opposite directions, locating where the electron-positron annihilation took place is possible, and hence, the location of the radiopharmaceutical. PET can be used to examine metabolite utilization. For example, brain glucose metabolism is typically examined using the radio-labeled tracer, [^{18}F]-fluorodeoxyglucose (^{18}FDG). In this way, PET can provide a direct measure of neuronal function. The main downfalls of this technique are cost, the need for a particle accelerator to produce short-lived radioisotopes, and poor spatial resolution in comparison to fMRI. PET can indirectly examine neuronal activity by measuring the regional cerebral blood flow (rCBF).

Single Photon Emission Computed Tomography, or SPECT, is similar to PET, but single gamma rays are emitted and the radiopharmaceuticals used have longer decay times (^{133}Xe, ^{99}Tc, ^{23}I) [49]. The signal from SPECT is detected by a photon absorbing collimator together with scintillator crystal and photomultiplier tube. The collimators detect the direction of the photons. These differences translate to a less expensive, but less sensitive and less detailed imaging modality than PET. SPECT images provide information relating rCBF and distribution of the radioactive tracer.

Structural information of soft tissues can be obtained using magnetic resonance imaging (MRI). MRI uses a magnetic field to manipulate the natural properties within the system. Magnetic resonance imaging of neuronal function, or fMRI, is a non-invasive technique that does not require the use of harmful radiation or contrast agents; as such, can be applied to pediatric research [50]. This technique is used to detect neuronal activity in the brain indirectly. The technique works under the premise that paramagnetic deoxygenated-hemoglobin acts as an endogenous MR contrast agent by altering the local magnetization relaxation times. Conversely, oxygenated hemoglobin is diamagnetic and does not contribute to relaxation. Upon functional activation, neurons take up more oxygen from their surroundings because of increased metabolic demand. At the same time, the local supply of oxygenated blood is increased in excess of the demand. The result is a net local increase in the concentration of oxyhemoglobin, giving rise to an increase in the MRI signal in the area of the activation. This imaging method is known as blood oxygenation level dependent (BOLD) imaging [51]. Sites of neuronal activation are identified by comparing images obtained during rest and stimulation. Support has grown for the theory that the BOLD signal is related more closely to the magnitude of synaptic events than neuronal firing rates [52]. FMRI has the best spatial resolution of the neuroimaging techniques. The temporal resolution, however, relies on the hemodynamic response. As such, fMRI is unable to detect changes on the very short neuronal response time scale.

Electroencephalography (EEG) and magnetoencephalography (MEG) record the electrical and magnetic field arising from neuronal activity, respectively. The EEG and event-related potential (ERP) methods have a temporal resolution on the order of 1-5 ms [53]. EEG scalp recordings of underlying brain activity can be made using over 100 electrodes, providing a direct measure of neuronal function. Distortion of neuronal potentials as the signal passes through the highly resistive skull limits the spatial resolution. Changes in the electrical signal vary with mental activity.

Thus, measuring the sub-second component processes of stimulus-related electrical brain activity is possible, using event-related potentials, to look at sensory, motor, and cognitive processing [53]. Functional networks can then be proposed between cortical regions by examining the EEG time series derived from the different electrodes. MEG, like EEG, does not provide adequate information regarding where the signal originates and is considerably more expensive. Although not truly 'neuroimaging' techniques, EEG and MEG provide a direct measure of neuronal activity with excellent temporal resolution; nevertheless, even with the current advances in the field, spatial resolution is poor, about 1 cm^2 [49]. Either EEG or MEG can be combined with other neuroimaging techniques like fMRI in hopes of improving both spatial and temporal resolution.

A LITERATURE SEARCH

A literature search was conducted to obtain a comprehensive list of publications involving fetal alcohol spectrum disorders, neuroimaging, and functional neuroimaging (n = 45) from 1990 through the first quarter of 2007. The current chapter focuses on functional neuroimaging of cognitive processes in FASD-affected individuals. Structural anomalies are presented in table 1 to link them to the functional neuroimaging findings. Only results for which volumes were corrected relative to either the whole brain or cerebellum are included; absolute volumetric measures were not listed. Only studies showing anatomical brain differences relative to normal controls are presented. Studies in which no significant structural differences were found were omitted.

Table 1. Review of structural imaging findings in FASD

Brain area affected	Structural abnormality	FAS No. in study (Age range) (yrs)	FASD* No. in study (Age range) (yrs)	Observed/Potential functional impairment	Refs
Frontal Lobe	Reduced volume	14(8-22)	7(8-22)	Executive Function, memory, motor, language, attention	(91)
Parietal	Narrowing/ reduced volume	14(8-22); 14(8-19)	7(8-22); 12(10-22)	Somatosensory, spatial perception, integration of auditory and visual information	(18, 91)
	Increase GM/ reduced WM	14(8-22); 14(8-22); 9(18-25)	7(8-22); 7(8-22);		(19, 91, 92)
Cortical sulci	Wide	5(12-14)	12(12-14)		(93)
Infer Parietal/ Superior Temporal	Less Asymmetry (NS)	14(8-22)	7(8-22y)	Language, comprehension, Receptive language, auditory	(94)
Temporal Lobe	Increased GM/ reduced WM	14(8-22)	7(8-22)	Emotions, visceral responses, learning, memory	(19)
Basal Ganglia (Caudate Nucleus)	Reduced volume/ Atrophy	6(8-19); 14(8-19); 5(12-14); 7(11-12)	12(10-22); 2(16); 12(12-14); 8(11-12); 4(9-12); 2 of 11(3-13)	Cognition, motor; Executive function, spatial learning, attention, perseveration, response inhibition	(18, 63, 68-70, 93)
Corpus Callosum	Shape features/ displacement/	15(18-36); 60(14-37); 30(18-36); 13(8-22);	15(18-36); 60(14-37); 30(18-37);	Verbal learning impairment;	(13, 20, 63, 65, 87, 95-98)
	Agenesis/ Atrophy	10(4-26); 9(0.5-20); 11(8-18); 2 of 3(11-29); 1 of 2(13-14y)	7(10-19); 2(8-18)	Learning, sensory, cognition, mnemonic information	
	Hypoplastic	10(4-26); 9(0.5-20); 5 (12-14); 1 of 10(14); 1 of 2(13-14)	12(12-14)		(13, 66, 87, 93, 99)
(Posterior - isthmus)	Reduced WM Greater diffusivity	9(18-25)	14(10-13)		(92) (100)

Brain area affected	Structural abnormality	FAS No. in study (Age range) (yrs)	FASD* No. in study (Age range) (yrs)	Observed/Potential functional impairment	Refs
Cerebellum	Atrophy		2 of 11 (3-13)	Motor equilibrium, coordination	(63)
Cerebellar Vermis	Reduced volume	6(8-22); 14(8-22); 3(14-21)	3(8-22y); 7(10-19); 7(14-21)	Learning, memory Attention, sensation, motivation, behaviour, autonomic activity	(97, 101, 102)
Hippocampus	Hypoplasia	5(12-14)	12(12-14)	Verbal memory, motor dexterity	(93)
	Reduced volume/ Agenesis	14(8-19); 5(12-14); 10(4-26); 1 of 3(29)	12(10-22); 12(12-14)	Learning, memory, emotional behaviour, regulation of autonomic nervous system	(13, 18, 65, 93)
Septum pellucidum	Agenesis	10(4-26); 9(0.5-20)		cognitive dysfunction, mental retardation, developmental delay	(13, 99)
Ventricles	dilation	10(4-26); 9(0.5-20); 1 of 11(3-13); 1 of 2(13-14); 3(14-21)	7(14-21)	N/A	(13, 63, 87, 99, 102)
Inferior olivary eminences	hypoplasia	10(4-26); 9(0.5-20); 1 of 3(15)		Motor coordination, equilibrium	(13, 65, 99)
Brain stem	Reduced volume	10(4-26); 9(0.5-20); 1 of 3(15)		N/A	(13, 65, 99)

The description of subjects in table 1 includes whether the study specifically examined individuals with FAS or included other diagnoses within the spectrum of the disorder (FASD). Diagnoses of ARND, partial FAS, fetal alcohol effects (FAE), and prenatal alcohol exposure (PAE) are labeled FASD. Affected brain regions were correlated with known cognitive functions. Where provided, the type of functional impairment is noted; otherwise, potential functional impairment is suggested.

All studies of functional neuroimaging findings (n = 5) were reviewed, and the regions of impairment were correlated with known MRI structural, metabolic, and psychological studies to provide additional information regarding cognitive impairment. Papers on behavioral and psychological assessment of individuals with FASD are not included; where appropriate, however, reference is made to behavioral studies to correlate the functional neuroimaging findings.

Functional MRI data analysis was performed, and functional activity overlaid on the rendered images, using statistical parametric mapping (SPM) [54], as described previously [24].

Magnetic Resonance Imaging (MRI)

Of the manuscripts relating to the neuroimaging of individuals prenatally exposed to alcohol, the overwhelming majority use MRI to examine structural features of the brain and include several recent review articles [21,55-60]. Table 1 outlines the major structural abnormalities found in individuals with FASD, the cognitive impairment noted during the studies and/or inferred from known cognitive and behavioral functions of the affected region.

An overall reduction in brain size is apparent in individuals with FASD. Due to the condition of microcephaly and reduction in stature in these subjects, the results are not significant (NS) when comparing brain volume to the cranium size, or specific brain regions normalized to the entire brain or cerebellum. Several authors, however, report significantly reduced corrected brain volume or atrophy for the basal ganglia, corpus callosum, inferior parietal lobe, cerebellum, hippocampus, and brain stem. Diffusion MRI studies show increased grey matter and or reduced white matter in the corpus callosum, inferior parietal and temporal lobes. Several studies showed an enlargement of cortical sulci, the septum pellucidum, and ventricles. Hypoplasia was observed in the corpus callosum, cerebellar vermis, and inferior olivary eminences.

Functional Neuroimaging

Of the five studies that apply functional neuroimaging methods to individuals with FASD, three use SPECT and one uses PET to determine cerebral perfusion data. Regional CBF, measured by PET and SPECT, is considered a reliable index of neuronal activity [61,62]. The only study that examined task-dependent brain function is the fMRI examination of working memory in FASD. Table 2 outlines the functional neuroimaging findings from the literature related to the brain region impaired in FASD.

Table 2. Review of functional neuroimaging findings in FASD

Method	Diagnosis (age years)	Observations Brain region abnormality/Significant differences	Conclusion Dysfunction/Impairment	Ref
PET ^{18}FDG	19 FAS (16-30)	FAS: Decreased rCBF in thalamus (left and right) and basal ganglia (left and right caudate heads, right caudate, putamen body)	Thalamus: distractibility, impulsiveness; Basal Ganglia: motor incoordination, clumsiness	[22]
SPECT ^{99}Tc-HMPAO	11 FAS (3-13)	FAS: FC: left-right dominance lacking left parieto-occipital: mild hypoperfusion FC: slight hyperperfusion	Left hemisphere: arithmetic, logic, grammar	[63]
SPECT ^{123}I Nor-β-CIT	10 FAS, 2 FAE + ADHD (5-16)	SERT: FAS < controls – particularly medial frontal cortex DAT: basal ganglia: FAS > control	Executive dysfunction related to serotonergic function	[66]
SPECT Neurolite	3 FAS (6-29) 2/3ADHD	Temporal: ≥ 25% reduction in CBF (n = 3) FAS (n = 2): Left hypoperfusion	Temporal: emotion, learning, memory; Left hemisphere: arithmetic, logic, grammar	[65]
fMRI Working memory task	Children: 5 ARND, 6 PFAS, 3 FAS (7-12);	Children: FASD > control (C): inferior-middle frontal (GFi, GFm), orbital (GO), inferior slices of anterior cingulate (AC); FASD: Decreased GFi activity with task difficulty C > FASD superior slices of AC, superior slices of frontal cortex (FC), parietal cortex (PC) C: Increased GFi activity with task difficulty	prefrontal, middle frontal and orbital cortex	[24]
	Adults: 6 ARND, 1 pFAS, 3 FAS (18-33)	FASD > C GFi, GFm C: GFi, GFm: greater activity with task difficulty Overall Brain activity: FASD < C All subjects: Increased GFi activity with task difficulty	Impaired working memory function, executive function	
	All subjects: Child and Adult	Activity in DLPFC and AC; FASD > C: GFi, GFm, GO Increasing activity with task difficulty in PC, FC at superior levels		

Table 3. Neuronal/electrical recordings in individuals with FAS compared to normal controls (C)

Method	Diagnosis (age)	Observations - Brain region abnormality – Significant differences	Ref
ERP Oddball and noise paradigm	18 FAS (4-15y) 18 C	Parietal: FAS greater P300 latency to noise burst P300 – cognitive information processing – encoding, selecting, memorizing, decision making, etc.	[88]
EEG	18 FAS (4-15y) 18 C	9/18 FAS: immature/poorly developed, low voltage or amplitude less alpha and lower alpha freq (7.5-12 HZ); reduction in mean power; excessive slowing (left hemisphere parieto-occipital)	[89]
EEG	2 FAS (13y, 14y)	EEG moderately abnormal mainly posterior: dominant rhythm: theta 4-6 Hz, occasional delta 1-2 Hz No focal abnormality	[87]
EEG	5 FAS (4-7y) 11 C (4-6y)	FAS: increased power during quiet sleep – verbal, quantitative, general cognitive and memory scores reduced. No difference in REM sleep – no motor score difference	[103]
EEG	11 FAS (3-13y)	No focal abnormalities except: 2/11 paroxysmal 4Hz theta activity bioccipitally 1/11 asymmetric EEG spikes and slow waves in left parietooccipital	[63]

Table 3 summarizes EEG and ERP studies of individuals with FASD compared to healthy controls. These findings provide information regarding fast events but not anatomical specificity. Nonetheless, valuable information is gained from these direct measures of neuronal function. In addition, they can be correlated with neuroimaging modalities, such as fMRI, to provide information related to timing of cognitive processes and localization of brain function.

Functional Neuroimaging of FASD using PET

The structural and functional brain integrity of non-retarded (mean full scale IQ 80.2) young adults (n = 19; 16-30 years) with FAS was examined by Clark et al [22]. MR images were acquired to determine the structural integrity of the brain. The subject with the lowest IQ showed structural abnormality that included thinning of the corpus callosum and a small ventricular system (table 1). PET was used to determine the functional brain integrity. Injection of ^{18}FDG was used to measure regional rates of glucose metabolism (rCMR$_{glc}$) in 27, 1.2 cm^2 regions of interest, compared with age-matched normal subjects (n = 15). Absolute regional metabolic rates were compared by t-test, and individual rate differences removed by standardizing rCMR$_{glc}$ to the basal metabolism. Whereas no differences were observed for the absolute metabolic rates, five areas were found to be significantly reduced relative to the cerebellum for the standardized rates: the right and left thalamus, right and left caudate heads and right caudate/putamen body.

Functional Neuroimaging of FASD using SPECT

Riikonen et al [63] used MRI, EEG and SPECT to examine morphological and brain perfusion vulnerabilities in children (n = 11; 3-13 years) with FAS. Morphological anomalies were apparent in six subjects (see table 1). All children had language difficulties and attention deficits, and several had or showed risk factors for dyslexia or dyscalculia. Two had moderate learning disability (IQ 40-46), whereas the rest had mild learning disability (IQ 68-85) or normal intelligence (IQ >85). Six FAS subjects were anesthetized and of these, three were pre-sedated with diazepam for the SPECT study. Six cortical regions were defined on both sides of the brain from frontal to occipital and the left-right index of the average radioactivity calculated for each region and hemisphere on the axial slices. Similarly, axial slices of the striatum were used to calculate the left-right index in symmetrical regions of interest. For ethical considerations, no healthy control volunteers were subjected to SPECT; MRI, however, was conducted in six normal subjects (3-23 years) for comparison.

Compared with the published results from normal children, children with FAS showed significantly reduced rCBF in the left compared with the right cortex. In particular, mild hypoperfusion was observed in the left parieto-occipital and frontal regions in children with FAS, which is opposite to that found in healthy children of the same age [63, 64]. The authors suggest that the normal left-right dominance that is lacking points to impaired function of the left hemisphere.

Bhatara et al [65] reported three cases using SPECT imaging to examine brain function in sedated individuals with FAS who had previously undergone MRI and shown several structural brain abnormalities (see table 1). For ethical considerations, no SPECT studies were performed on healthy children; instead, data were compared with prior SPECT results from two normal adults (29 and 35 years old). Axial slices were examined for left-right differences in radioactive counts.

Subject 1, a 15-year old with ADHD and full IQ scale of 72, did not show left-right hemispheric differences in CBF, but the right CBF was 25% lower than the ipsilateral occipital and cerebellar regions. Subject 2, an 11-year old with ADHD and full scale IQ of 85, showed no general right-left differences, but CBF was greater than 25% lower in the temporal lobes than in the ipsilateral cerebellum, bilaterally. Subject 3, a 29 year old with full scale IQ of 77, showed left-right hemispheric differences, with lowest counts in the right frontal region, followed by the right temporal and parietal areas. A bilateral decrease was observed in the temporal lobe compared with the cerebellum.

Overall, CBF was reduced by at least 25% in all three subjects in the temporal region compared with the cerebellum. In comparison, CBF was reduced 4-7% in control subjects, suggesting temporal lobe dysfunction in subjects with FAS.

Riikonen et al [66] examined deep serotonergic and dopaminergic metabolism and structures (see table 1) in children with FASD and ADHD (n = 12; 5-16 years) with mean IQ of 76.2, using SPECT and MRI, respectively [66]. Four of these subjects were classified as mild to moderate mental retardation. SPECT was performed with 10 children. Again, because of ethical constraints, no normal children were subjected to SPECT studies, but the results from affected individuals were compared with age-matched patient controls. Normal healthy children were not used for comparison regarding structural findings, but the clinical population was stipulated as having 'normal' MRI findings. No significant differences in relative brain volumes were found in any of the regions examined.

Serotonin and dopamine (SERT and DAT) neuro-transmission, known to be affected by prenatal alcohol exposure, were examined [66]. The bilateral regions of interest selected for the SPECT were the midbrain, medial frontal cortex (MFC), temporal poles, and striatum, with the cerebellum as the reference region. SPECT showed lower SERT binding in the MFC and higher DAT binding in basal ganglia in controls. The left-right dominance lacking in the previous SPECT studies was not observed. Serotonin levels in children with FASD were 20% lower than in controls, especially in the MFC anterior cingulate region, and had increased dopamine transporter binding.

Functional Neuroimaging of FASD Using fMRI

Malisza et al (24) conducted fMRI experiments in 24 individuals with FASD (n = 14; 7-12 years and n = 10; 18-33 years) and age- and sex-matched healthy control subjects to determine if any difference could be observed between children and adults with FASD and healthy controls. Subjects completed a series of n-back tasks to examine the functional activation of spatial working memory. The FMRI tasks required the subject to indicate spatial locations of a colored circle during presentation (n = 0, control task), at the end of a brief delay during which blank circles were presented (n = 1, simplified 1-back task), or after presentation of one additional stimulus (n = 1, 1-back task). In addition, all participants completed three standard psychological tests before the imaging session: a Self Ordered

Pointing Task (SOPT), a Continuous Performance Task (CPT), and the Wisconsin Card Sorting Task (WCST).

Consistent activations were observed at p < 0.001 in regions of the brain associated with working memory and attention, namely dorsolateral prefrontal cortex and anterior cingulate, and in the visual cortex in healthy volunteers. Children with FASD displayed greater inferior-middle frontal lobe activity, whereas greater superior frontal and parietal lobe activity was observed in control subjects. Control children also showed an overall increase in frontal lobe activity with increasing task difficulty, whereas children with FASD showed decreased activity. The adults with FASD demonstrated less functional brain activity overall, but greater inferior-middle frontal lobe activity during the simpler tasks, relative to controls. Control adults demonstrated greater inferior frontal activity with increasing task difficulty, whereas this pattern was not consistently observed in adults with FASD. In all four groups, activity increased with task difficulty in the parietal and frontal regions at more superior slice levels.

Figure 1 demonstrates the regions of fMRI activity (p < 0.01 uncorrected) from all child subjects in the groups who performed with greater than 50% task accuracy in both the n = 0 and 1-back tasks, following subtraction of the control (n = 0) task activations from the 1-back tasks. Figure 2 shows the corresponding data in adults (p<0.01, uncorrected). Subjects were also required to perform the psychological tests satisfactorily in order to be included in the group analysis. Controls were matched to age and sex and were required to meet the performance inclusion criteria mentioned as well.

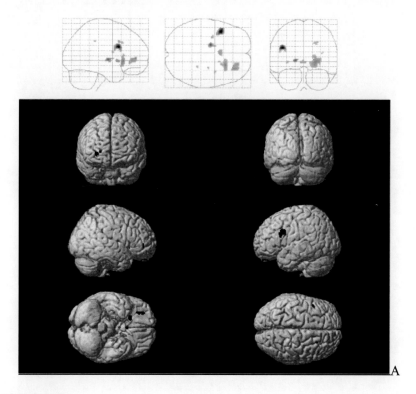

Figure 1. (Continued).

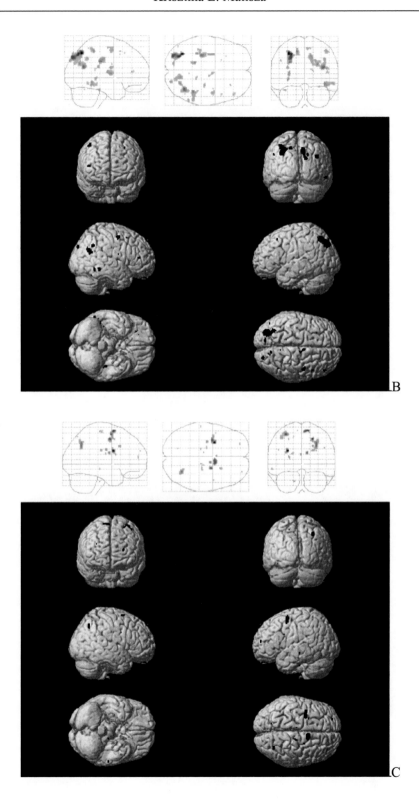

Figure 1. (Continued).

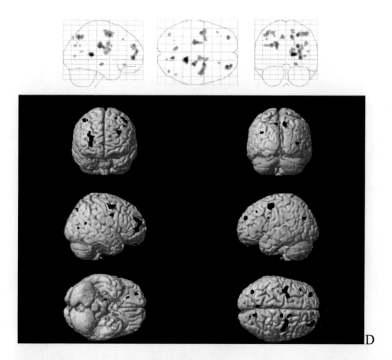

Figure 1. One sample T-tests in the child subject groups showing group fMRI activity from 1-back tasks. Functional MRI regions of activity depicted are at a level of $p < 0.01$ for the performance of the simplified 1-back task following subtraction of control (n = 0) task with (A) FASD (n = 9) and (B) controls (n = 8), and for the performance of continuous 1-back task following subtraction of the control (n = 0) task with (C) FASD (n = 7) and (D) control (n = 8) subjects.

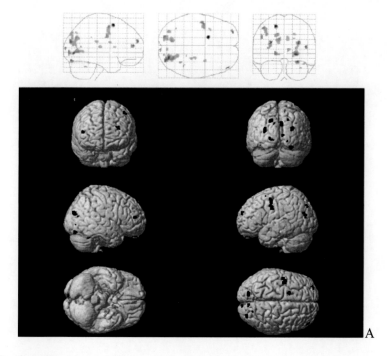

Figure 2. (Continued).

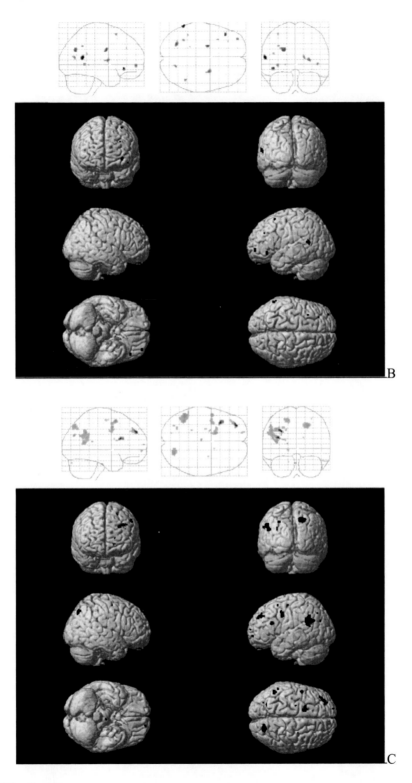

Figure 2. (Continued).

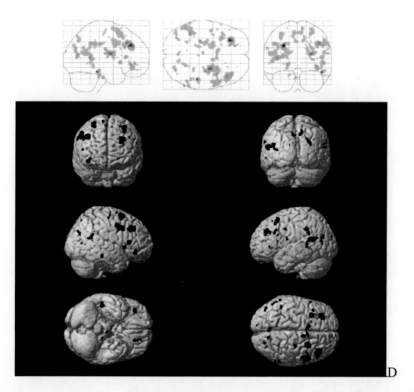

Figure 2. One sample T-tests in the adult subject groups showing group fMRI activity from 1-back tasks. Functional MRI regions of activity depicted are at a level of p < 0.01 for the performance of the simplified 1-back task following subtraction of control (n = 0) task with A) FASD (n = 10) and B) controls (n = 9), and for the performance of continuous 1-back task following subtraction of the control (n = 0) task with C) FASD (n = 6) and D) control (n = 6) subjects.

DISCUSSION

The findings of Clark et al [22] relate to the sensory-motor pathway and point to a subtle dysfunction of the sensory pathway to the cortex. The thalamus is a collection of nuclei that serve as the main relay center between the cortex and lower structures, such as the basal ganglia, cerebellum, brainstem, and spinal cord. The three classes of thalamic nuclei include the specific sensory relay nuclei that transmit all sensory information, except olfaction, to the cortex, motor nuclei that pass information from the frontal cortex to the basal ganglia and cerebellum, and non-specific association nuclei that link cortical association regions and the limbic system with association cortices [67]. The caudate receives input from the cerebral cortex, sensorimotor cortex, intralaminar nuclei of the thalamus, and substantia nigra. The caudate is involved in motor function and possibly cognitive functions.

The putamin is also involved in motor function. Clark et al [22] suggest that the dysfunction of this sensory gateway is consistent with clinical descriptions of distractibility and impulsiveness in FAS children because basal ganglia estimates were found to be significantly lower in these subjects. The basal ganglia has been implicated in affective and motivation functions, as well as in executive functioning, spatial learning, attention, perseveration, and response inhibition [58,68-70]. Dysfunction of these brain regions is consistent with problems associated with motor function, coordi-nation, or clumsiness observed in subjects with FASD.

Riikonen et al [63] relate ADHD in FAS to frontal lobe perfusion asymmetry. The frontal region is implicated in executive functioning, attention and response inhibition [24,71-75]. The SPECT findings suggest that normal frontal left-right dominance is lacking in children with FAS [63]. In normal children greater than three years of age, the CBF in the left hemisphere of the brain is significantly higher than in the right [64]. In children with FAS, a reduction in perfusion in the parieto-occipital region is consistent with cognitive, logical, and grammatical dysfunction [76,77].

The left parietotemporal region is associated with dyslexia, dysphasia and dyscalculia [76-78]. Bhatara et al [65] also note a lack of normal left-right dominance in two children with FAS. The temporal lobe dysfunction observed may be the source the inappropriate behavioral responses found in FASD affected individuals. In addition to problems with facial recognition and perception of emotions, temporal lobe dysfunction is implicated in sexuality, visual perception, emotion, sense of self, and behaviors affecting an individual's ability to comprehend situations and consequences adequately [79]. The PET studies of children with autism have shown hypoperfusion in the temporal lobe, which supports the cognitive dysfunctions outlined above [80]. Riikonen et al [66,81] used SPECT to examine serotonin and dopamine transporter binding that plays a role in neuronal maturation and production of synapses. Changes in SERT and DAT binding may result in loss of those synapses and affect behaviors upon which they depend.

The MFC was particularly affected in FAS individuals. Selective deficiency of dopamine at the synaptic levels in the MFC is consistent with executive dysfunction, problems with attention, excessive motor activity, impulsivity, memory problems, spatial learning, and problems with response inhibition [24,65,73]. These observations are supported by the fMRI studies using working memory tasks, demonstrating frontal lobe dysfunction, particularly in the medial frontal cortex in subjects with FASD [24].

In addition, EEG studies of individuals with a family history of alcoholism in adolescence, a condition to which children with FASD are predisposed, were shown to have frontal brain asymmetries [82]. These EEG studies showed alcoholism is localized to the left hemisphere [82]. This result is consistent with previous SPECT findings regarding hypoperfusion in the left hemisphere of the brain in FAS subjects [63,65]. Left-right asymmetry was not confirmed in one study [66]. Other SPECT studies suggest dysfunction and reduced rCBF in the inferior and medial frontal brain region in alcoholics during detoxification [83,84]. These regions are known to affect executive function, working memory and response inhibition. In addition, Riikonen et al [66] note that decreased SERT and increased DAT binding are typically found in type 2 alcoholics. Common inappropriate behaviors exhibited by children with FAS are also characteristics of such alcoholics, including antisocial personality, early onset of instability to abstain from alcohol, impulsiveness and fighting.

All children with FAS in the study by Riikonen et al [66] also had comorbid diagnoses of ADHD. SPECT studies in children with ADHD have shown higher rCBF in the anterior cingulate and lower rCBF in the superior parietal lobe in children who respond to methylphenidate, compared with those who do not. These regions are involved in working memory function, executive function, and attention [72]. Increased DAT density was also found in SPECT studies of adults with ADHD [85].

The fMRI study by Malisza et al (24,25,34,86) showed that subjects with FASD did not perform statistically worse on any of the psychological tasks with the exception of response latency during a CPT that measures sustained attention. In addition, only subjects who performed the task adequately (> 50% correct responses) were included in the analysis. Significant activity was observed in the anterior cingulate in all subjects, an area of the brain known to be involved in attention. The results corroborate the conclusion that FASD individuals were paying attention during the fMRI tasks. The findings also allow for greater certainty in the fMRI results of the block tasks because the subjects were matched to performance accuracy. Therefore, the delayed response rate was more likely indicative of impaired working memory processing and not of problems with inattention.

Due to the nature of FASD, the small subject numbers, age ranges, and the tasks employed, the fMRI results are quite variable. Although the tasks examine working memory specifically, they also have components of attention, response selection, saccadic eye movement, motor, sensory and visual response, spatial memory, and spatial perception, resulting in a great amount of functional activity during task performance. The large amount of inter-subject variability resulted in data that are difficult to analyze and interpret by group comparisons confidently.

Nonetheless, the fMRI was performed to provide a measure of functional activity between the FASD and control populations. The group data presented, however, are composed only of the subjects and age- and sex-matched controls who met the inclusion criteria specified previously. Despite these drawbacks, at least two distinct brain regions demonstrate differential activity between the affected populations and the control subjects (figures 1 and 2). The results suggest impairment in spatial working memory in subjects with FASD that does not improve with age, and that fMRI may be useful in evaluating brain function in these individuals.

Individuals with FASD exhibit a wide range of anatomical abnormalities and cognitive deficits. Whereas anatomical abnormalities are easily measurable, cognitive deficits, which are also apparent in individuals without the facial dysmorphology, are much more difficult to characterize. It is well known that CNS damage and cognitive functional problems exist as a result of prenatal alcohol exposure, despite an individual not having a specific diagnosis of FAS. Both structural and cognitive dysfunction may vary with the severity of the syndrome and is dependent upon several factors, including the amount, duration, and fetal developmental period of prenatal alcohol exposure [12].

Despite this variability and small subject numbers, functional neuroimaging studies provide a good start in evaluation of cognitive brain dysfunction in FASD affected populations. The differences in fMRI task performance remain a major concern in any affected population. Full event-related fMRI studies, including larger group sizes to provide adequate statistical power, are required to address the cognitive dysfunctions associated with FASD. In particular, self-paced events would provide the means for subjects to respond to individual stimuli or events at their own pace, reducing or eliminating concerns of the delayed response times observed in affected individuals. Although the implementation and analysis of these types of studies are difficult, greater confidence will be derived form the results and the many different ways in which this data can be analyzed, eliminating the confounding issues with blocked data.

Although sparse, the neuroimaging data acquired using PET, SPECT, and fMRI suggest impairment in the prefrontal, orbital, and middle frontal cortices, thalamus, basal ganglia, parieto-occipital, parieto-temporal, and temporal brain regions. These findings either were correlated to or may correspond to dysfunction in the areas of working memory, executive function, attention, motor coordination, arithmetic, logic, grammar, emotion, and learning. Anatomical MRI findings have shown a reduced volume of the frontal cortex and basal ganglia, and increased gray matter and reduced symmetry (although this asymmetry is not significant) in the temporal lobe of FASD-affected individuals (table 1).

The results of EEG studies suggest that compared with controls, differences in neuronal activity exist in subjects with FASD in the posterior part of the brain, including the parieto-occipital region, which is involved in visual processing and spatial perception (table 3) [63,87-89]. The study looking at an oddball and noise paradigm showed greater P300 latency in FASD compared with typical controls [88]. P300 latency is involved in cognitive information processing, such as encoding, selecting, memorizing, and decision-making. This finding is consistent with the fMRI results in which FASD subjects show significantly delayed response times in comparison with healthy controls [24]. Surprisingly, Kaneko et al [88] did not see differences in N100 amplitude, which is related to attention deficits, in FASD subjects compared with controls but the authors suggest that the reason may result from differences in problems of attention or pathways between these groups.

Whereas the determination of perfusion through PET and SPECT may relate to neuronal function, specific tasks were not evaluated in any of these neuroimaging studies [22,63,65,66]. To date, the only functional neuroimaging study to evaluate specific task performance with brain function in FASD used fMRI [24]. Clearly, a more concentrated effort is required to map brain function in FASD-affected individuals. One of the greatest problems encountered is the variability of the results because of the nature of the disorder. Well-designed experiments are required to examine the multiple cognitive deficits apparent in FASD.

One main drawback and potential reason for the few functional neuroimaging studies in this subject population is the difficulty in imaging individuals, in particular children, with FASD. For example, the use of sedation or anesthesia to restrict motion was deemed necessary to obtain good SPECT images [63,65,66]. This requirement further confounds the data as sedation may alter neuronal function. Chloral hydrate, a γ-amino-butyric acid (GABA)-mimetic, has been shown to induce neuronal injury and cell death in the brain of juvenile animal models, and can interact with other glutamatergic receptors as well [90]. As indicated by Bhatara et al [65] sedation with chloral hydrate is not always successful, leading to additional sedation or anesthesia, further complicating functional neuroimaging. Furthermore, studies using PET and SPECT are invasive procedures requiring the use of radioactive markers. This drawback limits their use, resulting in a lack of data from healthy control subjects, especially pediatric populations, who are excluded for ethical considerations. In contrast, fMRI provides a means to examine neuronal function indirectly and non-invasively, without the use of harmful radiation.

Finally, it is noteworthy that co-morbidities are common in subjects with FASD. In particular, an overlap of symptoms between ADHD and FASD frequently results in difficulty in diagnosis or even in misdiagnosis. Very few studies have examined the link between FASD and ADHD, but the effects of these co-morbidities must be considered when analyzing neuro-imaging data.

Despite the availability of techniques for well over a decade, functional neuroimaging of cognitive function in FASD is in its infancy. If identifiable differences in brain function exist between control subjects and FASD affected populations, between subtypes of FASD, and between FASD comorbid with other conditions, such differences could provide the objective information regarding CNS function that is required to distinguish them clinically. Additionally, behavioral testing and brain activity patterns can clearly indicate cognitive deficits in these subject populations. This can enhance a physicians' ability to make accurate clinical diagnoses and offers increased potential for early and tailored intervention.

CONCLUSIONS

Significant numbers of MRI anatomical studies of FASD exist, but very little functional neuroimaging studies have been performed to date. This lack is likely due to the perception that this subject population is uncooperative and difficult to image. Many areas of the brain are affected by prenatal exposure to alcohol, and much remains to be determined regarding brain function in individuals with FASD. Functional neuroimaging tasks must be designed to evaluate the different brain regions and cognitive functions that are affected in this population. Existing functional neuroimaging studies provide a good starting point. Understanding the CNS impairment in FASD and mapping of brain function can help evaluate education and support programs for affected individuals. The knowledge gained may also assist with accurate clinical diagnosis, especially in difficult-to-diagnose cases that include individuals who do not possess the physical features usually associated with FAS, and/or have symptoms similar to or are co-morbid with other disorders or diseases.

ACKNOWLEDGMENTS

I would like to thank Dr. A. Chudley, Dr. S. Longstaffe, Dr. D. Shiloff, Dr. L. Jakobson, Ms. A. A. Allman and Mr. D. Foreman for assistance with the FASD fMRI studies. Dr. Chudley is deserving of a very special thank you for being a strong motivating force behind the FASD studies in Manitoba. I gratefully acknowledge Dr. M. Malainey for helpful discussions and editing.

REFERENCES

[1]   Chudley AE, Longstaffe S. Fetal Alcohol Syndrome and Fetal Alcohol Spectrum Disorder. In: Chassidy SB, Allanson JE, eds. *Management of genetic syndromes*. 2nd ed. New York, NY, USA: Wiley-Liss; 2005:225-37.

[2]   Williams RJ, Odaibo FS, McGee JM. Incidence of fetal alcohol syndrome in northeastern Manitoba. *Can. J. Public Health* 1999;90(3):192-4.

[3]   Loock C, Conry J, Cook JL, Chudley AE, Rosales T. Identifying fetal alcohol spectrum disorder in primary care. *CMAJ* 2005;172(5):628-30.

[4]   Astley SJ, Clarren SK. Diagnosing the full spectrum of fetal alcohol-exposed individuals: introducing the 4-digit diagnostic code. *Alcohol Alcohol* 2000;35(4):400-10.

[5]   Chudley AE, Conry J, Cook JL, Loock C, Rosales T, LeBlanc N. Fetal alcohol spectrum disorder: Canadian guidelines for diagnosis. *CMAJ 2005*; 172(5 Suppl):S1-S21.

[6]   Nanson JL, Hiscock M. Attention deficits in children exposed to alcohol prenatally. *Alcohol Clin Exp. Res.* 1990;14(5):656-61.

[7]   Oesterheld JR, Kofoed L, Tervo R, Fogas B, Wilson A, Fiechtner H. Effectiveness of methyl-phenidate in Native American children with fetal alcohol syndrome and attention deficit/hyper-activity disorder: a controlled pilot study. *J. Child Adolesc. Psychopharmacol* 1998;8(1):39-48.

[8]   Roebuck TM, Mattson SN, Riley EP. Behavioral and psychosocial profiles of alcohol-exposed children. *Alcohol Clin. Exp. Res.* 1999;23(6):1070-6.

[9]   Barinaga M. A critical issue for the brain. *Science* 2000;288:2116-9.

[10]   Davis MI, Szarowski D, Turner JN, Morrisett RA, Shain W. In vivo activation and in situ BDNF-stimulated nuclear translocation of mitogen-activated/extracellular signal-regulated protein kinase is inhibited by ethanol in the developing rat hippocampus. *Neurosci. Lett* 1999;272(2):95-8.

[11]   Mitchell JJ, Paiva M, Walker DW, Heaton MB. BDNF and NGF afford in vitro neuroprotection against ethanol combined with acute ischemia and chronic hypoglycemia. *Dev. Neurosci.* 1999;21(1): 68-75.

[12]   Clarren SK. Neuropathology in fetal alcohol syndrome. In: West JR, ed. *Alcohol and brain development.* New York, NY, USA: Oxford Univ Press, 1986:158-66.

[13]   Swayze VW, 2nd, Johnson VP, Hanson JW, Piven J, Sato Y, Giedd JN et al. Magnetic resonance imaging of brain anomalies in fetal alcohol syndrome. *Pediatrics* 1997;99(2):232-40.

[14]   Smith DE, Foundas A, Canale J. Effect of perinatally administered ethanol on the develop-ment of the cerebellar granule cell. *Exp. Neurol* .1986;92(3):491-501.

[15]   Miller MW, Potempa G. Numbers of neurons and glia in mature rat somatosensory cortex: effects of prenatal exposure to ethanol. *J. Comp. Neurol.* 1990;293(1):92-102.

[16]   Goodlett CR, Leo JT, O'Callaghan JP, Mahoney JC, West JR. Transient cortical astrogliosis induced by alcohol exposure during the neonatal brain growth spurt in rats. *Brain Res. Dev Brain Res.* 1993;72(1):85-97.

[17]   West JR, Hamre KM. Effects of alcohol exposure during different periods of development: changes in hippocampal mossy fibers. *Brain Res.* 1985;349 (1-2):280-4.

[18]   Archibald SL, Fennema-Notestine C, Gamst A, Riley EP, Mattson SN, Jernigan TL. Brain dysmorphology in individuals with severe prenatal alcohol exposure. *Dev. Med. Child Neurol.* 2001; 43(3):148-54.

[19]   Sowell ER, Thompson PM, Mattson SN, Tessner KD, Jernigan TL, Riley EP et al. Voxel-based morphometric analyses of the brain in children and adolescents prenatally exposed to alcohol. *Neuroreport* 2001;12(3):515-23.

[20]   Bookstein FL, Sampson PD, Streissguth AP, Connor PD. Geometric morphometrics of corpus callosum and subcortical structures in the fetal-alcohol-affected brain. *Teratology* 2001;64(1):4-32.

[21] Roebuck TM, Mattson SN, Riley EP. A review of the neuroanatomical findings in children with fetal alcohol syndrome or prenatal exposure to alcohol. *Alcohol Clin. Exp. Res.* 1998;22(2):339-44.

[22] Clark CM, Li D, Conry J, Conry R, Loock C. Structural and functional brain integrity of fetal alcohol syndrome in nonretarded cases. *Pediatrics* 2000;105(5):1096-9.

[23] Malisza KL. Evaluation of spatial working memory function in children and adults with FASD: A functional magnetic resonance imaging study. *Seventh Fetal Alcohol Can Expertise Res. Roundtable 2006,* Moncton, NB, 2006.

[24] Malisza KL, Allman AA, Shiloff D, Jakobson L, Longstaffe S, Chudley AE. Evaluation of spatial working memory function in children and adults with fetal alcohol spectrum disorders: a functional magnetic resonance imaging study. *Pediatr. Res.* 2005;58(6):1150-7.

[25] Malisza KL, Allman AA, Shiloff D, Jakobson L, Longstaffe S, Chudley AE. Using fMRI to evaluate executive function in FASD. *Fifth Fetal Alcohol Can Expertise Res. Roundtable 2004*, Saskatoon, SK, 2004.

[26] Aronson M, Hagberg B. Neuropsychological disorders in children exposed to alcohol during pregnancy: a follow-up study of 24 children to alcoholic mothers in Goteborg, Sweden. *Alcohol Clin. Exp. Res.* 1998;22(2):321-4.

[27] Iosub S, Fuchs M, Bingol N, Gromisch DS. Fetal alcohol syndrome revisited. *Pediatrics* 1981;68(4): 475-9.

[28] Mattson SN, Riley EP. Implicit and explicit memory functioning in children with heavy prenatal alcohol exposure. *J. Int. Neuropsychol. Soc.* 1999;5(5):462-71.

[29] Uecker A, Nadel L. Spatial but not object memory impairments in children with fetal alcohol syndrome. *Am. J. Ment. Retard.* 1998;103(1):12-8.

[30] Connor PD, Sampson PD, Streissguth AP, Bookstein FL, Barr HM. Effects of prenatal alcohol exposure on fine motor coordination and balance: A study of two adult samples. *Neuropsychologia* 2006;44(5):744-51.

[31] Simmons RW, Thomas JD, Levy SS, Riley EP. Motor response selection in children with fetal alcohol spectrum disorders. *Neurotoxicol. Teratol.* 2006;28(2):278-85.

[32] Roebuck TM, Simmons RW, Mattson SN, Riley EP. Prenatal exposure to alcohol affects the ability to maintain postural balance. *Alcohol Clin. Exp. Res.* 1998; 22(1):252-8.

[33] Roebuck-Spencer TM, Mattson SN, Marion SD, Brown WS, Riley EP. Bimanual coordination in alcohol-exposed children: role of the corpus callo-sum. *J. Int. Neuropsychol. Soc.* 2004;10(4):536-48.

[34] Allman AA, Jakobson L, Shiloff D, Chudley AE, Longstaffe S, Malisza KL. *Executive function and spatial working memory in fetal alcohol syndrome.* Canadian Society for Brain, Behaviour and Congitive Science 13th Annual meeting 2003, Hamilton, ON, 2003.

[35] Casey BJ, Cohen JD, Jezzard P, Turner R, Noll DC, Trainor RJ, et al. Activation of prefrontal cortex in children during a nonspatial working memory task with functional MRI. *Neuroimage* 1995;2(3):221-9.

[36] Casey BJ, Cohen JD, O'Craven K, Davidson RJ, Irwin W, Nelson CA, et al. Reproducibility of fMRI results across four institutions using a spatial working memory task. *Neuroimage* 1998; 8(3):249-61.

[37] Barch DM, Braver TS, Nystrom LE, Forman SD, Noll DC, Cohen JD. Dissociating working memory from task difficulty in human prefrontal cortex. *Neuropsychologia* 1997;35(10):1373-80.

[38] Braver TS, Cohen JD, Nystrom LE, Jonides J, Smith EE, Noll DC. A parametric study of prefrontal cortex involvement in human working memory. *Neuroimage* 1997;5(1):49-62.

[39] Cohen JD, Perlstein WM, Braver TS, Nystrom LE, Noll DC, Jonides J, et al. Temporal dynamics of brain activation during a working memory task. *Nature* 1997;386(6625):604-8.

[40] Courtney SM, Ungerleider LG, Keil K, Haxby JV. Object and spatial visual working memory activate separate neural systems in human cortex. *Cereb Cortex* 1996;6(1):39-49.

[41] Smith EE, Jonides J, Koeppe RA. Dissociating verbal and spatial working memory using PET. *Cereb Cortex* 1996;6(1):11-20.

[42] Coles CD, Platzman KA, Lynch ME, Freides D. Auditory and visual sustained attention in adolescents prenatally exposed to alcohol. *Alcohol Clin. Exp. Res.* 2002;26(2):263-71.

[43] Coles CD, Platzman KA, Raskind-Hood CL, Brown RT, Falek A, Smith IE. A comparison of children affected by prenatal alcohol exposure and attention deficit, hyperactivity disorder. *Alcohol Clin. Exp. Res.* 1997;21(1):150-61.

[44] Mattson SN, Calarco KE, Lang AR. Focused and shifting attention in children with heavy prenatal alcohol exposure. *Neuropsychology* 2006;20(3): 361-9.

[45] Streissguth A, Bookstein FL, Sampson PD, Barr HM. Attention: prenatal alcohol and continuities of vigilance and attentional problems from 4 through 14 years. *Dev. Psychopath* 1995;7:419-46.

[46] Kopera-Frye K, Carmichael Olson H, Streissguth AP. Teratogenic effects of alcohol on attention. In: Burack JA, Enns JT, eds. *Attention, development and psychopathology.* New York, NY, USA: Guilford, 1997:171-204.

[47] Streissguth AP, Barr HM, Sampson PD, Parrish-Johnson JC, Kirchner GL, Maritin DC. Attention, distraction and reaction time at age 7 years and prenatal alcohol exposure. *Neurobehav Toxicol. Teratol.* 1986;8(6):717-25.

[48] O'Malley KD, Nanson J. Clinical implications of a link between fetal alcohol spectrum disorder and attention-deficit hyperactivity disorder. *Can J. Psychiatry* 2002;47(4):349-54.

[49] Sommer FT, Hirsch JA, Wichert A. Theories, data analysis, and simulation models in neuroimaging: An overview, Exploratory analysis and data modeling in functional neuroimaging. Cambridge, Massachusetts, USA: MIT Press, 2003:1-13.

[50] Marshall J, Martin T, Downie J, Malisza K. A comprehensive analysis of MRI research risks: in support of full disclosure. *Can. J. Neurol. Sci.* 2007;34(1):11-7.

[51] Ogawa S, Menon RS, Tank DW, Kim SG, Merkle H, Ellermann JM et al. Functional brain mapping by blood oxygenation level-dependent contrast magnetic resonance imaging. A comparison of signal characteristics with a biophysical model. *Biophys. J.* 1993;64(3):803-12.

[52] Logothetis NK, Pauls J, Augath M, Trinath T, Oeltermann A. Neurophysiological investigation of the basis of the fMRI signal. *Nature* 2001; 412(6843):150-7.

[53] Gevins AS, M.E.; Mcevoy, L.K EEG and ERP Imaging of Brain Function. In: Polich J, ed. *Detection of Change: Event-Related Potential and fMRI Findings.* Norwell, MA: Kluwer, 2003:133-5.

[54] Friston KJ, Jezzard P, Turner R. Analysis of functional MRI time-series. *Human Brain Mapping* 1994;1:153-71.

[55] Riley EP, McGee CL, Sowell ER. Teratogenic effects of alcohol: a decade of brain imaging. *Am. J. Med. Genet C Semin. Med. Genet.* 2004;127(1): 35-41.

[56] Toga AW, Thompson PM, Sowell ER. Mapping brain maturation. *Trends Neurosci.* 2006;29(3): 148-59.

[57] Spampinato MV, Castillo M, Rojas R, Palacios E, Frascheri L, Descartes F. Magnetic resonance imaging findings in substance abuse: alcohol and alcoholism and syndromes associated with alcohol abuse. *Top Magn Reson Imaging* 2005;16(3):223-30.

[58] Spadoni AD, McGee CL, Fryer SL, Riley EP. Neuroimaging and fetal alcohol spectrum disorders. *Neurosci. Biobehav. Rev.* 2007;31(2): 239-45.

[59] McGee CL, Riley EP. Brain imaging and fetal alcohol spectrum disorders. *Ann. Ist Super Sanita* 2006;42(1):46-52.

[60] Chen WJ, Maier SE, Parnell SE, West JR. Alcohol and the developing brain: neuroanatomi-cal studies. *Alcohol. Res. Health* 2003;27(2):174-80.

[61] Posner MI, Petersen SE, Fox PT, Raichle ME. Localization of cognitive operations in the human brain. *Science* 1988;240(4859):1627-31.

[62] Lou HC, Henriksen L, Bruhn P. Focal cerebral dysfunction in developmental learning disabilities. *Lancet* 1990;335(8680):8-11.

[63] Riikonen R, Salonen I, Partanen K, Verho S. Brain perfusion SPECT and MRI in foetal alcohol syndrome. *Dev. Med. Child Neurol.* 1999;41(10): 652-9.

[64] Chiron C, Jambaque I, Nabbout R, Lounes R, Syrota A, Dulac O. The right brain hemisphere is dominant in human infants. *Brain* 1997;120(Pt 6):1057-65.

[65] Bhatara VS, Lovrein F, Kirkeby J, Swayze V, 2nd, Unruh E, Johnson V. Brain function in fetal alcohol syndrome assessed by single photon emission computed tomography. *SDJ Med.* 2002; 55(2):59-62.

[66] Riikonen RS, Nokelainen P, Valkonen K, Kolehmainen AI, Kumpulainen KI, Kononen M et al. Deep serotonergic and dopaminergic structures in fetal alcoholic syndrome: a study with nor-beta-CIT-single-photon emission computed tomography and magnetic resonance imaging volumetry. *Biol. Psychiatry* 2005;57(12):1565-72.

[67] Orrison WWJ. Atlas of brain function New York, NY, USA: *Thieme Medical*, 1995.

[68] Mattson SN, Riley EP, Jernigan TL, Garcia A, Kaneko WM, Ehlers CL et al. A decrease in the size of the basal ganglia following prenatal alcohol exposure: A preliminary report. *Neurotoxicol. Teratol.* 1994;16(3):283-9.

[69] Mattson SN, Riley EP, Sowell ER, Jernigan TL, Sobel DF, Jones KL. A decrease in the size of the basal ganglia in children with fetal alcohol syndrome. *Alcohol Clin. Exp. Res.* 1996;20(6): 1088-93.

[70] Cortese BM, Moore GJ, Bailey BA, Jacobson SW, Delaney-Black V, Hannigan JH. Magnetic resonance and spectroscopic imaging in prenatal alcohol-exposed children: preliminary findings in the caudate nucleus. *Neurotoxicol. Teratol.* 2006; 28(5):597-606.

[71] Duckworth Warner T, Behnke M, Eyler FD, Padgett K, Leonard C, Hou W et al. Diffusion Tensor Imaging of Frontal White Matter and Executive Functioning in Cocaine-Exposed Children. *Pediatrics* 2006;118(5):2014-24.

[72] Cho S-C, Hwang J-W, Kim B-N, Lee H-Y, Kim H-W, Lee J-S et al. The relationship between regional cerebral blood flow and response to methylphenidate in children with attention-deficit hyperactivity disorder: Comparison between non-responders to methylphenidate and responders. *J. Psyhiatric. Res.* 2007;41:459-65.

[73] Okuda J, Fujii T, Yamadori A, Kawashima R, Tsukiura T, Fukatsu R et al. Participation of the prefrontal cortices in prospective memory: evidence from a PET study in humans. *Neurosci. Lett.* 1998;253(2):127-30.

[74] Faw B. Pre-frontal executive committee for perception, working memory, attention, long-term memory, motor control, and thinking: a tutorial review. *Conscious Cogn* 2003;12(1):83-139.

[75] Booth JR, Burman DD, Meyer JR, Lei Z, Trommer BL, Davenport ND et al. Neural development of selective attention and response inhibition. *Neuroimage* 2003;20(2):737-51.

[76] McDaniel KD, Wagner MT, Greenspan BS. The role of brain single photon emission computed tomography in the diagnosis of primary progressive aphasia. *Arch. Neurol.* 1991;48(12): 1257-60.

[77] Liesman G. Coherence of hemispheric function in developmental dyslexia. *Brain Cogn* 2002;48(2-3):425-31.

[78] Shalev RS. Developmental dyscalculia. *J. Child Neurol.* 2004;19(10):765-71.

[79] Rubia Vila FJ. The remarkable symptoms of the temporal lobe dysfunction. Anales de la real academia nacional de medicina 2001;118(3):583-95.

[80] Zilbovicius M, Boddaert N, Belin P, Poline J-B, Remy P, Mangin J-F et al. Temporal lobe dysfunction in childhood autism: A PET study. *Am. J. Psychiatry* 2000;157(12):1988-93.

[81] Mazer C, Muneyyirci J, Taheny K, Raio N, Borella A, Whitaker-Azmitia P. Serotonin depletion during synaptogenesis leads to decreased synaptic density and learning deficits in the adult rat: a possible model of neurodevelopmental disorders with cognitive deficits. *Brain Res.* 1997;760(1-2):68-73.

[82] Bauer LO, Hesselbrock VM. Lateral asymmetries in the frontal brain: Effects of depression and a family history of alcholism in female adolescents. *Alcohol Clin. Exp. Res.* 2002;26(11):1662-8.

[83] Noel X, Paternot J, Van der Linden M, Sferrazza R, Verhas M, Hanak C et al. Correlation between inhibition, working memory and delimited frontal area blood flow measured by 99MTc-bicisate SPECT in alcohol-dependent patients. *Alcohol Alcoholism* 2001;36(6):556-63.

[84] Tutus A, Kugu N, Sofuoglu S, Nardali M, Simsek A, Karaaslan F et al. Transient frontal hypoperfusion in Tc-99m hexamethylpropylene-amineoxime single photon emission computed tomography imaging during alcohol withdrawal. *Biol. Psychiatry* 1998;43(12):923-8.

[85] Dougherty DD, Bonab AA, Spencer TJ, Rauch SL, Madras BK, Fischman AJ. Dopamine transporter density in patients with attention deficit hyperactivity disorder. *Lancet* 1999;354 (9196):2132-3.

[86]   Malisza KL, Allman AA, Shiloff D, Stroman PW, Jakobson L, Longstaffe S et al. Functional MRI of fetal alcohol syndrome. *11th Proc. Int Society Magnetic Resonance Med 2003*, Toronto, ON, 2003:544.

[87]   Mattson SN, Riley EP, Jernigan TL, Ehlers CL, Delis DC, Jones KL et al. Fetal alcohol syndrome: a case report of neuropsychological, MRI and EEG assessment of two children. *Alcohol Clin. Exp. Res.* 1992;16(5):1001-3.

[88]   Kaneko WM, Ehlers CL, Philips EL, Riley EP. Auditory event-related potentials in fetal alcohol syndrome and Down's syndrome children. *Alcohol Clin. Exp. Res.* 1996;20(1):35-42.

[89]   Kaneko WM, Phillips EL, Riley EP, Ehlers CL. EEG findings in fetal alcohol syndrome and Down syndrome children. *Electroencephalogr Clin. Neurophysiol.* 1996;98(1):20-8.

[90]   Mellon RD, Simone AF, Rappaport BA. Use of anesthetic agents in neonates and young children. *Anesth Analg* 2007;104(3):509-20.

[91]   Sowell ER, Thompson PM, Mattson SN, Tessner KD, Jernigan TL, Riley EP et al. Regional brain shape abnormalities persist into adolescence after heavy prenatal alcohol exposure. *Cereb Cortex* 2002;12(8):856-65.

[92]   Ma X, Coles CD, Lynch ME, Laconte SM, Zurkiya O, Wang D et al. Evaluation of corpus callosum anisotropy in young adults with fetal alcohol syndrome according to diffusion tensor imaging. *Alcohol Clin. Exp. Res.* 2005;29(7):1214-22.

[93]   Autti-Ramo I, Autti T, Korkman M, Kettunen S, Salonen O, Valanee L. MRI findings in children with school problems who had been exposed prenatally to alcohol. *Devl. Med. Child Neurol.* 2002;44:98-106.

[94]   Sowell ER, Thompson PM, Peterson BS, Mattson SN, Welcome SE, Henkenius AL et al. Mapping cortical gray matter asymmetry patterns in adolescents with heavy prenatal alcohol exposure. *Neuroimage* 2002;17(4):1807-19.

[95]   Bookstein FL, Sampson PD, Connor PD, Streissguth AP. Midline corpus callosum is a neuroanatomical focus of fetal alcohol damage. *Anat. Rec.* 2002;269(3):162-74.

[96]   Bookstein FL, Streissguth AP, Sampson PD, Connor PD, Barr HM. Corpus callosum shape and neuropsychological deficits in adult males with heavy fetal alcohol exposure. *Neuroimage* 2002; 15(1):233-51.

[97]   Sowell ER, Jernigan TL, Mattson SN, Riley EP, Sobel DF, Jones KL. Abnormal development of the cerebellar vermis in children prenatally exposed to alcohol: size reduction in lobules I-V. *Alcohol Clin. Exp. Res.* 1996;20(1):31-4.

[98]   Riley EP, Mattson SN, Sowell ER, Jernigan TL, Sobel DF, Jones KL. Abnormalities of the corpus callosum in children prenatally exposed to alcohol. *Alcohol Clin. Exp. Res.* 1995;19(5):1198-202.

[99]   Johnson VP, Swayze VW, II, Sato Y, Andreasen NC. Fetal alcohol syndrome: craniofacial and central nervous system manifestations. *Am. J. Med. Genet* 1996;61(4):329-39.

[100] Wozniak JR, Mueller BA, Chang PN, Muetzel RL, Caros L, Lim KO. Diffusion tensor imaging in children with fetal alcohol spectrum disorders. *Alcohol Clin. Exp. Res.* 2006;30(10):1799-806.

[101] O'Hare ED, Kan E, Yoshiii J, Mattson SN, Riley EP, Thompson PM et al. Mapping cerebellar vermal morphology and cognitive correlates in prenatal alcohol exposure. *Neuroreport* 2005;16 (12):1285-90.

[102] Fagerlund A, Heikkinen S, Autti-Ramo I, Korkman M, Timonen M, Kuusi T et al. Brain metabolic alterations in adolescents and young adults with fetal alcohol spectrum disorders. *Alcohol Clin. Exp. Res.* 2006;30(12):2097-104.

[103] Ioffe S, Chernick V. Prediction of subsequent motor and mental retardation in newborn infants exposed to alcohol in utero by computerized EEG analysis. *Neuropediatrics* 1990;21:11-7.

In: Alcohol-Related Cognitive Disorders
Editors: L. Sher, I. Kandel, J. Merrick pp. 57-66

ISBN: 978-1-60741-730-9
© 2009 Nova Science Publishers, Inc.

Chapter 3

THE HUMAN FETUS AND MATERNAL ALCOHOL CONSUMPTION

Peter G. Hepper

ABSTRACT

Studies examining maternal alcohol consumption during pregnancy have mainly examined the effects on the individual after birth. The observation of the fetus during pregnancy, the time period of exposure, can enable a better understanding of the effects of alcohol on the fetus. Because the behavior of the fetus is directly reflective of the functioning of its central nervous system, the effect of alcohol on neural system functioning and integrity may be assessed. This paper reviews the few studies that have examined the effects of alcohol on the behavior of the human fetus. Studies reveal that chronic and acute alcohol exposure influences behavior and, significantly, at lower doses than are considered important when evaluating effects after birth. There appears to be a dose-dependent effect, and the influence of alcohol on the behavior of the fetus persists after alcohol has been cleared from the mother's blood stream. Possible mechanisms of action include a direct effect of alcohol on the developing nervous system; and, an indirect effect of alcohol induced disruption of normal behavioral patterns central to the development of the brain and CNS. Observing the fetus's behavior may thus enable the mechanisms underlying alcohol-induced effects on the individual to be better understood.

INTRODUCTION

It is widely accepted that consumption of alcohol by women during their pregnancy can result in harmful affects on the fetus, evidenced by adverse health and well-being after birth [1]. Initial reports regarding the effects of prenatal exposure to alcohol, concentrating on women drinking heavily during pregnancy [2,3], have documented individuals exhibiting poor growth, a characteristic facial appearance, and the presence of cardiac and neural anomalies. This constellation of effects was subsequently termed Fetal Alcohol Syndrome [3]. Now recognized is that this syndrome is at one end (the most severe) of a spectrum of effects that may arise from prenatal exposure to alcohol [4]. At lower doses of alcohol consumption during pregnancy, neurobehavioral effects are often reported in the absence of the full syndrome. Such effects are often exhibited as behavioral disorders, cognitive deficits, and social problems [4,5] There is little dispute that these effects result from exposure to alcohol whilst in the womb. The observed neurobehavioral outcomes arise from some permanent influence of alcohol during the prenatal period on the development and functioning of the individual's central nervous system. The vast majority of studies of the effects of maternal consumption of alcohol during pregnancy report observations after birth, long after the time of exposure. Although these clearly indicate the long-term effects of prenatal alcohol exposure, such studies do not provide information on how alcohol influences neurobehavioral function and development at the time of exposure. Such information may be crucial in understanding the effect(s) of alcohol on the developing brain. Recent advances in studying the function of the fetus's central nervous system through observation of its behavior may enable a more detailed assessment to be made of how alcohol may adversely affect development, in particular neurobehavioral function.

BEHAVIOR OF THE HUMAN FETUS

Fetal behavior can be defined as any observable action or reaction (to an external stimulus) by the fetus [6]. The behavior of the fetus can be evaluated through the maternal perception of movements or Doppler ultra-sound recordings of fetal movements [6]. Yet, the clearest observations of the fetus's behavior can be achieved through the use of ultrasound [7]. In recent years, the advent of real-time, 4-D, ultrasound [8] has provided an even clearer window on the behavior and development of the fetus. Behavior can be spontaneous, that is endogenously generated by the fetus itself, or elicited, that is occurs in response to an external stimulus [6].

The behavior of the fetus has been reviewed in detail elsewhere [7,9], and only a brief overview is provided here. The first spontaneous movements of the fetus occur around 7-8 weeks of gestation. As observed using ultrasound, these movements appear to begin in the back or spine, are slow, and can result in the passive displacement of the arms and legs [10]. Over the course of the next few weeks, a wide range of movements develops, and over 20 different movement patterns have been identified (see table 1). By about 20 weeks of gestation the fetus displays most of the individual movements that it will produce during its time in utero and exhibits motor patterns similar to those observed in pre-term and term infants.

As the fetus develops, its movements become organized into periods of activity and inactivity. This culminates at the end of pregnancy with the emergence of behavioral states [11]. Four states are identified in the human fetus—quiet sleep, active sleep, quiet awake, active awake—precursors of the behavioral states seen in newborns [11]. These states are defined by three variables: the presence or absence of eye movements; the presence or absence of body movements; and, fetal heart rate pattern. These combine in a stable fashion as the fetus develops and from 36 weeks of gestation, individual states persist for relatively long periods of time. The transition from one state to the next is rapid, with the variables that define a particular state changing almost simultaneously. After 36 weeks of gestation, the fetus spends very little time in 'no state'. It is suggested that the appearance of behavioral states marks a further maturation of brain development and function [11]

Table 1. The gestational age at which behaviours are first observed in the fetus [7,9,10] Behaviour Gestational Age (wks)

Behaviour	Gestational Age (wks)
Just discernible movement	7
Startle	8
General movement	8
Hiccup	9
Isolated arm movement	9
Isolated leg movement	9
Isolated head retroflexion	9
Isolated head rotation	9-10
Isolated head anteflexion	10
Fetal breathing movements	10
Arm twitch	10
Leg twitch	10
Hand-face contact	10
Stretch	10
Rotation of fetus	10
Jaw movement	10-11
Yawn	11
Finger movement	12
Sucking and swallowing	12
Clonic movement arm or leg	13
Rooting	14
Eye movements	16

In terms of elicited movements, the fetus first responds to auditory stimuli at around 24-26 weeks of gestation [12] and to visual stimuli at 26-28 weeks of gestation [13]. Studies of exteriorized fetuses have demonstrated that the first motor responses of the fetus occur to touch around the lips at 8 weeks gestation and by 14 weeks most of the body is responsive to tactile stimulation [14].

FETAL BEHAVIOR AND NEURAL INTEGRITY

Observations of the behavior of the fetus offer an opportunity to assess the functioning of the fetal brain and central nervous system [6]. An individual's behavior is a product of the functioning of its central nervous system, thus by examining behavior, making inferences about the functioning of the central nervous system, including the brain, is possible. Despite advances in mapping the human genome and physiological techniques to study brain function (fetal MEG, fetal fMRI), observations of behavior still provide the best opportunity to assess the functioning and integrity of the brain. Indeed, to assess brain function, observing the output of this organ, i.e. behavior, is essential.

Atypical behaviors [6] have been observed in fetuses with chromosomal abnormalities, neural tube defects, fetal compromise (e.g. intra-uterine growth retardation), or in response to maternal illness (e.g. diabetes). Both the spontaneous and elicited behavior of the fetuses is influenced by fetal neural abnormalities [6,7,9]. For example, fetuses with trisomy 18 exhibit abnormal eye movements and rest-active cycles, and, fetuses with trisomy 21 exhibit altered habituation patterns compared to unaffected fetuses [6]. Moreover, the analysis of behavior enables the severity of effect to be determined [6].

Assessing brain function from observation of behavior in the fetus has another significant advantage, particularly in the case of exposure to teratogens [6]. The behavior emitted by the fetus is independent of any recall of the extent of exposure, e.g. in the case of alcohol, the amount consumed by the mother. Rather than relying on estimates of exposure, observations of behavior enable the effect of this exposure to be documented directly. This aspect assumes further importance when considering the effects of alcohol due to the reported individual differences in the effects of alcohol consumption in different pregnancies. Offspring of mothers who drank the same amount of alcohol may exhibit different levels of effect. Thus, observing behavior enables a direct assessment of any adverse effect rather than relying on statements concerning consumption. Finally, because the observation of behavior indicates the functioning of the brain at that time, developing interventions to address any effects arising from alcohol exposure at a time when the brain is at its most plastic may be possible in future years.

In summary, as the behavior of the fetus is a direct reflection of CNS functioning and integrity, observation of the behavior of the fetus provides the opportunity to examine the functioning of its CNS and to assess the influence of exposure to alcohol (or indeed any other substance) on the fetal brain and CNS.

MATERNAL ALCOHOL CONSUMPTION AND FETAL BEHAVIOR

The effects of alcohol consumption during pregnancy have been extensively studied with respect to the individual after birth, yet very few studies have been undertaken on the fetus. Case studies have reported that chronic [15] and acute [16] consumption of alcohol disrupts the normal behavior patterns exhibited by the fetus. A fetus observed at 38 and 40 weeks of gestation [15] exhibited abnormal organization of fetal behavioral states. This fetus exhibited a greater time in no-state and changed directly from 'quiet sleep' to 'active' without the more usual transition through 'active sleep' [11]. This latter aspect has been observed only in this case and not in other normal pregnancies or in those with other complications. The woman in this case was reported as drinking "10 glasses of beer or more" during the first 12 weeks of pregnancy, and between "2 and 10 glasses of beer a day during the following months". She was hospitalized at 36 weeks of gestation, and thus it is unlikely that she consumed alcohol immediately before the study of her fetus. This observation suggests that chronic high levels of alcohol consumption during pregnancy exert an effect on fetal behavior.

A second case study reported the behavior of the fetus of a mother with a history of drinking during pregnancy, and in this observation recorded behavior during and after an acute bout of intoxication at 37 weeks of gestation [16]. The fetus was observed for 60 minutes when the mother was intoxicated, a blood alcohol level of 322mg/dl at the start of the observation and 282mg/dl by the end. Behavior was compared with a second observation 24 hours later, when the mother had a blood alcohol level of less than 10 mg/dl. The fetus exhibited a reduced incidence of body and breathing movements when the mother was intoxicated compared to when she was not (0.11% cf 5.53%, 30.80% cf 67.60%, respectively). The observations of this fetus are quite interesting. At this age, one would expect that the fetus would exhibit breathing movements 30% to 40% of the time. Compared with a control group of fetuses not exposed to alcohol, an observation of 30% incidence of breathing would appear normal (see later in this paper). The authors reported evidence in the newborn infant of facial dysmorphology consistent with Fetal Alcohol Syndrome. Indeed the mother had been previously admitted to hospital during this same pregnancy with extremely high blood alcohol levels (339 and 353 mg/dl at 21 and 28 weeks gestation). It would appear likely that this fetus was exposed to high levels of alcohol. This will be returned to later.

ACUTE EFFECTS OF ALCOHOL ON FETUS

Studies examining the behavior of the fetus following the acute maternal consumption of low levels of alcohol have been conducted in late gestation, after 36 weeks. All consistently report that consumption of alcohol exerts an 'immediate' effect on behavior. Akay and Mulder [17] studied 28 fetuses between 37-40 weeks of gestation for 2 hours following maternal consumption of two glasses of white wine (11%v/v corresponding to 0.25g ethanol/kg maternal body weight) and again having consumed no alcohol. They report a rapid decline in breathing movements following maternal consumption of alcohol and, by 40 minutes, breathing was almost abolished. This persisted for the two hours of observation.

McLeod et al [18] observed 11 fetuses between 37-40 weeks of gestation following maternal consumption of ethanol diluted in soda water (15% solution at 0.25g ethanol/kg maternal body weight). Again, mothers served as their own controls, being observed in an identical procedure not having consumed alcohol. Breathing and body movements were recorded for 3.5 hours after the mother drank the alcohol (or control non-alcoholic soda). Maternal ethanol concentrations peaked around 30 minutes after drinking alcohol and fetal breathing movements were abolished by 30 minutes after alcohol consumption. There was no effect on body movements. Interestingly, even though maternal blood ethanol levels indicated no ethanol was present by the end of the observation (3.5 hours later), fetal breathing movements were still absent. Fox et al (19) asked seven mothers to drink one ounce of 80% proof vodka in 90ml of ginger ale, when 37-39 weeks pregnant (0.25 g ethanol/kg maternal body weight). A separate group of controls drank only ginger ale. Again, fetal breathing movements were abolished within 30 minutes after maternal consumption of alcohol. The authors reported that breathing resumed later during the observation, but did not record at what time.

A final study examined the effects of acute exposure on behavioral states [20]. Mothers (n=28), between 37-40 weeks of gestation, consumed two glasses of white wine (11% v/v) corresponding to 0.25 mg alcohol/kg maternal body weight. The fetuses, serving as their own controls, were observed in the absence of exposure to alcohol. Observations of behavior for two hours, using ultrasound, documented fetal heart rate, eye movements, and body movements to evaluate the effect of alcohol on fetal behavioral state. Consistent with previous studies, fetal breathing movements were completely suppressed by the consumption of alcohol. Moreover, alcohol consumption reduced fetal eye movements, and as a consequence, the behavioral state organization of the fetus was disrupted.

Studies of the acute effects of maternal alcohol consumption are important as they demonstrate that alcohol consumed by the mother exerts an effect on fetal behavior. The studies are consistent in reporting that alcohol suppresses fetal breathing movements and disrupts behavioral state organization. The reduction in breathing movements persists even after no alcohol remained in the mother's blood stream. There is some evidence for a dose-dependent effect as 1 oz of alcohol suppressed breathing for less time than did 1.9 oz (ref [19] cf ref [18]). These studies demonstrate that low levels of alcohol, 1-2 glasses of wine, exert a prolonged effect on the behavior of the fetus. Thus, there can be no doubt of the potential for alcohol to influence the functioning of the fetus's nervous system. The question remains as to what levels and duration of consumption are required before a permanent effect on the nervous system occurs.

CHRONIC EFFECTS OF ALCOHOL ON FETUS

Two studies have examined the effects of alcohol on the behavior of the fetus in pregnant women drinking low-medium levels of alcohol but who had no alcohol in their body at the time of observation. Thus, the chronic (permanent) effects of alcohol could be observed as opposed to any acute effect. These studies observed the fetal startle response. Both the spontaneous and elicited startles were observed.

Spontaneous startles emerge at approximately eight weeks gestation and decrease in incidence from approximately nine weeks gestation [21]. Such startles appear as rapid movements lasting about one second, initiated in the limbs and spreading through the body [21]. This pattern of behavior is thought to represent a primitive state of the nervous system and as the fetus matures and its nervous system becomes more developed, more sophisticated movement patterns prevail. In particular, the development of inhibitory pathways may contribute to the decreased incidence of startle behavior with advancing gestation.

Later in pregnancy (from approximately 24-26 weeks gestation), a 'startle' response may be observed following the presentation of a loud sound or vibroacoustic stimulus [12]. This 'elicited' startle is similar in appearance to spontaneously occurring startles observed earlier in gestation and is observed as a rapid movement of the body, especially the upper body or arms, and occurs in response to a stimulus [12]. The startle is probably the precursor of the startle response seen after birth occurring following a stimulus or event that makes us 'jump'.

Both spontaneous and elicited startles are influenced by the development of the nervous system, but in opposing directions. As the nervous system develops, the incidence of spontaneous startles decreases, whereas elicited startles become more developed (occurring more rapidly and directly following presentation of a stimulus). Thus not only do they provide an insight into the current functioning of the fetus's nervous system but also enable observations to be made about its development.

An initial study [22] examined the spontaneous fetal startle at 18-20 weeks of gestation and the elicited fetal startle at 25 weeks of gestation in mothers who drank alcohol (n=20) and mothers who did not drink alcohol (n=50). Mothers in both groups were observed at 18-20 weeks for 45 minutes using ultrasound and the number of spontaneous startles exhibited recorded. Significantly, more startles were exhibited by fetuses of mothers who drank compared with mothers who did not drink. At 25 weeks, the same fetuses were observed but this time their response to loud sound was examined (an elicited startle). Fetuses of mothers who drank were significantly less likely to startle in response to the sound than fetuses of mothers who did not drink. No alcohol was present in the blood of the women when tested, thus the effect was not due an acute effect. The mean number of units (+/- s.d.) of alcohol per week consumed by women in this study was 2.43 +/- 1.37. No correlation was found between the amount drunk and the effect on the fetus. A second study followed up this finding by observing spontaneous startles longitudinally across gestation [23]. Fetuses were observed for 45 minutes at 20, 25, 30, and 35 weeks of gestation. Twenty-three mothers drank alcohol, an average of 4.2 +/- 1.9 units of alcohol per week, and thirty-three mothers did not drink alcohol. The study found that consistent with the results of the previous study, exposure to alcohol increased the incidence of startle behavior across gestation in fetuses exposed to alcohol compared with fetuses not exposed to alcohol. The difference between the number of startles exhibited by fetuses exposed and those not exposed to alcohol decreased with advancing gestation. That is, exposure to alcohol appeared to delay the normal decrease in the incidence of startles observed with development in those fetuses exposed to alcohol. As development progressed, the behavior of those fetuses exposed to alcohol 'caught' up with the behavior of fetuses not exposed to alcohol, i.e. they exhibited fewer spontaneous startles. However at 35 weeks gestation, despite a significant catch up, the number of startles exhibited was still significantly different between fetuses exposed and not exposed to alcohol. Fetuses of mothers exposed to alcohol exhibited more spontaneous startles than did fetuses of mothers not exposed to alcohol. This result is perhaps indicative of a permanent effect on the fetal nervous system.

SUMMARY OF EFFECTS ON FETUS

Overall, the results indicate that low levels of alcohol exert an effect on fetal behavior. Such effects are most likely mediated by alcohol (or its breakdown products) influencing the functioning of its brain and central nervous system. Studies of the effects of acute exposure indicate that maternal consumption of 1-2 units of alcohol rapidly suppresses the behavior of her fetus. Research examining the effects of chronic consumption indicate that, at low levels of exposure (2-5 units per week), fetuses demonstrate a developmental delay in their behavior, indicative of a delay in the functional development of their nervous system and this delay could result in a permanent effect. Moreover, the effect is apparently dose dependent, in that any effect on behavior persists for longer at higher doses of alcohol exposure.

All these studies of both acute and chronic exposure have used women who drink little during their pregnancy, usually four glasses of wine per week or less. All studies are consistent in their observation that alcohol suppresses breathing, with the exception of one case study [16] which, in comparison with controls could be argued to have found no effect on breathing. A significant difference between the results of this study and those of the others was that this individual possibly exhibited Fetal Alcohol Syndrome; in all the other studies, there was no hint of this possibility. That this fetus was exposed to alcohol at a much higher level than fetuses in the other studies suggests that this difference may account for the difference in findings. Although one must be cautious in not over-interpreting the results of a single case study, this study may point to an effect arising from increased tolerance to alcohol through continual exposure and that continual exposure alters the behavior of the fetus.

Also noteworthy is that the effects on behavior persisted long after the alcohol had been removed from the maternal blood stream. Thus, fetal exposure to alcohol is not restricted only to the period that ethanol can be found present in the mother's blood stream. Fetal exposure may persist because the fetus is unable to clear the ethanol from its system as quickly as its mother can or through a reservoir of pooled alcohol in the amniotic fluid.

Studies of acute exposure indicate that the fetus is affected by even one glass of alcohol in the short term. Thus, it is not possible to say that one glass (unit) of alcohol does not affect the fetus—it does. How this relates to the neurobehavioral effects observed after birth is unknown. Generally, studies observing the fetus report effects at lower doses than those observed after birth. This observation may mean the effects are transient and do not exert a long term effect. Possibly, the effects observed after birth are the cumulative result of multiple brief exposures prenatally. Observations of the fetus may provide highly sensitive evaluations of the effects of alcohol exposure and provide an opportunity to document the effects of alcohol on the developing brain and its function.

TWO ROUTES OF ALCOHOL MEDIATED EFFECTS

Exposure to alcohol can exert its affect in two broad ways. First, a teratogenic effect on the developing nervous system may occur [24]. Alcohol or its break-down products directly interact with the neural substrates of the fetus and change their integrity and function. This mode of action raises particular concerns for 'binge' drinking, in that high exposures occur in a short space of time, despite perhaps average levels, when taken over the week, being low. A second mechanism of action could be due to the persistent changes in behavior resulting from alcohol exposure. Now recognized is that prenatal development is not just under genetic control but also experiential factors exert an effect and that the sensory environment, motor behavior, actions, and reactions of the fetus all contribute to the normal developmental processes [14]. The effects of a continual disruption of these processes are unknown. For example, a single unit of alcohol on a daily basis would continually disrupt breathing, eye movements, and potentially other behavioral processes, for two hours or more. What effect this may have on development is unknown but raises the significant question that repeated exposure to low doses of alcohol, by continually disrupting normal behavioral and neural processes, could also have an adverse effect on fetal development, and attention must be paid to this issue.

CONCLUSIONS

In conclusion, because it is developing at its most rapid rate during the fetal period, the central nervous system can be considered at greater risk for damage at this time. The observation of the behavior of the fetus may be a (the most) sensitive means of detecting the effects of alcohol on the developing individual. Studies of the behavior of the fetus indicate that small amounts of alcohol (one unit) exert an effect on the fetus, disrupting its normal behavior. Fetal exposure to alcohol via maternal consumption has the potential to cause permanent damage through a teratogenic effect or via continual disruption of normal developmental processes. At what level of consumption such potential risk becomes real is presently unknown. The evidence, however, does suggest one statement that can be made with regard to drinking during pregnancy, namely that one unit of alcohol exerts an effect on fetal behavior and the fetal nervous system.

REFERENCES

[1]   O'Leary C. *Fetal alcohol syndrome: A literature review.* Canberra, AU: Commonwealth Australia, 2002.

[2]   Lemoine P, Harousseau H, Borteyru JP, Menuet JC. Les enfants de parents alcooliques Anomalies observees: A propos de 127 cas. *Quest Medical* 1968;21:476-82.

[3]   Jones KL, Smith DW. Recognition of the fetal alcohol syndrome in early infancy. *Lancet* 1973; 2:999-1001.

[4]   Riley EP, McGee CL. Fetal alcohol spectrum disorders: an overview with emphasis on changes in brain and behavior. *Exp. Biol. Med.* 2005;230: 357-65.

[5]   Kelly SJ, Day N, Streissguth AP. Effects of prenatal alcohol exposure on social behavior in humans and other species. *Neurotoxicol. Teratol.* 2000;22:143-9.

[6]   Hepper PG. The behavior of the foetus as an indicator of neural functioning In: Lecanuet JP, Fifer WP, Krasnegor NA, Smotherman WP, eds. *Fetal development: A psychobiological perspective.* Hillsdale, NJ: Lawrence Erlbaum, 1995:405-17.

[7]   Nijhuis JG, ed. *Fetal behavior. Developmental and perinatal aspects.* Oxford, UK: Oxford Univ, 1992.

[8]   Kurjak Λ, Carrera JM, Medic M, Azumendi A, Andonotopo W, Stanojevic M. The antenatal development of fetal behavioral patterns assessed by four-dimensional sonography. *J. Mat. Fetal Neonat. Med.* 2005;17:401-16.

[9]   Lecanuet J-P, Fifer W, Krasnegor N, Smother-man, W. eds. *Fetal Development. A Psychobio-logical Perspective.* Hillsdale, NJ: Lawrence Erlbaum, 1995.

[10] Prechtl HFR. Assessment of fetal neurological function and development. In: Levene M, Bennett M, Punt J, eds. *Fetal and neonatal neurology and neurosurgery.* Edinburgh, Scotland, UK: Churchill Livingstone, 1988:33-40.

[11] Nijhuis JG, Martin CB, Prechtl HFR. Behavioral states of the human fetus. In: Prechtl HFR, ed. Continuity of neural functions from prenatal to postnatal life. *Clin. Dev. Med.* London, UK: Blackwell,1982:65-78.

[12] Hepper PG, Shahidullah S. The development of fetal hearing. *Fet. Mat. Med. Rev.* 1994;6:167-79.

[13] Polishuk W, Laufer N, *Sadovsky E. Fetal reaction to external light*. Harefuah 1975;89:395. [Hebrew].

[14] Hepper PG. Fetal psychology. An embryonic science. In: Nijhuis JG, ed. Fetal Behavior. *Developmental and perinatal aspects*. Oxford, UK: Oxford Univ, 1992:129-56.

[15] Mulder EJH, Kamstra A, O'Brien MJ, Visser GHA, Prechtl HFR. Abnormal fetal behavioral state regulation in a case of high maternal alcohol intake during pregnancy. *Ear. Hum. Dev*. 1986;14:321-6.

[16] Castillo RA, Devoe LD, Ruedrich DA, Gardner P. The effects of acute alcohol intoxication on biophysical activities: A case report. *Am. J. Obstet. Gynecol*. 1989;160:692-3.

[17] Akay M, Mulder EJH. Investigating the effect of maternal alcohol intake on human fetal breathing rate using adaptive time-frequency analysis methods. *Ear. Hum. Dev*. 1996;46:153-64.

[18] McLeod W, Brien JF, Loomis C, Carmichael L, Probert C, Patrick J. Effects of maternal ethanol ingestion on fetal breathing movements gross body movements and heart rate at 37 to 40 weeks gestational age. *Am. J. Obstet. Gynecol*. 1983;145:251-7.

[19] Fox HE, Steinbrecher M, Pessel D, Inglis J, Medvid L, Angel E. Maternal ethanol ingestion and the occurrence of human fetal breathing movements. *Am. J. Obstet Gynecol*. 1978;132:354-58.

[20] Mulder EJH, Morssink LP, van der Schee, Visser GHA. Acute maternal alcohol consumption disrupts behavioral state organization in the near-term fetus. *Ped. Res*. 1998;44:774-9.

[21] De Vries JIP, Visser GHA, Prechtl HFR. The emergence of fetal behavior I: Qualitative aspects. *Ear. Hum. Dev*. 1982;7:301-22.

[22] Little JF, Hepper PG, Dornan JC. Maternal alcohol consumption during pregnancy and fetal startle behavior. *Physiol. Behav*. 2002;76:691-4.

[23] Hepper PG, Dornan JC, Little JF. Maternal alcohol consumption during pregnancy may delay the development of spontaneous fetal startle behavior. *Physiol. Behav*. 2005;83:711-4.

[24] Chen WA, Maier SE, Parnell SE, West JR. Alcohol and the developing brain: neuroanatomical studies. *Alch. Res. Health* 2003;27:174-180.

In: Alcohol-Related Cognitive Disorders
Editors: L. Sher, I. Kandel, J. Merrick pp. 67-89

ISBN: 978-1-60741-730-9
© 2009 Nova Science Publishers, Inc.

Chapter 4

FETAL ALCOHOL SYNDROME SPECTRUM DISORDERS: DIAGNOSIS, SURVEILLANCE AND SCREENING

Christine Cronk and Marianne Weiss

ABSTRACT

Fetal Alcohol Spectrum Disorder (FASD) is a prevalent preventable disorder with a significant societal burden related to the cognitive and behavioral disabilities associated with this disorder. This chapter reviews published work on FASD diagnosis, surveillance and screening programs. Challenges inherent to FASD diagnosis remain, and complicate attempts to estimate FAS prevalence. In addition, the drive toward diagnostic accuracy has led to formulation of screening protocols for children at school ages after many disabilities associated with FASD are established.

We present the design and selected findings from a regional multi-stage screening project piloted in Wisconsin. Small for gestational age (SGA) newborns with birth head circumference less than 10th percentile were selected in the first screening stages. Those meeting these criteria were evaluated for growth, development and FAS facial features at about two years of age. Of newborns meeting the initial screening criteria, 30% demonstrated growth deficits and developmental delays at about 2 years of age. Children with any FAS facial feature (of 177 children assessed, n=13 with 2 or 3 facial findings, n=77 with one facial finding) showed greater deficits in growth and a greater proportion were developmentally delayed. These findings demonstrate the potential value of embedding screening for FAS within a multistage screening method to identify infants at risk for developmental delay. Because this model would be a part of larger population screening for developmental delay, cost efficiencies could be achieved. Problems relating to protection and confidentiality that inevitably accompany screening to identify FASD would also be reduced in a screening model that focuses on identification of children at risk for developmental delay rather than confirmation of the etiologic source of the delays.

INTRODUCTION

Fetal alcohol spectrum disorder (FASD) is likely the most prevalent preventable cause of childhood disability, cognitive limitation and behavioral disorder in the US, and the increase in alcohol consumption rates by pregnant women and women of child-bearing age (including any use, chronic use and binge drinking) suggest that population risks for this disorder may be increasing [1-3]. Costs of care for FASD (annually $2.8 billion 1998 dollars, with a lifetime cost for one individual of $2 million [4]) are likely to increase.

Identification and diagnosis of children with FASD is complex, and has been influenced by social and policy considerations [5,6]. In spite of the investment of researchers and public health agencies, problems with FASD diagnosis remain, creating barriers to optimum secondary prevention and treatment. Surveillance for FASD that could improve accuracy of prevalence estimates has remained challenging and inhibited public health planning and efficient resource allocation for families with FASD affected children. Finally, because of problems with diagnosis and imprecision of prevalence estimates, implementation programs for screening children (as opposed to the relatively less complex screening to identify women at risk for prenatal alcohol use) have been difficult to support.

This chapter traces the evolution of FASD diagnosis and reviews methods and data from surveillance studies estimating FASD prevalence. We then report on published findings from FASD screening programs and selected findings from a regional screening project piloted in Wisconsin. We highlight findings about growth deficits present at birth in relation to developmental findings at two years of age, and the relation of growth and development for children with some or all of the facial features associated with FASD. These findings suggest the potential value of early screening particularly for secondary prevention of developmental delay. We maintain that the drive for diagnostic accuracy evident in the historical definitions of FAS, FAE, ARBD, ARND, and finally FASD have made early identification of children with FASD more difficult. Because the diagnostic certainty for FASD is diminished during infant and toddler years, there is the perception that screening should be delayed until school years when the physical and behavioral features of this disorder are more clearly manifested. Intervention efforts initiated at this time are less effective [7]. On the other hand, despite the uncertainty of etiology and therefore diagnosis, two key features of FAS (intrauterine growth deficit and microcephaly) can be applied early in life and result in identification of children with a higher probability of developmental and physical growth delays regardless of the ultimate etiology. Treatment for developmental delay does not rely on diagnostic certainty. Thus in contrast to delaying screening until school age after the onset of learning and behavior problems, early screening and appropriate intervention could ultimately reduce the individual and societal burdens of this condition.

HISTORY AND IMPORTANCE OF FASD DIAGNOSIS

Though no systematic description of clinical findings appeared in the medical literature until later, the association of mental retardation with alcoholism in the mother was suspected and investigated more than 200 year ago. The gin epidemic in eighteenth century England (occurring when taxes on gin were lowered to revive the grain market) resulted in increased availability of gin to the poor, and many thought, led to an increase infant mortality and mental disability in offspring of female inebriates [6].

Fetal alcohol syndrome (FAS) was first systematically described and named in 1972 and 1973 [8-10] by Jones and coinvestigators in Washington, though an earlier description of the syndrome in *Ouest Medical* in 1968 actually preceded these reports [11]. Work has followed documenting additional cases [12-14], an expanded list of physical abnormalities, and a range of neurodevelopmental and behavioral manifestations of FASD [15-18]. Other human, animal and bench research investigating dose effects and potential ecogenetic influences have also appeared [6]. The drive behind these investigations derives in part from the focus on the effects of teratogens in the environment, the growing medicalization of prenatal care, and emphasis on the individual responsibility of the mother to avoid risks associated even with small amounts of alcohol intake [5].

FASD DIAGNOSIS

Diagnosis of FASD remains complex for many reasons: (a) No diagnostic test can confirm FAS, so it is a co-occurrence of traits that defines the syndrome; (b) While the combination of cardinal facial features of the syndrome are distinctive, no individual feature is pathognomonic of FASD, and many characterize other syndromes. In particular, retarded body and head growth typify many congenital and perinatal abnormalities [19,20]; (c) Some of the traits of the disorder overlap with features within the range of normal (for example, the presence of epicanthal folds, or the familial inheritance of flat philtrum) [21]; (d) As with the other features of FASD, only the co-occurrence of the constellation of behavioral abnormalities observed in these children is distinctive though not unique to FASD [22-26]; (e) The syndrome has a broad range of expressivity likely arising from variation in timing, level and pattern of alcohol intake, other interacting cofactors (e.g. substance use, poor nutrition) and maternal/fetal factors affecting susceptibility to alcohol effects [27,28]; (f) Though some studies document consistency of phenotype across the lifespan [29], others suggest that the features of the syndrome change with age [30,31]; (g) Documentation of maternal alcohol exposure during pregnancy is complex. Prenatal alcohol use is underreported, probably by a factor of three or more [28]; accurate quantification of levels of alcohol exposure is difficult, and the impact of drinking pattern (e.g., bingeing versus chronic heavy alcohol use) is documented in animal studies, and presumed for humans [32]. FASD is a frequent concern for children in foster placement where exposure cannot be well documented [33].

These complications led to the formation of a National Academy of Science Institute of Medicine (IOM) expert panel to standardize the criteria for making the diagnosis of FASD [28]. The IOM instituted the concept of a spectrum of disorders secondary to prenatal alcohol exposure that was intended to improve diagnostic precision, lead to better prevention, treatment and intervention for these children, and assist with public health planning. Key issues considered by the IOM panel included:

- Whether a history of exposure to alcohol should be required for the
- diagnosis of FAS

- Which physical features should be used to define the disorder
- Whether behavioral or cognitive features should be used to define the disorder
- Whether differing criteria should be specified in making the diagnosis across the life span

A particular concern of the panel was the common use of the term FAE (fetal alcohol effects) to characterize children without all the necessary features of FAS, but with a set of behavioral outcomes typical for children affected by alcohol. The term FAE was first used to describe findings in animal studies.[34,35]. Its use to refer to cognitive and behavioral effects of alcohol in the absence of other features of FAS enhanced the imprecision of FAS diagnosis, and some suggested that it be dropped (36). The panel also addressed many other issues that complicate diagnosis including measuring alcohol intake, presence of confounding risks (e.g. cocaine use), uncertainty of the harm level of differing exposures, and lifespan changes in diagnostic features.

The IOM panel created a set of diagnostic categories with alcohol exposure and the facial phenotype for FAS considered central to diagnosis. Types and criteria for the IOM classifications within FASD are reproduced in table 1.

Astley and Clarren [37] had concerns about the IOM criteria, particularly their lack of specificity and qualitative rather than quantitative definition; the poorly specified causal link between Alcohol Related Neurological Defects (ARND) (see table 1) and Alcohol Related Birth Defects (ARBD) and documented alcohol exposure (classifications substituting for FAE and intended to improve diagnostic precision); and the fact that the broad range of cognitive and behavioral abnormalities did not play into the IOM diagnostic criteria.

As an alternative to this 'gestalt' diagnostic approach, they developed a quantitative diagnostic system based on insights from previous work and explicit evaluation of findings for more than 1,000 patients seen at the Washington State FAS Diagnostic and Prevention Network (DPN). Each diagnostic category is associated with a four digit code reflecting the magnitude of expression of four key diagnostic features of FASD: (a) growth deficiency, (b) facial phenotype, (c) CNS abnormalities, and (d) prenatal alcohol exposure. Lip and philtrum conformation is rated using a 5-point Likert scale photographic reference. Palpebral fissure length (PFL) is measured and a z-score computed using reference data [38].

Based on the combination of ratings for all elements used in this system, a child can be placed into one of 22 categories (from FAS alcohol exposed to Normal/no alcohol exposure). A 2004 revision and is available as a downloadable pdf file [39]. Associated tools, software and training resources are referenced in this guide and available at http://depts.washington.edu/fasdpn

Hoyme and colleagues [19,40] agreed that the IOM criteria were vague, but criticized the Astley/Clarren system for its unwieldy complexity, persisting ambiguities, vagueness regarding neurobehavioral findings, and lack of integration of family and genetic background. These authors offered an alternative scoring system which was based on examination of 164 Native American and South African children examined independently by two dysmorphologists and other professionals.

As part of this system, they assigned a dysmorphology score based on 25 abnormalities weighted according to their frequency of observed association with FAS.

Table 1. Institute of Medicine (1996) diagnostic criteria for fetal alcohol syndrome and alcohol-related effects [28]

FAS with confirmed maternal alcohol exposure

A. *Confirmed maternal alcohol exposure*
B. *Evidence of characteristic pattern of facial anomalies including*
•   Flat upper lip
•   Short palpebral fissures
•   Flattened philtrum
•   Flat midface
C. *Evidence of growth retardation in at least one of the following:*
•   Low birth weight for gestational age
•   Decelerating weight overtime not due to nutrition
•   Disproportional low weight to height
D. *Evidence of CNS neurodevelopmental abnormalities in at least one of the following:*
•   Decreased cranial size at birth
•   Structural brain abnormalities
•   Neurological hard or soft signs

FAS without confirmed maternal alcohol exposure (B-D above)

Partial FAS with confirmed maternal alcohol exposure
A. *Confirmed maternal alcohol exposure*
B. *Evidence of some of the components of the pattern of characteristic facial anomalies*
Either
C. *Evidence of growth retardation (see C above) OR*
D. *Evidence of CNS neurodevelopmental abnormalities (see D above) OR*
E. *Evidence of a complex pattern of behavior or cognitive abnormalities* inconsistent with developmental level and not explainable by family background or environment alone (learning difficulties, deficits in school performance, poor impulse control, problems with social perception, deficits in higher level of receptive and expressive language, poor capacity for abstraction or metacognition, specific deficits in math skills or problems in memory, attention or judgment

Alcohol Related Effects: Clinical conditions in which there is a history of maternal alcohol exposure

•   Alcohol-related birth defects (ARBD)-Congenital anomalies with documented association
•   Alcohol-related neurological defects (ARND)

Evidence of CNS neurodevelopmental abnormalities in at least one of the following *(see D above)*
Evidence of a complex pattern of behavior or cognitive abnormalities *(see E above)*

In the Hoyme system, an FAS diagnosis requires abnormalities in all domains (facial dysmorphology, growth and CNS structure or function); ARBD requires confirmed maternal alcohol use, a typical facies (two of the cardinal features), and one or more specific structural anomalies; and ARND requires confirmed maternal alcohol exposure in combination with a characteristic pattern of behavioral or cognitive abnormalities typical of prenatal alcohol exposure, not documented in other family members, and not explained by postnatal influences. Hoyme's system was subsequently used in diagnosing FASD in a Finnish sample [41].

Astley [42] criticized the system introduced by Hoyme and colleagues for what she saw as key violations of the quantitative approach of the Astley/Clarren 4 digit code system including:

- Requiring only two rather than three facial features to diagnose full FAS
- Requiring a head circumference less than 10th percentile rather than using the more conventional cut off for microcephaly (less than 3rd percentile)
- Requiring that CNS evidence be structural instead of either structural or functional
- Specifying that 'excessive' rather than any prenatal alcohol exposure be documented
- Not specifying the severity of the functional abnormalities required to meet the diagnostic criteria
- Not specifying the number of domains in which functions must be impaired

Astley also pointed out that the validation sample for this diagnostic system included only Native Americans and South Africans, and phenotypic variations in eye, lip and philtrum in these groups differ materially from those of US populations. To illustrate these difficulties further, Astley used Hoyme's diagnostic criteria to classify children from the DPN database. A large number met Hoyme's facial criteria (i.e. two of the three cardinal facial features) (n=330 of 952 DPN cases). But only 39 of these 330 children were diagnosed with full FAS using all criteria specified in the Hoyme system.

Astley classified the 952 cases using both the 4-Digit Code and the Hoyme diagnostic criteria for full FAS. We summarize the numbers reported by Astley showing agreement between the two systems in Table 2. A total of 57 children were diagnosed as FAS by one or other system. Positive agreement was poor (17 children, 30%).

Table 2. Data reported by Astley (42) comparing numbers of children diagnosed with FAS by the Astley and Clarren (19) and Hoyme diagnostic systems [39]

		Astley Clarren System		
		No	Yes	Total
Hoyme	No	895	22	917
system	Yes	18	17	35
Total		913	39	952

To achieve consistency across clinicians diagnosing FASD, national recommendations have been formulated by the Public Health Agency of Canada and by the Centers for Disease Control and Prevention in the US. The Canadian FAS diagnostic guide [20] specifies that:

- A comprehensive, multidisciplinary evaluation (including a physician, psychologist, occupational therapist and speech-language pathologist) is necessary to make an accurate diagnosis and recommendation for management
- Screening and referral should be carried out with all pregnant and postpartum women using standardized alcohol use evaluation tools
- Referral for possible FASD should be made when the following are present
  - Three cardinal facial features of FAS
  - Evidence of significant prenatal exposure to alcohol
  - One or more facial features with growth deficits plus known or probable significant prenatal alcohol exposure
  - One or more facial features with one or more CNS deficits plus known or probable significant prenatal alcohol exposure
  - One or more facial features with pre- or postnatal growth deficits (or both) and one or more CNS deficits plus known or probable significant prenatal alcohol exposure

Similarly, the CDC produced a set of recommendations for standardized diagnosis in the US [31]. They defined FASD (a collection of diagnostic categories, not a diagnosis that can be assigned to an individual child) as the range of effects that can occur in a person whose mother drank alcohol during pregnancy including physical, mental, behavior and learning disabilities including lifelong implications. The key criteria for full FAS specified were:

- All three facial features using the Astley/Clarren lip philtrum guide, and measured PFL
- Confirmed growth abnormalities relative to age, sex, gestational age and race/ethnicity specific reference data
- CNS abnormalities including
  - Measured age, sex adjusted head circumference <10th percentile
  - Clinically meaningful brain abnormalities observable through imaging
  - Functional abnormalities documented by substantially reduced test performance for either global cognitive functioning or functional deficits less than 1 SD below normal in three domains (determined by a qualified professional)

Importantly, because of insufficient scientific evidence, this set of recommendations does not specify subcategories within the FASD spectrum apart from full FAS.

The most widely used diagnostic systems discussed above have not used promising methods based on specialized assessments requiring use of photographs [43], additional anthropometric equipment, or more time-consuming craniofacial measurements. Vitez and coworkers [44,45] developed a scoring system using photographs and morphometric analysis which successfully discriminated alcohol-exposed offspring. The system developed by Hoyme [19] has some similarities with this system. Moore and colleagues [46,47] tested use of 21 craniofacial dimensions measured directly on subjects. Using stepwise discriminant function analysis two dimensions (head circumference and bigonial diameter) discriminated children diagnosed with FAS, five measures discriminated full from partial FAS (head circumference, bigonial breadth, midfacial depth, bizygomatic breadth and maxillary arc), and six variables discriminated alcohol-exposed children from controls (minimal frontal breadth, bigonial breadth, midfacial depth, PFL, head circumference and maxillary arc). These studies do indicate that the effects of alcohol on craniofacial growth and development are more global (affecting midfacial development underlaid by deficient or abnormal development of the brain). These authors suggest that use of multiple measurements would potentially allow detection of the range of phenotypic effects of alcohol from subtle to full FAS.

In spite of its potentially great value for early identification and intervention, accurate diagnosis of FAS in the neonatal period has been discouraged because of difficulties in accurate measurement of the facial features, head size (due to delivery related deformations of the skull), and the fact that some infants with FAS have normal birth size and do not manifest growth failure until after birth [48]. But several studies have suggested approaches to assessment near birth. Ernhart and colleages [49] used birth weight <10th percentile for gestational age, the presence of four anomalies including at least one craniofacial anomaly specific to FAS, and one neurologic anomaly to identify newborns with potential FAS. Coles and coinvestigators (50) used an index based on maternal risk variables, maternal prenatal alcohol exposure, microcephaly, and neurodevelopmental evaluation, and concluded that it is possible to identify at risk neonates using the risk index.

As this section suggests, there is general agreement about the cardinal diagnostic features of FAS/FASD, but differing approaches to achieving diagnostic certainty and precision. Diagnostic certainty is best achieved for full FAS during childhood when physical and behavioral traits of the syndrome are most clearly evident, and ultimately requires ascertainment of prenatal alcohol exposure. However, by the age at which the FASD diagnosis is most accurate, the optimal time for initiation of early intervention has passed. Thus children who do not meet diagnostic criteria but have neurologic or behavioral patterns consistent with prenatal exposure may be bypassed by the diagnostic process. Surveillance and prevalence estimation efforts are compromised by this same diagnostic dilemma.

SURVEILLENCE AND ESTIMATING FAS PREVALENCE

Because of the difficulties in establishing a FAS diagnosis, estimating FAS prevalence has been challenging. Initially, clinic-based studies were used to estimate the occurrence of FAS. Abel [27] analyzed clinic-based studies and documented rates between 0 and 30 per 10,000 live births, with increased rates among persons of low socioeconomic status (SES), African Americans and American Indians. When the samples from these collected studies were combined, the worldwide incidence was 9.7 per 10,000 live births (95 cases out of 97,756 individuals) with US rates substantially higher (19.5 per 10,000) than those from other countries (0.8 per 10,000), possibly due to heightened awareness of FAS in the US. The incidence of FAS estimated from studies of women who are heavy drinkers was 4.6% (162 cases out of 3,761).

But clinic-based studies have many biases. Surveillance has been the most promising approach to estimating population prevalence of this disorder. However, FASD surveillance has proved challenging because of the complexities involved in diagnosis (see above) and the consequent need for specialized skills in arriving at a diagnosis. Because national or state level surveillance systems often rely either on passive reporting (i.e. reports submitted by clinicians or reported electronically from hospitals to a central registry) or active ascertainment (where trained abstractors collect recorded information from one or more sources such as medical or educational records), diagnostic consistency and accuracy cannot be assured. Surveillance for many birth defects is accomplished by mandated reporting usually for children in the first two to six years of life, or by multiple source methods involving medical, birth, death, fetal death, hospital discharge, school and other records. The National Birth Defects Prevention Network publishes prevalence estimates for a range of conditions in states with birth defects registries. There is great variation in sources and inclusion criteria among states. Some have specific active surveillance for FAS while others rely on passive reports. Of 35 registries, 24 reported prevalence figures for FAS for the period 1999-2003 ranging from 0 to 3.14 per 10,000 live births [51]. In general, state registries without special procedures for identifying FAS have been found to have low reliability. Fox and Drueschel [52] compared cases reported to the New York State Congenital Malformations Registry (CMR) by physicians or hospitals (passive reporting) with those actively ascertained through the Fetal Alcohol Syndrome Surveillance Network (FASSNet), a CDC-funded initiative. Of 33 cases reported for 1995 through 1998 to the CMR, 19 were confirmed by FASSNet, and 24 cases not reported to the CMR were ascertained by FASSNet. Of cases ascertained on the basis of an ICD9 code of 760.71 (the code most specific to this condition), more than 40% were false positives because this code can be applied to children with prenatal alcohol exposure without examination of the child.

Specialized surveillance for FASD has most often used linked multiple source methodologies. Egeland and coworkers [53] used a capture/recapture method from Indian Health Service (IHS) Medicaid claims, pediatric practices (using the ICD-9 760.71 codes) and an active FAS screening program in Alaska. Cases were verified by a chart review and the number of unique and common cases from screening versus physician diagnosis evaluated. They found that IHS screening identified 66% of the cases with better ascertainment among older than younger children. Birth and death certificates did not contribute additional cases. Bergeson and coworkers (54) used ICD9 code 760.71 from birth and death certificates, Medicaid claims files, and the IHS to identify FAS cases. Ascertainment was best for IHS patients, and worst in birth certificate identified cases.

Miller and coworkers [55] used an existing state registry as the basis of a multiple source methodology including enhanced surveillance at two sites and active medical record surveillance to identify FAS cases among births in Colorado from 1992-94. Based on abstracted information, 173 potential FAS cases were identified. Twenty-seven percent of these were identified by more than one source. Enhanced surveillance had the highest sensitivity. However, with the exception of genetic clinics, the positive predictive value of the sources used was low (less than 30%). Of the 173 cases, 78 were evaluated as 'definite' cases by a geneticist. About 85% of the 'definite' cases were diagnosed as FAS, though only 67% of definite cases received an unequivocal FAS diagnosis in the source document. Among the probable and possible FAS cases evaluated by a geneticist, only 23% had some FAS or related diagnosis confirmed. The results of this effort suggest that FAS diagnosis must involve expert physician evaluation.

In 1997, in an attempt to determine the prevalence of FAS more precisely, the Centers for Disease Control and Prevention worked with five US states to develop a multiple source method for ascertaining FAS (Fetal Alcohol Syndrome Surveillance Network, FASSNet). This group first developed a surveillance case definition (i.e. a definition that could be employed using only records but no direct diagnostic encounter with children) with two categories, confirmed and probable, as reproduced in table 3. The FASSNET system recognized the possibility that prenatal alcohol exposure is under-reported, and therefore classified children based on face, CNS, and growth criteria.

Table 3. FAS Surveillance Network (FASSNet) case definition categories [56]

Case Definition Category	Face	CNS	Growth
Confirmed FAS phenotype with or without maternal alcohol exposure	Abnormal facial features consistent with FAS as reported by a physician OR	Head circumference ≤10th percentile at birth or any age OR	Intrauterine weight or height ≤10th percentile for gestational age OR
	Two of the following: Short palpebral fissures Abnormal philtrum Thin upper lip	Standardized measure of intellectual function ≤ standard deviation below the mean OR	Postnatal weight or height ≤ 10th percentile for age OR
		Developmental delay or mental retardation diagnosed by a qualified examiner (e.g. psychologist or physician) OR	Postnatal weight for height ≤ 10th percentile for age
		Attention deficit disorder diagnosed by a qualified evaluator	
Probable FAS phenotype with or without confirmed maternal alcohol exposure	Required; facial features same as above	Must meet either CNS or growth criteria	as outlined above

In four of the states (Alaska, Arizona, Colorado, and New York) records from hospitals, birth defects surveillance programs, genetic clinics, developmental clinics, early intervention programs, Medicaid files and others were used, and a software program developed to guide abstractors through record evaluation [56]. Multiple records (e.g. medical and school records) for a given individual were linked. Case status was determined using a computer algorithm. In the fifth state (Wisconsin), a screening rather than a surveillance process was used (see below Screening for FAS).

In the four states using the surveillance methodology, records of 1,489 children were reviewed, with multiple sources available for 90% of cases. A total of 185 of these children met the case definitions for confirmed (n=142) or probable (n=43) FAS. There were 437,252 total births yielding a birth prevalence of 2.6 to 4.5 per 10,000 live births with the rate in Alaska (14.9 per 10,000 births) significantly higher than this. Ethnic-specific rates ranged from 1.8 per 10,000 live births to 32 per 10,000 live births for Native Americans. These rates are similar to those reported in other population based prevalence studies of FAS, even though a different case definition and ascertainment methods were used [57].

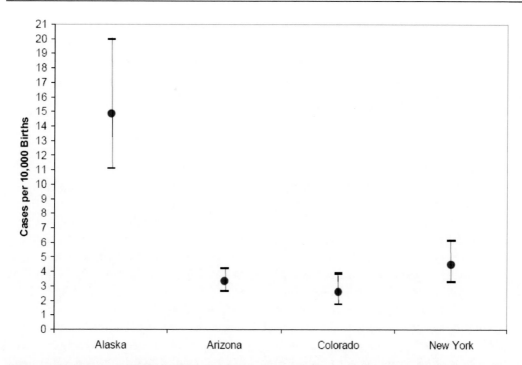

Figure 1. Rates per 10,000 live births (± 95% Poisson CI) for FAS computed using data from 4 States funded by 1997 CDC initiative, Fetal Alcohol Syndrome Surveillance Network ,(FASSNet) using multi-source ascertainment [56].

Surveillance systems use retrospective methods to enumerate cases, and data from these systems are used for public health program and policy development, and resource allocation. However, because careful surveillance case definitions for full FAS (as used by FASSNet) require the presence of some of the cardinal facial features of the syndrome, most ascertained cases are at an age beyond infancy when early intervention is best instituted. As discussed above, when this approach is used for screening, it supports greater diagnostic certainty, but is not optimal for instituting secondary prevention for disabilities associated with FAS.

SCREENING FOR FAS

Screening involves the use of quick, simple testing procedures to identify individuals with a disease or condition so that prevention or intervention efforts can be instituted. Screening of childbearing age or pregnant women is the only approach to primary prevention of FASD [58,59]. Screening methods focused on infants or children with FAS have also been developed. Most have targeted early school aged children and have used two stage processes.

Clarren and coinvestigators tested the feasibility of FAS screening of first graders in elementary schools in Washington state using specially trained school or public health nurses [60]. They focused on first graders because, in contrast to newborns, the features of FASD are more readily identified, and this is the first point after the birth event when the majority of children come in contact with a single system through which the screening can be implemented. The screening protocol was staged. In stage 1, children meeting one of three criteria were selected based on the following criteria: a) height and/or weight less than 10th percentile and one key FAS facial feature; b) normal size with one or more key FAS facial feature, and teacher concerns about behavioral and developmental problems associated with FAS; c) recorded reference to alcohol exposure during gestation in the child's educational records. In stage 2, children meeting these criteria were formally assessed at a special diagnostic clinic. One hundred twenty-four (124) of 3,740 children screened positive in stage 1. Of these only about half completed the evaluation in the special diagnostic clinic. Seven previously undiagnosed children were identified as FAS or atypical FAS, and 19 had other FASD diagnoses. The remainder had isolated findings associated with FASD or some other diagnosis. The investigators concluded that this experience supported further consideration of school entry screening, though barriers to such a program would arise depending upon the way the screening is presented and if active rather than passive consent is sought.

A photographic screening method was developed and used with children in foster care [33]. Standardized photographs were taken either by trained university students during a home visit, or by families provided with directions on how to complete the photographs. The photographs were assessed using the Astley-Clarren diagnostic system criteria [39]. A measurement of head circumference and a review of foster care educational and health records was also completed. Children screening positive were referred for a full diagnostic evaluation. When compared with the full diagnostic system, this screening method was 100% sensitive and 99.8% specific with a positive predictive value positive of 85.7%. The prevalence of FAS in the screened population was 10-15 times higher than in the general population, and the investigators concluded that screening children in foster care is likely to be highly beneficial, particularly for advising foster parents, school personnel and health care providers who will be working with the child.

Burd and colleagues developed an FAS screen including 32 items (primarily physical abnormalities) frequently documented in their patient series. This inventory consisted of features that could be reliably measured by individuals with limited training in a short time (15 minutes or less per case) thus excluding difficult to measure features such as PFL (61). Children scoring >20 were referred to a local dysmophologist, and, in some cases, additional information was collected from school and medical records and by maternal interview. From 1992 through 2000, 1,384 kindergarten children were screened with 69 screening positive on the FAS inventory; seven were confirmed to have FAS or partial FAS by a dysmorphologist [62,63]. This screen was completed within the school without additional financial, logistical or technical support.

A screening program was completed in elementary schools in two parts of South Africa with suspected high rates of FAS using a two-stage screening/case finding approach [64,65]. In stage 1, children with weight, height and/or head circumference values less than the WHO/Fels standards were selected. In stage 2, facial and other phenotypic abnormalities were identified, including the cardinal features of FAS using measurements of the eye and qualitative assessment of lip and philtrum. Thirty-two schools with 1,822 children between 5 and 10 years of age participated. Of these, 67 (3.7%) received a diagnosis of FAS.

Finally, Duimstra et al [66] piloted a multi-level FAS screening project in four American Indian communities. These investigators also used a staged screening approach, but one instituted within the first years of life. Low birth weight infants whose mothers used alcohol during pregnancy were identified using birth records, and then evaluated by a dysmorphologist during a follow up clinic visit occurring between 5 and 18 months of age. They ultimately identified four FAS infants out of a total of 1,022 initially in the pool (39 per

10,000 live births). The Wisconsin Fetal Alcohol Syndrome Screening Project was based in part on this design.

WISCONSIN FETAL ALCOHOL SYNDROME SCREENING PROJECT (WFASSP)

The Wisconsin Fetal Alcohol Syndrome Screening Project [67] used a prospective, multi-source, multi-stage system to identify children who met diagnostic criteria for fetal alcohol syndrome. This approach was originally used to determine the prevalence of FAS in Southeastern Wisconsin, and was an alternative approach to the multi-source, record-based ascertainment method used by the four other states funded under this CDC initiative (56). Advantages of this approach include:

- Unbiased ascertainment: Screening of a full birth cohort holds the potential for identifying children without clearly apparent risks (e.g. offspring of upper socioeconomic status women who drank during pregnancy)
- Age standardized ascertainment: Some studies indicate that the FAS facial phenotype varies throughout childhood (7;36). Evaluation within a limited age range (in this case 20-30 months) limits age-related differences in the facial phenotype
- Early screening/secondary prevention of disabilities: Screening at birth and early childhood offers the potential for earlier intervention for developmental delay and behavioral disorders. The major sources of burden from FAS are mental retardation, learning disabilities, mental health problems and disrupted school experiences. Later in life, these problems lead to a host of other difficulties including trouble with the law, confinement, inappropriate sexual behavior, and problems with drugs and alcohol. Streissguth and coworkers [7] document that early detection and intervention with children with FAS was a strong universal protective factor for all of the secondary disabilities evaluated.

The WFASSP used features of FAS diagnostic criteria developed by FASSNet that could be applied without evidence of prenatal alcohol exposure,in a staged screening process. In the first step (Screen 1) infants less than 10th percentile for gestational age and sex-adjusted birth weight [68] were selected using the electronic birth file from the Wisconsin Bureau of Health Information and Policy. Screen 2 involved abstraction of birth medical records of infants identified in Screen 1 to identify those with a birth head circumference less than gestation age specific 10th percentile [69]. Evidence of maternal alcohol use was recorded if available but was not used as a screening criterion. In screen 3, FAS facial features, postnatal growth (height, weight and head circumference) and infant development (using the Denver Developmental Screening Test II (DENVER II) [70]) were assessed at approximately 2 years of age. Exams were completed in the child's home or in an infant developmental assessment lab by teams of nurses trained by a dysmorphologist, anthropometrist and specialist certified in administering the DENVER II. Facial features were assessed using the Astley-Clarren lip-philtrum chart [39] (with scores of 4 or 5 considered a positive finding). PFL was measured using a clear plastic ruler following the method described by Hall [38]. Details of the methods are reported elsewhere [67].

Figure 2 gives the numbers of infants/children passing through each screen level. The birth cohort for the project consisted of infants born in 1998 and 1999 in 22 birth hospitals to mothers resident in an eight county Southeast Region of Wisconsin which includes urban, suburban, and rural households. Of cases eligible for participation in Screen 3, 177 (29%) agreed to be seen, and 438 (71%) were lost to follow-up. About half of those lost to follow up (n=308) could not be located, 130 (21%) parents refused, and 18 (0.3%) were excluded for other reasons (died, moved).

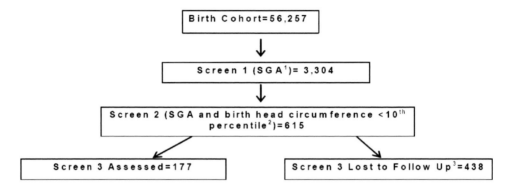

Figure 2. Flow Diagram giving numbers screened at each for the WFASSP Screens.

The 177 children evaluated in screen 3 had fewer demographic and pregnancy risk factors than those lost to follow-up and a lower rate of smoking, alcohol, and illicit drug use. Thirteen children evaluated in Screen 3 met the case criteria for FAS. Three of these children had evidence of alcohol exposure during pregnancy in the electronic birth or neonatal medical record.

GROWTH AND DEVELOPMENT CORRELATES OF SCREEN 3 EVALUATION

We were most interested in evaluating the utility of the first two screens in identifying growth and developmental problems at follow up where intervention could be instituted. We also wished to assess the degree to which the presence of FAS phenotypic features was related to developmental outcomes.

The average age of children seen for follow-up and included in the analysis was 28 months (range 21-41 months). Seven children were untestable on the DENVER II, and recumbent length could not be measured in six children due to refusal, irritability, or sleepiness at the time of testing. Inter-observer errors for anthropometric measurements were 0.12 cm for recumbent length, 0.04 kg for weight and 0.11 cm for head circumference. On average, length, weight, head circumference and weight for length z scores were reduced by 0.5 to 0.8 SD relative to reference data for normal children (between 20th and 30th percentiles). In general, the children seen in Screen 3 were similar to the full birth cohort.

About 40% of the mothers of these children were unmarried; 20% had less than a high school education. Most had received timely prenatal care.

Growth and Developmental Delays for Children Seen in Screen 3

All of the children included in the group seen for Screen 3 clinical evaluation had gestation age-specific birth weight and head circumference less than 10th percentile documented at birth, based on data collected in Screens 1 and 2. Nearly one third (31.6%) of these children had suspected delays on the DENVER II, with language and gross motor skills more frequently affected. Most (66%) had delays on more than one subscale. Almost half of the children seen for screen 3 evaluation had age and sex-specific growth less than 10th percentile. Children with suspected developmental delays were more likely to have at least one physical growth delay.

Growth and Developmental Delays for Children FAS Cardinal Facial Features

The next tables and figures document growth and developmental status of children according to whether they had none (49.2%), one (43.2%) or two or three (7.4%) of the cardinal FAS facial features (i.e. PFL less than 10th percentile, and Astley-Clarren rating of 4 or 5 for philtrum or lip) at Screen 3 follow-up (see table 4). A greater proportion of children with two or three FAS facial findings had prenatal alcohol exposure documented in birth records (about 30% versus 3-5% for the other groups). However, no differences among the groups for other risk factors for postnatal growth and development were apparent.

Table 4. Number and percentage of children seen for follow up in the WFASSP by number of FAS facial features present at Screen 3 follow up examination. WFASSP=Wisconsin Fetal Alcohol Syndrome Screening Project

Number of Facial Features	Number of children	Percent
None	87	49.2
Any one	77	43.4
Any two	6	3.4
All three	7	4.0

Children with none, one, or multiple FAS facial features all had similar z scores at birth, that is, all were relatively equally growth retarded in gestation specific length, weight and head circumference. At follow-up around two years of age, all remained smaller than average in each dimension (corrected for gestational age) (figure 3). Children with any FAS facial feature were significantly smaller and lighter with smaller head circumferences than those without FAS facial features. Nearly half of the children with any facial finding and more than

75% of those with two or three facial findings for FAS had suspected delays on the DENVERII (see figure 4).

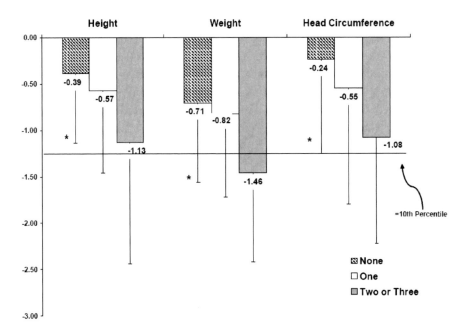

Figure 3. Average z scores for birth and follow up height/length, weight and head circumference by number of FAS facial features present at follow up in the WFASSP.

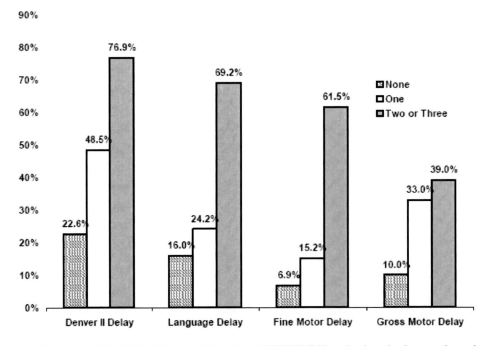

Figure 4. Percent of WFASSP children with delayed DENVERII and subscales by number of FAS facial features present at follow up in the WFASSP.

DISCUSSION

Our findings suggest that a screening program deployed near birth, with follow up in infancy or toddlerhood has the potential of identifying both children with prenatal alcohol exposure and those who will be developmental delayed regardless of etiology, thus offering the promise that early intervention can be initiated and disabilities prevented or limited. Developmental problems observed in FASD children are similar to those seen in children with other etiologies [71]. As Coles points out, children who qualify for services do so because of their specific disabilities, not because they carry an FASD diagnosis [72]. Moreover, though some interventions designed for children with FAS have been developed or are in the planning stages [73] (and http://www.cdc.gov/ncbddd/fas/intervening.htm), resources tailored to FASD specific disabilities are not widely available in most communities [72]. Studies of early intervention programs for biologically vulnerable infants have repeatedly demonstrated their success, particularly in the face of additional social/environmental risk factors [74-76]. It is notable that only a quarter of the children found to be delayed during Screen 3 assessment were enrolled in services at the time of their evaluation. Levental [74] found that the most socially and economically disadvantaged infants benefited most from early intervention services, but received the fewest services during their first five years of life. Many infants and young children with developmental delays or risk factors for poor developmental outcomes are not identified in a timely manner. When they are identified, they are often not referred to appropriate early intervention services or early childhood development programs [77]. Palfrey [78] found that of children enrolled in special education, only about 5% were identified at birth, and only 30% before the age of 5 years. Moreover, identification occurred later in children of lower socioeconomic status.

King points out that pediatric practitioners are best positioned to improve children's developmental outcomes by identifying and referring children with evidence for delays [77], and there is little negative impact of false positives on developmental assessments [79]. Early developmental monitoring of infants with the combination of features used in WFASSP study could improve referral to early intervention and reduce long-term consequences and costs of developmental delay.

The fact that children with even one FAS facial feature have suspected developmental delays and growth deficiencies at follow up indicates either prenatal alcohol exposure or disrupted embryogenesis due to some other influence. Careful evaluation by a dysmorphologist would likely identify additional phenotypic anomalies associated with another multiple minor congenital anomaly syndrome.

A Model for Early FAS Screening

This discussion illustrates the continuing challenges of FAS diagnosis and surveillance which in turn affect public health programs for its prevention and treatment. The lack of agreement about the specifics for diagnosing FASD [19,42], and the difficulties in achieving objective, unbiased, consistent ascertainment in surveillance systems limits the reliability and precision of FASD population prevalence estimates.

The greatest promise for reducing the health and social burdens of FASD is the institution of early screening programs that will assure prevention of secondary disabilities [7,49,60,61]. The WFASSP was originally conceived as a screening program fully instituted within the first months of life. The first two screen levels (i.e. identification of birth weight and head circumference less than gestational age specific 10th percentile) can be completed through a centralized flagging process within state vital records systems. Many states have systems in place to assure follow up for infants identified as high risk at birth (e.g. with a metabolic disorder, abnormal hearing screen, low birth weight, or congenital infections). Assessments specific to identification of FASD could include those used in the WFASSP Screen 3 or elements from stage 1 of one of the other screening programs described above. Developmental delays and some behavioral problems in FASD children become apparent early in life [50,80].

Follow up assessments of growth, development and phenotype could be completed by public health nurses or primary care providers with limited training. Web-based training modules and videotapes developed for the WFASSP incorporated instruction in anthropometric measurements of length and head circumference, qualitative phenotypic assessment, measurements of PFL, use of the Astley/Clarren lip/philtrum charts [39] and use of the DENVERII. Training of primary care providers has been demonstrated to be feasible. Jones and colleagues found that pediatricians can be trained to identify children with the extremes of the FASD after an intensive two day training (81). For this screening program to work, an efficient referral system to neurodevelopmental and dysmorphology evaluation would need to be in place.

Because this model would be embedded in population screening for developmental delay, cost efficiencies could be achieved in spite of the relatively high per case cost of identifying children with FASD [82]. In addition, a model that focuses on identification of infants at risk for developmental delay regardless of etiology would avoid problems relating to protection and confidentiality that inevitably accompany screening to identify and label children with FASD [71]. These problems were encountered in our project (with 40% of those located for screen 3 follow up refusing to be seen). In the Washington screening project, only about half of those screening positive in stage 1 completed the follow up exam in one of the two school districts, and there was a reduced response rate when active consent was required in the second school district [60].

Prospective screening using the data available in the birth record with periodic assessment for additional features of FASD offers an approach that is likely to yield diagnosis at the earliest possible time. It also provides the opportunity for timely intervention in anticipation of the associated developmental and physical growth sequelae or as they can be reliably identified. Using birth weight and head circumference in initial screening will assist with early identification of both FASD children and children at-risk for developmental and physical growth delays from other and unidentifiable etiologies.

In either case, early intervention is the treatment approach of choice. Multi-level screening supports the diagnostic process and improved surveillance while promoting early identification of at risk children for whom activation of appropriate services offers the possibility of improved outcomes.

ACKNOWLEDGMENTS

This study was funded in part by Centers for Disease Control and Prevention Cooperative Agreement U50/CCU514563 to the Wisconsin Center for Health Information and Policy. The authors would like to acknowledge the collaboration of Dr. Sandra Mahkorn, Mr. Randall Glysch, and Ms. Sara Zirbel on some aspects of this work. Dr. Richard Pauli and Raymond Kessel at the University of Wisconsin Madison had significant input into the design of the WFASSP, and Dr. Pauli trained the assessors and developed the training materials for providers.

REFERENCES

[1] Alcohol consumption among women who are pregnant or who might become pregnant--United States, 2002. *MMWR* 2004;53(50):1178-81.

[2] Alcohol consumption among pregnant and childbearing-aged women--United States, 1991 and 1995. *MMWR* 19972;46(16):346-50.

[3] Sociodemographic and behavioral characteristics associated with alcohol consumption during pregnancy--United States, 1988. *MMWR* 1995;44(13):261-4.

[4] Lupton C, Burd L, Harwood R. Cost of fetal alcohol spectrum disorders. *Am. J. Med. Genet.* C 2004;127(1):42-50.

[5] Armstrong EM. Diagnosing moral disorder: the discovery and evolution of fetal alcohol syndrome. *Soc. Sci. Med.* 1998;47(12):2025-42.

[6] Golden J. *Message in a Bottle: The making of fetal alcohol syndrome.* Cambridge: Harvard Univ Press, 2005.

[7] Streissguth AP, Bookstein FL, Barr HM, Sampson PD, O'Malley KD, Young JK. Risk factors for adverse life outcomes in fetal alcohol syndrome and fetal alcohol effects. *J. Dev. Behav. Pediatr.* 2004;25(4):228-38.

[8] Jones KL, Smith DW, Ulleland CN, Streissguth P. Pattern of malformation in offspring of chronic alcoholic mothers. *Lancet* 1973;1(7815):1267-71.

[9] Jones KL, Smith DW. Recognition of the fetal alcohol syndrome in early infancy. *Lancet* 1973;2(7836):999-1001.

[10] Ulleland CN. The offspring of alcoholic mothers. *Ann. NY Acad. Sci.* 1972;197:167-9.

[11] Lemoine P, Harousseau H, Borteyru JP, Menuet JC. Children of alcoholic parents--observed anomalies: discussion of 127 cases. *Ouest. Med.* 1968;8:476-82.

[12] Smith DW. The fetal alcohol syndrome. *Hosp. Pract.* 1979;14(10):121-8.

[13] Mulvihill JJ, Klimas JT, Stokes DC, Risemberg HM. Fetal alcohol syndrome: seven new cases. *Am. J. Obstet. Gynecol.* 1976;125(7):937-41.

[14] Hanson JW, Jones KL, Smith DW. Fetal alcohol syndrome. Experience with 41 patients. *JAMA* 1976;235(14):1458-60.

[15] Adnams CM, Kodituwakku PW, Hay A, Molteno CD, Viljoen D, May PA. Patterns of cognitive-motor development in children with fetal alcohol syndrome from a community in South Africa. *Alcohol Clin. Exp. Res.* 2001;25(4):557-62.

[16] Carter RC, Jacobson SW, Molteno CD, Chiodo LM, Viljoen D, Jacobson JL. Effects of prenatal alcohol exposure on infant visual acuity. *J. Pediatr.* 2005;147(4):473-9.

[17] Coles CD, Platzman KA, Raskind-Hood CL, Brown RT, Falek A, Smith IE. A comparison of children affected by prenatal alcohol exposure and attention deficit, hyperactivity disorder. *Alcohol Clin. Exp. Res.* 1997;21(1):150-61.

[18] Willford J, Leech S, Day N. Moderate prenatal alcohol exposure and cognitive status of children at age 10. *Alcohol Clin. Exp. Res.* 2006;30(6):1051-9.

[19] Hoyme HE, May PA, Kalberg WO, Kodituwakku P, Gossage JP, Trujillo PM, et al. A practical clinical approach to diagnosis of fetal alcohol spectrum disorders: Clarification of the 1996 institute of medicine criteria. *Pediatrics* 2005;115(1):39-47.

[20] Chudley AE, Conry J, Cook JL, Loock C, Rosales T, LeBlanc N. Fetal alcohol spectrum disorder: Canadian guidelines for diagnosis. *CMAJ* 2005;172(5 Suppl):S1-S21.

[21] Hall BD. Photographic analysis: a quantitative approach to the evaluation of dysmorphology. *J. Pediatr.* 1996;129(1):3-4.

[22] Mattson SN, Riley EP. A review of the neurobehavioral deficits in children with fetal alcohol syndrome or prenatal exposure to alcohol. *Alcohol Clin. Exp. Res.* 1998;22(2):279-94.

[23] Mattson SN, Riley EP, Delis DC, Stern C, Jones KL. Verbal learning and memory in children with fetal alcohol syndrome. *Alcohol Clin. Exp. Res.* 1996;20(5):810-6.

[24] Mattson SN, Riley EP. Implicit and explicit memory functioning in children with heavy prenatal alcohol exposure. *J. Int. Neuropsych. Soc.* 1999;5(5):462-71.

[25] Schonfeld AM, Mattson SN, Lang AR, Delis DC, Riley EP. Verbal and nonverbal fluency in children with heavy prenatal alcohol exposure. *J. Stud. Alcohol* 2001;62(2):239-46.

[26] Thomas SE, Kelly SJ, Mattson SN, Riley EP. Comparison of social abilities of children with fetal alcohol syndrome to those of children with similar IQ scores and normal controls. *Alcohol Clin. Exp. Res.* 1998;22(2):528-33.

[27] Abel EL. An update on incidence of FAS: FAS is not an equal opportunity birth defect. *Neurotoxicol. Teratol.* 1995;17(4):437-43.

[28] Institute of Medicine. Fetal alcohol syndrome: Diagnosis, epidemiology, prevention, and treatment. Washington, DC: Nat Acad Press, 1996.

[29] Astley SJ, Clarren SK. Measuring the facial phenotype of individuals with prenatal alcohol exposure: correlations with brain dysfunction. *Alcohol Alcoholism* 2001;36(2):147-59.

[30] Streissguth AP, Aase JM, Clarren SK, Randels SP, LaDue RA, Smith DF. Fetal alcohol syndrome in adolescents and adults. *JAMA* 1991;265(15):1961-7.

[31] Bertrand J, Floyd LL, Weber MK. Guidelines for identifying and referring persons with fetal alcohol syndrome. *MMWR Recomm. Rep* 2005;54(RR-11):1-14.

[32] Gatford KL, Dalitz PA, Cock ML, Harding R, Owens JA. Acute ethanol exposure in pregnancy alters the insulin-like growth factor axis of fetal and maternal sheep. *American Journal of Physiology - Endocrinol Metab* 2007;292(2):E494-E500.

[33] Astley SJ, Stachowiak J, Clarren SK, Clausen C. Application of the fetal alcohol syndrome facial photographic screening tool in a foster care population. *J. Pediatr.* 2002;141(5):712-7.

[34] Armant DR, Saunders DE. Exposure of embryonic cells to alcohol: contrasting effects during preimplantation and postimplantation development. [Review] [115 refs]. *Semin Perinat* 1996;20(2):127-39.

[35] Nagahara AH, Handa RJ. Fetal alcohol exposure alters the induction of immediate early gene mRNA in the rat prefrontal cortex after an alternation task. *Alcohol Clin. Exp. Res.* 1995;19(6):1389-97.

[36] Aase JM, Jones KL, Clarren SK. Do we need the term "FAE"? *Pediatrics* 1995;95(3):428-30.

[37] Astley SJ, Clarren SK. Diagnosing the full spectrum of fetal alcohol-exposed individuals: introducing the 4-digit diagnostic code. *Alcohol Alcoholism* 2000;35(4):400-10.

[38] Hall JG, Froster-Iskenius UG, Allanson JE. *Handbook of normal physical measurements.* New York: Oxford Univ Press, 1989.

[39] Astley SJ. *Diagnostic guidelines for fetal alcohol spectrum disorders: The 4-Digit diagnostic code*, 3rd ed. Seattle: Univ Washington, 2004.

[40] Manning MA, Eugene HH. Fetal alcohol spectrum disorders: a practical clinical approach to diagnosis. *Neurosci. Biobehav. Rev.* 2007;31(2):230-8.

[41] Autti-Ramo I, Fagerlund A, Ervalahti N, Loimu L, Korkman M, Hoyme HE. Fetal alcohol spectrum disorders in Finland: clinical delineation of 77 older children and adolescents. *Am. J. Med. Genet A* 2006;140(2):137-43.

[42] Astley SJ. Comparison of the 4-digit diagnostic code and the Hoyme diagnostic guidelines for fetal alcohol spectrum disorders. *Pediatrics* 2006;118(4):1532-45.

[43] Astley SJ, Clarren SK. A case definition and photographic screening tool for the facial phenotype of fetal alcohol syndrome. *J. Pediatr.* 1996;129(1):33-41.

[44] Vitez M, Koranyi G, Gonczy E, Rudas T, Czeizel A. A semiquantitative score system for epidemiologic studies of fetal alcohol syndrome. *Am. J. Epidemiol.* 1984;119(3):301-8.

[45] Vitez M. Facial effects of fetal alcohol exposure: assessment by photographs and morphometric analysis. *Am. J. Med. Genet* 1987;28(4):1017-8.

[46] Moore ES, Ward RE, Jamison PL, Morris CA, Bader PI, Hall BD. The subtle facial signs of prenatal exposure to alcohol: An anthropometric approach. *J. Pediatr.* 2001;139(2):215-9.

[47] Moore ES, Ward RE, Jamison PL, Morris CA, Bader PI, Hall BD. New perspectives on the face in fetal alcohol syndrome: What anthropometry tells us. *Am. J. Med. Genet* 2002;109(4):249-60.

[48] Fetal alcohol syndrome--United States, 1979-1992. *MMWR* 1993;42(17):339-41.

[49] Ernhart CB, Greene T, Sokol RJ, Martier S, Boyd TA, Ager J. Neonatal diagnosis of fetal alcohol syndrome: not necessarily a hopeless prognosis. *Alcohol Clin. Exp. Res.* 1995;19(6):1550-7.

[50] Coles CD, Kable JA, Drews-Botsch C, Falek A. Early identification of risk for effects of prenatal alcohol exposure. *J. Stud. Alcohol.* 2000;61(4):607-16.

[51] Birth defects surveillance data from selected states, 1999-2003. *Birth Defects Res. A Clin. Mol. Teratol.* 2006;76(12):894-960.

[52] Fox DJ, Druschel CM. Estimating prevalence of fetal alcohol syndrome (FAS): effectiveness of a passive birth defects registry system. *Birth Defects Res. A Clin. Mol. Teratol.* 2003;67(9):604-8.

[53] Egeland GM, Perham-Hester KA, Gessner BD, Ingle D, Berner JE, Middaugh JP. Fetal alcohol syndrome in Alaska, 1977 through 1992: an administrative prevalence derived from multiple data sources. *Am. J. Public Health* 1998;88(5):781-6.

[54] Linking multiple data sources in fetal alcohol syndrome surveillance--Alaska. *MMWR* 1993;42(16):312-4.

[55] Miller LA, Shaikh T, Stanton C, Montgomery A, Rickard R, Keefer S, et al. Surveillance for fetal alcohol syndrome in Colorado. *Pub. Health Rep.* 1995;110(6):690-7.

[56] Fetal alcohol syndrome--Alaska, Arizona, Colorado, and New York, 1995-1997. *MMWR* 2002;51(20):433-5.

[57] Surveillance for fetal alcohol syndrome using multiple sources -- Atlanta, Georgia, 1981-1989. *MMWR* 1997;46(47):1118-20.

[58] Burd L, Klug MG, Martsolf JT, Martsolf C, Deal E, Kerbeshian J. A staged screening strategy for prenatal alcohol exposure and maternal risk stratification. *J. R. Soc. Health* 2006;126(2):86-94.

[59] Floyd RL, O'Connor MJ, Bertrand J, Sokol R. Reducing adverse outcomes from prenatal alcohol exposure: a clinical plan of action. *Alcohol Clin. Exp. Res.* 2006;30(8):1271-5.

[60] Clarren SK, Randels SP, Sanderson M, Fineman RM. Screening for fetal alcohol syndrome in primary schools: a feasibility study. *Teratology* 2001;63(1):3-10.

[61] Burd L, Cox C, Wentz M, Ebertowski J, Martsolf JT, Kerbeshian J, et al. The FAS screen: a rapid screening tool for fetal alcohol syndrome. *Addict. Biol.* 1999;4:329-36.

[62] Poitra BA, Marion S, Dionne M, Wilkie E, Dauphinais P, Wilkie-Pepion M, et al. A school-based screening program for fetal alcohol syndrome. *Neurotoxicol. Teratol.* 2003;25(6):725-9.

[63] Burd L, Olson M, Juelson T. A strategy for community-based screening for fetal alcohol syndrome. In: Tremblay RE, Barr RG, Peters RDeV, editors. *Encyclopedia on Early Childhood Development* [online] .Montreal, Quebec: Centre Excellence Early Childhood Dev, 2003:1-7.

[64] May PA, Brooke L, Gossage JP, Croxford J, Adnams C, Jones KL, et al. Epidemiology of fetal alcohol syndrome in a South African community in the Western Cape Province. *Am. J. Public Health* 2000;90(12):1905-12.

[65] Fetal alcohol syndrome--South Africa, 2001. *MMWR* 2003;52(28):660-2.

[66] Duimstra C, Johnson D, Kutsch C, Wang B, Zentner M, Kellerman S, et al. A fetal alcohol syndrome surveillance pilot project in American Indian communities in the Northern Plains. *Pub Health Rep.* 1993;108(2):225-9.

[67] Weiss M, Cronk CE, Mahkorn S, Glysch R, Zirbel S. The Wisconsin Fetal Alcohol Syndrome Screening Project. *WMJ* 2004;103(5):53-60.

[68] Alexander GR, Kogan MD, Himes JH. 1994-1996 U.S. singleton birth weight percentiles for gestational age by race, Hispanic origin, and gender. *Mat. Child Health J.* 1999;3(4):225-31.

[69] Lubchenco LO, Hansman C, Boyd E. Intrauterine growth in length and head circumference as estimated from live births at gestational ages from 26 to 42 weeks. *Pediatrics* 1966;37(3):403-8.

[70] Frankenburg WK, Dodds J, Archer P, Shapiro H, Bresnick B. The Denver II: a major revision and restandardization of the Denver Developmental Screening Test. *Pediatrics* 1992;89(1):91-7.

[71] Smith IE. FAE/FAS: Prevention, intervention and support services. Commentary on Burd and Juelson, Coles, and O'Malley and Streissgut. In: Tremblay RE, Barr RG,

Peters RDeV, eds. Encyclopedia on Early Childhood Development [online] .Montreal, Quebec: Montreal, Quebec: *Centre Excellence Early Childhood Dev*, 2003:1-8.

[72] Coles C. Individuals affected by Fetal Alcohol Spectrum Disorder (FASD) and their families : Prevention, intervention and support. In: Tremblay RE, Barr RG, Peters RDeV, eds. Encyclopedia on Early Childhood Development [online]. Montreal, Quebec: *Centre Excellence Early Childhood Dev*, 2003:1-5.

[73] Kalberg WO, Provost B, Tollison SJ, Tabachnick BG, Robinson LK, Eugene HH, et al. Comparison of motor delays in young children with fetal alcohol syndrome to those with prenatal alcohol exposure and with no prenatal alcohol exposure. *Alcohol Clin. Exp. Res*. 2006;30(12):2037-45.

[74] Leventhal T, Brooks-Gunn J, McCormick MC, McCarton CM. Patterns of service use in preschool children: correlates, consequences, and the role of early intervention. *Child Dev*. 2000;71(3):802-19.

[75] Berlin LJ, Brooks-Gunn J, McCarton C, McCormick MC. The effectiveness of early intervention: examining risk factors and pathways to enhanced development. *Prev. Med*. 1998;27(2):238-45.

[76] Hill JL, Brooks-Gunn J, Waldfogel J. Sustained effects of high participation in an early intervention for low-birth-weight premature infants. *Dev. Psychol*. 2003;39(4):730-44.

[77] King TM, Glascoe FP. Developmental surveillance of infants and young children in pediatric primary care. *Curr. Opin. Pediatr*. 2003;15(6):624-9.

[78] Palfrey JS FAU, Singer JD FAU, Walker DK FAU, Butler JA. Early identification of children's special needs: a study in five metropolitan communities. *J. Pediatr*. 1987;111(5):651-9.

[79] Glascoe FP. Are overreferrals on developmental screening tests really a problem? *Arch. Pediatr. Adolesc. Med*. 2001;155(1):54-9.

[80] Van Der LM, Van DK, Kleinhout M, Phaff J, De Groot CJ, De GL, et al. Infants exposed to alcohol prenatally: outcome at 3 and 7 months of age. *Ann. Trop. Paediatr* 2001;21(2):127-34.

[81] Jones KL, Robinson LK, Bakhireva LN, Marintcheva G, Storojev V, Strahova A, et al. Accuracy of the diagnosis of physical features of fetal alcohol syndrome by pediatricians after specialized training. *Pediatrics* 2006;118(6):e1734-e1738.

[82] Riley EP. FAE/FAS: Prevention, intervention and support services. Commentary on Burd and Juelson, Coles, and O'Malley and Streissguth. In: Tremblay RE, Barr RG, Peters RDeV, eds. Encyclopedia on Early Childhood Development [online] Montreal, Quebec: *Centre Excellence Early Childhood Dev.*, 2003:1-7.

In: Alcohol-Related Cognitive Disorders
Editors: L. Sher, I. Kandel, J. Merrick pp. 91-110

ISBN: 978-1-60741-730-9
© 2009 Nova Science Publishers, Inc.

Chapter 5

PRENATAL EXPOSURE TO ALCOHOL: LONG-TERM IMPAIRMENTS

Christie L. McGee and Edward P. Riley

ABSTRACT

Prenatal exposure to alcohol can lead to long-term impairments in cognition and behavior and represents a major public health concern. This chapter reviews studies examining the social and behavioral functioning of individuals with prenatal alcohol exposure. Social and behavioral functioning are important domains for study because deficits in these areas can lead to problems in everyday functioning and to maladjustment in later life. Most research with individuals with prenatal alcohol exposure has used caregiver or self-report questionnaires or semi-structured interviews to sample behavior. The vast majority of studies indicate significant difficulties with interpersonal functioning, internalizing and externalizing behavior problems, and high rates of psychopathology. Recent intervention studies conducted with individuals with prenatal alcohol exposure have shown promising results in improving the social skills and behavioral functioning in this population. Finally, this chapter concludes with recommendations for future studies in this area.

INTRODUCTION

Prenatal exposure to alcohol can result in long-term impairments in cognition and behavior. One consequence of prenatal alcohol exposure is the fetal alcohol syndrome (FAS), diagnosed by a constellation of symptoms, including specific dysmorphic facial features (i.e., smooth philtrum, thin upper vermillion, small palpebral fissures), growth retardation, and central nervous system dysfunction [1]. Fetal alcohol syndrome is a major public health concern with an estimated prevalence of 0.5 to 2.0 cases per 1000 live births [2] and an average annual cost of $3.6 billion in the United States [3].

However, FAS represents only a fraction of the problem. The effects of prenatal exposure to alcohol vary widely from FAS on the severe end of the spectrum to subtle physical, cognitive, or behavioral effects. The reasons for this disparity of outcome are not entirely understood, but they probably relate to the dose or the timing of exposure or to other maternal/fetal considerations. When the larger spectrum is considered, prevalence estimates are as high as 1 in 100 live births [4]. In addition, research has demonstrated that prenatal alcohol exposure can produce similar patterns of neurobehavioral dysfunction with or without the physical anomalies required for clinical recognition of FAS [5]. Children with histories of prenatal alcohol exposure tend to have reduced intelligence with IQ estimates averaging in the low 70s to the low 80s, although individual scores vary widely. In addition, impairments have been found in numerous cognitive domains including attention, language, visual-spatial skills, learning and memory, motor functioning, and executive skills. The pattern of performance across domains may be consistent with a generalized deficit in complex information processing (for a review see [6]).

As detailed in this review, individuals with a history of prenatal alcohol exposure have considerable difficulty interacting in social situations and regulating their behavior. Difficulties in these areas are likely due to a complex interplay of a variety of factors, including genetics, alcohol's teratogenic effects on brain development and cognition, early childhood social experiences, and social learning throughout the lifespan [7]. Some children with prenatal alcohol exposure also experience early chaotic living environments, which may limit their access to effective parenting and behavioral models. Social and behavioral functioning are important areas to study as they have implications for an individual's everyday functioning and ability to adapt to new situations. Difficulties in these areas can result in further problems and maladjustment later in life [8].

METHODOLOGICAL CONCERNS

Before reviewing the research on social and behavioral functioning in individuals with prenatal alcohol exposure, it is important to consider several methodological issues such as diagnostic terminology, subject recruitment, and behavioral sampling techniques.

While the diagnostic criteria for FAS have remained relatively consistent over the last 35 years, a number of diagnostic and non-diagnostic labels have been used with individuals having a history of prenatal alcohol exposure, particularly those who do not meet criteria for FAS (e.g., fetal alcohol effects (FAE), alcohol-related neurodevelopmental disorder (ARND), partial FAS (pFAS), alcohol-related birth defects (ARBD), prenatal exposure to alcohol (PEA), and fetal alcohol spectrum disorders (FASD)). The criteria used in applying these labels differ considerably and vary in their requirements for quantity and documentation of alcohol exposure. It is important to understand, for example, that a sample of children labeled as FAE may differ from children classified with ARND. Understanding this heterogeneity across studies is useful in resolving the discrepancies in findings and drawing inferences to the larger population. For consistency and parsimony, children will be referred to as having prenatal alcohol exposure (PAE) in this review, and diagnostic differences will be discussed when relevant.

Recruitment methodology is another important consideration when reviewing the PAE literature, as the nature of the sample and types of questions answered differ. In prospective designs, the subjects are identified before the outcome of interest occurs, and are often followed longitudinally. Typically, prospective recruitment entails screening pregnant women to identify those likely to give birth to offspring exposed to alcohol, or identifying exposed infants at the time of birth (or shortly thereafter). Such studies often represent population-based research, and the exposures are mostly at moderate or "social drinking" levels. In contrast, retrospective recruitment involves identifying subjects at some time after the alcohol exposure occurred. Such samples frequently contain a large number of "clinically referred subjects" who come to the study because of some clinically significant manifestation of PAE. Exposure levels tend to be heavier in retrospective studies.

Each ascertainment method has its advantages and disadvantages and implications for conclusions and generalizability. One advantage of prospective studies is that exposure measurement tends to be more accurate, and multiple dimensions of prenatal exposure are often assessed [9]. In addition, such designs offer greater control for confounding factors because environmental and demographic information can be collected more accurately at or near the time of exposure. Because of the more precise measurement and range of PAE, prospective designs allow for the investigation of dose-response relations, which represents a fundamental hypothesis in behavioral teratology. Longitudinal prospective designs also permit conclusions to be drawn regarding changes in outcome over time. The disadvantages of prospective designs include the expense and time it takes to conduct such studies, the small number of heavily exposed individuals often sampled, and the large number of subjects that must be recruited to detect effects related to PAE. In addition, the clinical signifi-cance of small effect sizes must be considered.

To detect adverse outcomes, oversampling individuals who have experienced high levels of exposure is frequently necessary; failure to do so can lead to inaccurate conclusions regarding the teratogenic capacity of an agent [10]. Retrospective studies generally involve comparing groups of heavily exposed individuals and non-exposed controls rather than treating alcohol as a continuous variable. The advantages of this methodology include reduced overall sample size required to detect effects, reduced time and cost to conduct the study, the ability to include distinct control or comparison groups, and increased sampling of more severe cases. Larger effect sizes and therefore clinically significant group differences are possible with this design. Such problems as subject attrition and instrument revisions rarely affect retrospective studies because most studies are cross-sectional in design. Whereas detecting effects with retrospective designs is often easier, there are disadvantages. One problem is reporting bias; patient reports of past behavior are often inaccurate. As antenatal reporting of alcohol consumption is more accurate than retrospective recall [11], the reliability of maternal alcohol consumption measures poses a major difficulty to retrospective studies. When children with a diagnosis of FAS are evaluated, the problem of reporting bias is largely circumvented because the characteristic facial features are indicative of such exposure. However, when children with PAE without FAS are included in the sample, there is more reliance on alcohol history. Retrospective studies also face ascertainment bias. Subjects are often recruited from specialty clinics or are referred to the study rather than by random selection, and thus are likely to have more problems than do non-referred clients.

The difference between prospective and retrospecttive designs is especially pertinent in the area of social and behavioral functioning. Children identified retrospectively are likely to be brought to the attention of clinicians and researchers if they have significant behavioral problems interfering with their everyday functioning, whereas prospective designs sample more widely, but may have less severely affected children. Thus, both designs are important and complement each other in improving our understanding of the difficulties faced in individuals with PAE.

Finally, the ways in which behavior is sampled can have a significant impact on the conclusions drawn and inferences made to the larger population. A range of assessment techniques can be used to sample behavior, including naturalistic observation, laboratory analog experiments, structured and semi-structured interviews, and self- or other-report questionnaires. Each technique has its advantages and limitations. Naturalistic observation involves observing individuals in their everyday environment and describing their behavior qualitatively and quantitatively. This approach involves the least intrusion, representing the most ecologically valid assessment and reducing reporting bias. However, naturalistic observation is subject to reactivity (behavioral change due to being observed) and observer bias and is limited in the quantity and range of behaviors likely to be displayed by the observed individual [12]. This method requires a significant time commitment and does not often capture behavioral variability that is due to environmental differences (e.g., time, situation).

Analog laboratory experiments provide the researcher with more control over the types of situations observed and the likely behaviors to be elicited. This approach is especially useful as situations can be manipulated to determine if environmental changes result in different behavioral manifestations. However, such manipulations, as well as the laboratory setting, may limit ecological validity. Similar to naturalistic observation, analog studies are limited in the range and variability of behavior to be sampled and caution must be exercised in generalizing behavior observed at one time point to a greater representation of the individual's behavioral style.

Interviews and questionnaires provide an opportunity to measure behavior across a wide range of domains and to assess an individual's general pattern of behavioral functioning, rather than relying on observation in a specific situation at a specific time. Interviews and questionnaires can be completed with the individual or an informant, generally a caregiver or teacher. Although reports of behavior collected through interview or questionnaire tend to be more general, they are also susceptible to reporting bias, and reports from multiple informants may not be concordant. In comparison with naturalistic and analog studies, the psychometric properties of questionnaires and structured interviews are better studied and standardized scores are often available. Furthermore, most questionnaires and interviews are fairly straightforward and require less time to complete and fewer resources. One benefit of semi-structured interviews over questionnaires is that researchers can probe subjects to obtain more information when the initial response is unclear or insufficient. However, some subjects may be more comfortable in endorsing sensitive topics and problematic behavior in a pencil and paper format than in discussing these issues with an interviewer. All these advantages and limitations must be weighed when evaluating studies investigating social and behavioral functioning, and multiple methods of sampling behavior may be necessary to describe and answer pertinent questions in these domains.

This review begins by focusing on adaptive and social functioning in individuals with PAE. Next, studies utilizing general scales of behavioral and emotional functioning will be discussed, followed by research examining rates and types of psychopathology seen in individuals with PAE. Studies looking at predictors and possible mechanisms in specific areas of behavioral and emotional functioning, such as depression, delinquency, substance use, quality of life, and caregiver stress will be reviewed. Finally, several recent empirically studied psychosocial and pharmacological interventions will be discussed.

ADAPTIVE AND SOCIAL FUNCTIONING

Adaptive functioning refers to an individual's ability to meet developmental expectations of personal independence and social responsibility [13]. Such behaviors are essential for functioning effectively and for adapting to environmental change. Adaptive functioning is commonly assessed though the Vineland Adaptive Behavior Scales (VABS [13]), a semi-structured interview completed by a caregiver or other informant. The VABS consists of four scales: communication, daily living skills, socialization, and motor skills. Retrospective studies have identified consistent deficits in adaptive functioning in individuals with PAE. Specifically, one study found a mean level of adaptive functioning of seven years in a sample of 61 adolescents and adults with PAE (mean chronological age 17 years) who were not mentally retarded [14]. The highest scores were in daily living skills (age equivalent of 9 years) and the lowest scores in socialization (age equivalent of 6 years). No individual met age expectations in the areas of communication or socialization. Studies with children have identified similar deficits in adaptive functioning and have found socialization to be the most impaired domain. Specifically, socialization scores decrease with age, suggesting that as expectations increase as children get older, children with PAE have more difficulty meeting these standards [15-16]. Children with PAE show this relation, even when compared with other clinically referred children without alcohol exposure, suggesting that age-related social impairments are above and beyond what would be expected based on the presence of problems requiring clinical intervention [16].

The relation between socialization scores on the VABS and IQ has also been examined [15]. Children with FAS had significantly lower socialization scores than an IQ-matched control group, indicating that deficits in social skills were beyond those expected based on lower intellectual functioning. This relation was examined within the three subscales of the socialization domain. Interpersonal functioning was specifically impaired in children with FAS relative to IQ-matched controls, whereas the two groups did not differ on the coping and play/leisure subscales. Data from a case study of two participants have suggested that adolescents with PAE may have problems interpersonally due to an increased difficulty of providing sufficient information to communicative partners [17]. In addition, one study [18] found that impaired executive functioning correlates with poorer social skills and increased maladaptive behaviors in children with PAE.

Whereas retrospective studies have consistently found impairments in adaptive functioning, especially in the social domain, one study of prospectively identified children found no significant differences with respect to level of alcohol exposure on the VABS at age 6, with all scores falling within the average range [19]. Besides the differences due to ascertainment (e.g., lower exposures, fewer children with FAS) and the nature of the population sampled (e.g., both exposed and control children were African American and from predominately low SES homes), one additional explanation for this discrepancy may be the young age of the children studied. As discussed above, retrospectively identified children with PAE show increased deficits in social functioning at older ages. Thus, children in the prospective study may have had fewer problems than did the older children in the retrospective studies due to their ability to meet the lower expectations at their age. Further studies using prospectively identified adolescents and young adults are needed to understand better the adaptive abilities of individuals with PAE.

In summary, retrospective studies have found consistent impairments in adaptive functioning in individuals with PAE, with specific deficits in interpersonal functioning that become more pronounced with higher age-related expectations. Such deficits persist into adulthood and often result in difficulty getting along with others, difficulty making or keeping friends, and feelings of isolation and loneliness [20]. Research with children identified prospectively has not found impaired adaptive functioning, but age, the nature of the population sampled, and the level of exposure may account for the discrepancy. The findings of impaired social functioning in humans are consistent with the results of animal studies—for a review see [7]. Studies using animal models provide a more powerful indication that the deficits observed are initiated by the alcohol insult rather than abnormal environments. In addition, many of the structures suggested to be involved in social cognition such as the amygdala, prefrontal cortex, hippocampus, hypothalamus, ventral striatum, and parietal regions [21] have been found to be disrupted by prenatal alcohol exposure [22, 23].

BEHAVIORAL FUNCTIONING

General Behavior and Emotion Rating Scales

As children display a wide range of behavior that varies by situation, the predominant method of behavioral sampling is through questionnaires and standardized interviews completed by a caregiver or other informant, such as the child's teacher. The most common measure of behavioral functioning in children and adolescents is the Child Behavior Checklist [CBCL [24]], which asks parents to rate the frequency of specific problem behaviors and provides standardized scores in a range of problem areas. An analogous version, the Teacher Report Form [TRF [25]], completed by the child's teacher, is also available. Retrospectively identified children with PAE are generally rated by their caregivers and teachers as having significant behavioral problems as measured by the CBCL or TRF [26-27]. When compared with non-exposed children matched on IQ, children with heavy levels of exposure had significantly higher externalizing and total problem scores on the CBCL [26]. On the individual problem scales, alcohol-exposed children were rated as having more difficulty than their IQ-matched peers on the social, thought, attention, aggression, and delinquency problem scales. The mean scores for the PAE group were clinically elevated on the attention, aggression, and social problem scales, indicating significant problems in these areas. These findings are consistent with results from retrospectively identified children with PAE followed longitudinally in Berlin [27]. Scores from both the CBCL and TRF in this sample showed pronounced, clinically significant peaks for the attention and social problems scales that were consistent over time. At a 20-year follow-up of this cohort [28], young adults had elevated scores on the thought disorder, attention problems, intrusive behavior, and aggressive behavior scales of the Young Adult Behavior Checklist completed by a caregiver or relative. The results demonstrate that for individuals with PAE, behavior problems are significant and persistent across the lifespan.

Prospective studies have also found alcohol-related behavior problems in children and adolescents with PAE, but the results have been less consistent. A large prospective study [29] examined the behavioral func-tioning of over 450 adolescents at age 14 and found a significant dose-response relation between alcohol exposure and behavioral problems measured by the CBCL and interviews with the adolescent and caregiver. A binge pattern of drinking related more strongly to behavior problems than did a steady drinking pattern, and the most salient behavioral variables included the CBCL delinquency scale and related antisocial behavior problems.

A study with younger children also found a dose-response relation between alcohol and behavior problems at ages 6 to 7, with the effect being observed at average alcohol levels as low as one drink per week for some behaviors [30]. Children with both low and moderate/heavy exposures differed significantly from controls on ratings of aggressive behavior and externalizing problems, whereas the moderate/heavy group had significantly higher scores on the delinquency and total problems scales. A large number of potential covariates were also examined, and PAE remained a significant predictor of child behavior problems after controlling for exposure to other substances, maternal variables, child age and gender, family structure and socioeconomic status, and continued alcohol and drug use in the home. Whereas PEA remained significant, maternal psycho-pathology accounted for a significant amount of variance in child behavior, and boys tended to display more externalizing behavior and attention problems than girls.

One prospective study, however, found mixed results, with discrepant ratings between teachers and caregivers [31]. Teachers rated children whose mothers drank throughout pregnancy as having more problems and less social competence than did children of mothers who did not drink or stopped drinking during the second trimester of pregnancy. In contrast, all mothers, regardless of drinking history, rated their children similarly. Possible explanations for this discrepancy include lower caregiver expectations, maternal psychopathology, or situational specificity of behavioral problems.

Children with PAE have also been compared to children with Attention Deficit/Hyperactivity Disorder (ADHD) using the CBCL, as a number of symptoms overlap between these groups. Many alcohol-exposed individuals meet the criteria for ADHD, although several studies have identified different cognitive patterns between the two groups (e.g., 32). Still unclear, however, is whether children with PAE differ from children with ADHD on the CBCL. One study found that whereas both groups were impaired relative to typically developing controls, no differences existed between children with ADHD and children with PAE [33]. In contrast, another study [32] found that children with ADHD were rated as having more problems on the CBCL than both children with PAE and non-exposed controls, who did not differ from one another. However, when children with FAS were considered apart from the other alcohol-exposed children, they had significantly higher scores than did the alcohol-exposed children without FAS and controls, but had lower scores than the ADHD group. One methodological difference between these studies is that one involved a retrospective design, whereas the other was prospective. Clinically identified children with PAE had similar levels of behavior problems on the CBCL as did children with ADHD, whereas prospectively identified children with lower levels of exposure had fewer problems than did children with ADHD.

Although studies examining group differences between children with PAE and those with ADHD on the CBCL have yielded mixed results, one study identified sets of items from the CBCL that distinguish children with PAE from those with ADHD and typically developing controls [34]. Seven items distinguished children with PAE from typically developing controls (acts young, restless or hyperactive, impulsive, can't concentrate, lying or cheating, lack of guilt, and disobedience), while two sets of items were able to distinguish between children with PAE and those with ADHD (no guilt, cruelty, and acts young OR acts young, cruelty, no guilt, lying or cheating, steals from home, and steals outside of the home). The authors suggest the utility of combining these items as a clinical screening tool for identifying potential cases of PAE or ADHD for further evaluation.

In addition to the CBCL and TRF, researchers have also examined caregiver ratings on several other measures. In one study [35], alcohol-exposed children were rated as having higher levels of anxiety, autistic behaviors, communication disturbances, disruptive and antisocial behavior, and more self-absorbed behavior than controls. Disruptive behavior problems were rated the highest of all problems and tended to increase with age. Another study [36] compared children with PAE with typically developing controls on the Personality Inventory for Children (PIC). Alcohol-exposed children had more problems than controls on all scales, and scores were in the clinical range on achievement, intellectual screening, development, delinquency, and psychosis. The most marked differences were on the delinquency and intellectual scales.

Maladaptive behavior problems appear to persist into older adolescence and adulthood. One study found that 62% of a sample of adolescents and adults with PAE had significant behavior problems, including poor concentration and attention, dependency, stubbornness, social withdrawal, teasing or bullying, crying or laughing too easily, impulsivity, anxiety, and antisocial behavior [14]. In summary, the findings from general behavioral and emotional rating scales have identified significant problems associated with PAE, regardless of ascertainment method. The most significant and consistent difficulties appear in the areas of attention, disruptive and delinquent behavior, and social problems. Poor behavioral regulation may be partially related to alcohol-induced dysregulation of the limbic-hypo-thalamic-pituitary-adrenocortical (LHPA) axis, which is involved in the stress response [37]. Further research comparing behavioral profiles of children with PAE and other diagnostic groups would be beneficial.

Psychopathology

In addition to parent report questionnaires of behavioral and emotional functioning, a number of studies have used semi-structured and structured interviews to assess the prevalence of psychopathology in individuals with PAE. Most studies report high rates of psychiatric diagnoses across the age range and co-morbidity is common. In a large study [20] of alcohol-exposed individuals (n = 415) between the ages of 6 and 51, 94% of the sample had experienced at least one mental health problem and 23% had been hospitalized in an inpatient psychiatric facility for treatment. Additional studies with children have found similar rates of psychopathology ranging from 87% to 97% of the alcohol-exposed sample meeting criteria for at least one psychiatric disorder [38-39]. ADHD appears to be one of the most prevalent disorders among children with PAE, and the rates of mood disorders and other disruptive behavior disorders are relatively high in comparison with rates in the general population. Two studies found that children with PAE had a higher likelihood than controls of meeting the criteria for more than one Axis 1 disorder, with 62% to 71% of children meeting the criteria for two or more co-morbid disorders [38-39].

One longitudinal retrospective investigation examined the persistence of behavior associated with psychopathology in individuals with FAS [27-28]. The rate of many maladaptive behaviors, including hyper-activity, inattention, stereotypies, sleeping problems, tics, head and body rocking, peer relationship difficulties, and phobic behaviors was increased. Moreover, an index of psychopathological behavior, created from the sum of symptom scores, correlated with FAS severity. Follow-up studies demonstrated the persistence of psychopathological symptoms from preschool through adolescence. Specifically, hyperactivity was persistent across the age range and was the most prevalent symptom reported. Emotional disorders, sleep problems, and abnormal habits and stereotypies also persisted, especially in school-age children.

More age-specific problems such as enuresis, encopresis, and eating problems remitted over time, whereas conduct disorders remained consistent due to a mixed pattern of remissions and new manifestations [27].

Studies with adults have also identified high rates of psychopathology. In one retrospective study (40), 92% of the sample (n = 25) met the criteria for at least one Axis 1 disorder. The most common diagnoses were alcohol and drug dependence (60%), depressive disorders (44%), and psychotic disorders (40%). In addition, 48% of the sample met criteria for an Axis 2 disorder with avoidant (29%), antisocial (19%), and dependent (14%) personality disorders having the highest prevalence. An examination of the psychiatric functioning of the large prospectively identified sample in Seattle (n = 431) at age 25 found relatively high rates of depressive disorders (39%), anxiety disorders (29%), and substance abuse or dependence (35%) [41]. On Axis 2, the prevalence of obsessive-compulsive personality disorder (16%) was also relatively high. In addition, in comparison with a steady drinking pattern, maternal binge drinking was associated with increased odds of having the following disorders: somatoform disorders, substance abuse or dependence, passive aggressive personality disorder, and antisocial personality disorder [41]. In summary, the prevalence of psychopathology is consistently high in the PAE population regardless of ascertainment method and co-morbidity is common. We should note, however, that one study examining the relation between PAE and adolescent psychiatric disorders failed to find an association when family history of alcoholism was controlled for [42]. Further studies should be conducted in this area to resolve this discrepancy.

PREDICTORS AND PATHWAYS TO BEHAVIOR

In addition to general assessments of behavior and psychopathology, a number of studies have assessed predictors and mechanisms involved in the development of specific problems, such as depression, delinquency, drug and alcohol use, poor quality of life, and caregiver stress.

Depression

Increased rates of depressive disorders are seen in individuals with PAE, and identifying the potential mechanisms in the development of depressive symptoms could result in earlier identification and more focused treatments. The early identification and effective treatment of depression would not only ameliorate the individual's current symptoms but also would result in fewer and less severe relapses. Two research groups have investigated the influence of a negative affect in infancy and caregiver-child attachment as potential mediators of the relation between PAE and depressive symptomatology [43-47]. In addition to identifying a direct relation between PAE and depressive symptoms at age 6, the results supported an indirect relation mediated by infant negative affect measured at 1 year of age [45]. The results of that study were explained entirely by the girls in this sample: girls with higher levels of PAE were more likely to display negative affect at 1 year of age and higher levels of depressive symptoms at age 6. Maternal depression was also associated with higher levels of child depression at age 6 in this sample [44]. Caregiver-child attachment was also examined in relation to infant negative affect and child depressive symptoms. Caregivers who made fewer attempts at engaging their infant during play had infants with greater negative affect, and girls tended to have more negative affect than boys [43]. Similarly, in a sample of 4 and 5 year olds, 80% of alcohol-exposed children were rated as having an insecure attachment, compared with only 35% of controls [46]. Alcohol exposure was related to more negative child affect, mothers with more negative children were less emotionally connected with their children, and those children had higher levels of depressive symptoms [46,47]. Mothers of children with PAE who gave high levels of emotional support had children with better coping skills and more secure attachments [46].

Several studies have identified high rates of suicidality in adults and adolescents with histories of PAE [20,48]. Risk factors for suicide are common in individuals with PAE, including impulsivity, co-morbid mood disorder, and substance abuse problems [48]. Furthermore, one study [48] noted that the lethality of a suicide attempt or self-harm behavior often does not correlate with the degree of intent in this population, suggesting the need for close monitoring irrespective of intellectual ability.

Research using animal models has suggested a number of mechanisms connecting PAE and alterations to neural substrates proposed to be involved in mood disorder pathology. Alcohol-related alterations to circadian rhythms may play an important role in the etiology of mood disorders, as well as disruptions in sleeping and eating, social deficits, and attention problems [49-50]. Specifically, circadian rhythms can be disrupted via several mechanisms, including alterations to the suprachiasmatic nuclei (SCN) of the hypothalamus and related brain areas, a reduction in the number of serotonergic neurons in the dorsal and median raphe nuclei, and the suppression of brain-derived neurotrophic factor expression in the SCN. The influence of maternal thyroid hormone deficiency on the development of depressive symptomatology in prenatally exposed offspring [51] has also been examined. The results suggest that some of the behavioral abnormal-ities observed in offspring with PAE are due to the suppressive effects of alcohol on the maternal and fetal hypothalamic-pituitary-thyroid axis. The administration of prenatal thyroid hormone reversed the observed abnormalities in behavior and gene expression in adult offspring with PAE. These studies demonstrate the utility of animal models for identifying the potential biological mechanisms relating PAE and behavioral dysfunction that may prove useful in developing treatments to ameliorate symptoms.

Conduct/Delinquency

Several studies have looked at predictors of delinquency and the prevalence of conduct disorder in children with PAE. The large Seattle study [20] on PAE found that of individuals older than 12 years, 60% had been in trouble with the law, 50% had displayed inappropriate sexual behavior, and 60% had a disrupted school experience (e.g., expelled, suspended, dropped out of school). Of those individuals experiencing trouble with the law, 35% had been incarcerated, and one third committed their first crime between the ages of 9 and 14. The most common crimes were theft, burglary, assault, damage to property, and drug violations. Behavior problems in school were common and included high rates of difficulty getting along with peers, being disruptive in class, disobeying school rules, and fighting. The preva-lence of PAE has also been examined in a community sample of adolescents in the criminal justice system and was found to be as high as 23% [52].

Two recent studies have examined various risk factors and predictors of delinquent behavior in children and adolescents with PAE. One retrospective study [53] found that children with PAE had higher rates of delinquent behaviors than non-exposed controls, and specific sociomoral values were predictive of delinquent behavior. Alcohol-exposed children had lower overall moral maturity than controls, and the sociomoral values of providing help to family and friends and refraining from stealing or breaking the law were predictive of delinquent behavior above and beyond the effects of group membership and age. Furthermore, children with PAE were more likely than controls to have probable conduct disorder.

In a large prospective study of predominantly African American youth of low socioeconomic background [54], adolescents with PAE did not differ from controls in the variety or frequency of delinquent behavior. The reason for the discrepancy between studies could be due to differences in the recruitment method, level of alcohol exposure, socioeconomic status, cultural norms, or instruments used. Although alcohol exposure did not significantly predict delinquent behavior in the prospective sample [54], a number of risk factors were consistent with increased frequency or a wider range of delinquent acts for all subjects. Specifically, higher levels of adolescent stress, self-reported alcohol and drug use, and verbal aggression predicted a higher frequency of delinquent behavior. Similarly, higher levels of stress, higher alcohol and drug use, and lower parental supervision were related to a wider range of delinquent acts.

Adolescent and Adult Substance Use

High rates of substance-related disorders occur in individuals with PAE. In the Seattle cohort [20], 35% of adolescents and adults with PAE were reported to have alcohol and drug problems and 23% had sought treatment for their problems. Similarly, in a retrospective study of adult adoptees [55], individuals with histories of PAE had higher symptom rates of nicotine, alcohol, and drug dependence than controls, after taking into account sex, parental substance use, diagnoses, birth weight, gestational age, and other environmental variables.

Research has identified a clear association between family history of alcoholism and offspring alcohol problems, supporting a genetic component of alcoholism [56]. Due to the occurrence of high family density of alcohol problems in families of individuals with PAE, the high rate of alcohol abuse and dependence in individuals with histories of PAE may be due to genetic vulnerability rather than to the prenatal exposure itself. To address this question, one research group examined drinking patterns and genetic and environmental predictors in a large prospective sample of individuals at ages 14 and 21 years [57-58]. At age 14 [57], 57% of alcohol-exposed adolescents reported having consumed alcohol in their lifetime and 25% reported drinking in the last month. PAE was a significant predictor of adolescent alcohol problems and accounted for more variance than did a family history of alcoholism. Furthermore, this relation was still significant after controlling for family history, prenatal nicotine exposure, parenting style, current parent drinking, household stress, and adolescent self-esteem. At age 21 [58], the same individuals reported an average 5.77 drinking episodes per month and 3.79 drinks per occasion. In addition, 36.5% reported binge drinking at least once in the past month and 8% met the cutoff for at least mild alcohol dependence. Similar to findings at age 14, PAE was associated with alcohol problems at age 21 even after controlling for family history, other prenatal exposures, and postnatal environmental factors like parental use of other drugs.

A study completed in Australia [59] found a similar relation between PAE and alcohol problems in alcohol-exposed individuals at age 21, with and without a family history of alcoholism. In addition, this study identified that early exposure during pregnancy was a stronger predictor of alcohol problems at 21 than was exposure in late pregnancy. Young adults whose mothers continued to drink during their childhood and adolescence were more likely to have a later onset of alcohol problems than young adults whose mothers had quit drinking. The authors suggest that this finding may reflect a possible contribution of genetic and/or environmental exposures during childhood and adolescence to alcohol use.

Quality of life

As adults, many individuals with PAE have a reduced quality of life. In one sample of 90 adults over age 21 [20], 83% were in a dependent living environment (e.g., group home, with relatives) and 79% had problems with employment. A large proportion had difficulty managing finances and making decisions on their own, and many had difficulty obtaining medical and social services. Alcohol-exposed individuals had more difficulty in holding down a job than in obtaining one, and their employment problems often included getting easily frustrated, poor task comprehension, poor judgment, social problems, unreliability, poor anger management, and problems with supervisors. In addition, almost half of the sample had become parents, and half of these individuals had been separated from their children. Protective factors for improved outcomes included early identification and diagnosis, a stable and nurturant home, no violence against self, and developmental disabilities services.

A 20-year follow-up of the Berlin cohort [28] also identified high rates of dependence and low occupational attainment. Specifically, only 14% of the sample was living independently and 16% lived with a partner or had their own family. Only 13% of subjects had ever held an "ordinary" job, which is disappointing when considering that 69% had had some preparatory job training, and 58% had either started or progressed to formal occupational training.

One study [60] investigated the quality of life of a small sample of women with histories of PAE. The women endorsed a lower quality of life relative to standardization samples and other at-risk populations. Similar to other studies, these women had high levels of mental health disorders and behavioral problems, and the authors suggest that the high levels of psychiatric distress might play a substantial role in the reduced quality of life reported among these women.

Caregiver Stress

The quantity and severity of problems experienced by individuals with PAE are likely to result in high levels of caregiver stress. A better understanding of the correlates of caregiver stress may aid in developing interventions for caregivers that could reduce this stress and allow for improved parent-child interactions. Two studies have looked at predictors of caregiver stress in parents of children with PAE. In one study [61], the biological parents of young children (ages 4-5) with moderate to heavy prenatal exposure had higher levels of child-domain stress than did the parents of children with light to no exposure. In addition, higher levels of stress were predicted by higher levels of child externalizing behaviors and fewer family resources. A second study [62] expanded on the previous findings by evaluating caregiver stress in biological, adoptive, and foster parents of school-aged children. The findings were similar to the previous study [61], with biological parent status and fewer family resources associated with higher levels of parent-domain stress. In addition, adoptive parent status was related to higher levels of child-related stress. Further studies are needed with adolescents and adults, especially as many alcohol-exposed adults remain dependent on relatives or other community caregivers.

PSYCHOSOCIAL AND MEDICAL INTERVENTIONS

Few studies have examined specific treatments and interventions designed for individuals with PAE. Several studies, however, have recently evaluated the effectiveness of specific interventions and additional studies are underway [63]. One well-designed study [64] examined the effectiveness of a 12-week parent-assisted friendship training group with school-aged children with PAE. In this intervention, groups were run simultaneously for parents and children. Children focused on specific social skills such as social network formation, informational exchange with peers, group entry, and conflict avoidance and negotiation. Skills were taught through simple rules, modeling, rehearsal, and performance feedback. Parents were instructed in how to assist their children in generalizing and maintaining the skills they were learning in group to the home environment.

Children and parents completed their homework assignments, and rehearsal at home was emphasized. The children who completed the intervention improved in their knowledge of appropriate social skills, and based on caregiver reports, demonstrated observable improvement in social skills and reductions in problem behaviors. Caregiver-reported social skills showed further improvement at the 3-month follow-up. Whereas the parents reported significant improvement with intervention, similar measures completed by the children's teachers showed little improvement. Possible reasons for this discrepancy include the tendency for the original baseline ratings of social skills by the teachers to be in the average range, few opportunities for observation in the classroom of the types of behaviors targeted by the intervention, and caregiver overestimation of improvement. Although plausible, the last reason is less likely due to the observed improvement in the children's knowledge of social rules of behavior [64].

A follow-up study examined the relation between medication status and outcomes in the parent-assisted friendship training group [65]. Parent and teacher reports were compared across four subgroups of children who were prescribed either stimulant or neuroleptic medication, neither, or both. The results indicated that children prescribed with neuroleptic medication showed greater improvement on all outcome measures when compared with children not prescribed with neuroleptics, whereas children prescribed with stimulants either failed to show improvement or showed poorer outcomes when compared with children not prescribed with stimulants. The results of this study have implications for medication management and indicate the benefits of physicians routinely asking about PAE to treat children with ADHD-like symptomatology more effectively.

As discussed above, adults with PAE often have difficulty in living independently, holding a job, and obtaining appropriate medical and social services. A pilot study was completed with 19 young women with PAE [66], using an intervention that was modified from an existing framework developed to assist women with young children access appropriate services and ensure adequate housing. The standard intervention uses paraprofessional case managers that assist clients in accessing and coordinating services among a multi-disciplinary network, ensuring that clients follow through with recommendations, and teaching clients to develop these skills on their own. The standard intervention was modified through targeted education to teach case managers and service providers about the effects of PAE and to provide case managers with strategies and materials to aide their clients. Improved outcomes included decreased alcohol and drug use, increased use of contraceptives, improved utilization of medical and mental health care, and stable housing. Clients with PAE had difficulty in learning the skills necessary to access services themselves, but demonstrated improved utilization with the aid of case managers.

In addition to psychosocial interventions, several studies have examined the effectiveness of medications in children with PAE. One study using a retrospective chart review methodology [67] identified 22 patients with PAE involved in a total of 66 medication trials. Due to co-morbidity, medications were often directed at more than one symptom. Different classes of medications varied in effectiveness. The most prescribed class of medications was stimulant medication. Out of 27 stimulant trials, 63% resulted in improvement, whereas nearly 30% were discontinued due to side effects. The response rates to trials of SSRIs (11), mood stabilizing anticonvulsants (8), and antipsychotics (6) were all above 80%. Tricyclic anti-depressants were not effective in any of the four trials administered. Two other studies have examined the effectiveness of stimulants in children with PAE. Although both studies demonstrated positive responses to stimulant medication [68-69], one study found a differential positive response of dextroamphetamine (Adderall) over methylphenidate (Ritalin; [68]). We should emphasize, however, that both studies had small sample sizes and may not be generalizable to the larger population of alcohol-exposed individuals. Further research is needed in the area of intervention design and effectiveness.

CONCLUSIONS AND FUTURE DIRECTIONS

In summary, children and adults with PAE have significant difficulties in the domains of social and behavioral functioning. In general, research has found impaired adaptive functioning, especially in the social domain. Social deficits are above and beyond what would be expected based on IQ and appear to increase with age as individuals have greater difficulty meeting age-related expectations. Children with PAE also display a wide range of behavior problems, including difficulties with attention, aggression, antisocial and delinquent behavior, and social problems. Maladaptive behavior is persistent and often continues into late adolescence and adulthood, frequently resulting in dependency, isolation, difficulty with employment, and poor quality of life. The prevalence of psychopathology is high across all ages and co-morbidity is common. In children, common diagnoses include ADHD, mood disorders, and other disruptive behavior disorders. In adulthood, substance abuse and dependence, depressive disorders, suicidality, and anxiety are elevated. Finally, recent studies have identified useful interventions for this population, although much more work in this area is needed.

Although discrepancies exist in the literature, most of these are likely due to the recruitment method, with prospective designs generally finding fewer and less significant impairments than retrospective designs. Nevertheless, a number of prospective studies have demonstrated alcohol-related behavioral problems and high rates of psychopathology. Their findings complement those of the retrospective studies and allow for greater confidence in the relation between alcohol exposure and the behavior problems found in clinically referred samples.

Whereas a considerable amount is known about the social and behavioral functioning in individuals with PAE, further research is needed in a number of areas. Additional studies using a prospective ascertainment method in the area of social functioning, especially with older samples, could help clarify the discrepancies found in the literature. A wider range of measures and behavioral sampling methods used in studies could also greatly expand and refine our knowledge of the social abilities in this population and may lead to more targeted interventions. For example, analog studies of social situations may improve our understanding of the social information processing and the problem-solving abilities of children with PAE. Expanding the sampling methodology of behavior problems and competencies would also assist in delineating common predictors and the mechanisms involved in their development. Furthermore, comparisons between individuals with PAE and related groups (e.g., ADHD) may aid in diagnostic specificity and in developing a behavioral profile or profiles consistent with this exposure. Designing studies to examine potential confounders, such as differences in living environment, lower cognitive functioning, and other environmental influences would greatly benefit the field. Finally, much research is needed in the area of intervention. Few interventions have been empirically tested with this population, and as evidenced above, are greatly needed. Empirically developed interventions based on specific cognitive and behavioral features associated with PAE may be especially useful. To be effective, any intervention used with individuals with PAE should be multidisciplinary and take into account the spectrum of challenges faced by this population.

REFERENCES

[1]   Hoyme HE, May PA, Kalberg WO, Kodituwakku P, Gossage JP, Trujillo PM, et al. A practical clinical approach to diagnosis of fetal alcohol spectrum disorders: Clarification of the 1996 Institute of Medicine criteria. *Pediatrics* 2005; 115(1):39-47.

[2]   May PA, Gossage JP. Estimating the prevalence of fetal alcohol syndrome: A summary. *Alcohol Res Health* 2001;25(3):159-67.

[3]   Lupton C, Burd L, Harwood R. Cost of fetal alcohol spectrum disorders. *Am. J. Med. Genet C Semin Med. Genet.* 2004;127(1):42-50.

[4]   Sampson PD, Streissguth AP, Bookstein FL, Little RE, Clarren SK, Dehaene P, et al. Incidence of fetal alcohol syndrome and prevalence of alcohol-related neurodevelopmental disorder. *Teratology* 1997;56(5):317-26.

[5]   Mattson SN, Riley EP, Gramling LJ, Delis DC, Jones KL. Neuropsychological comparison of alcohol-exposed children with or without physical features of fetal alcohol syndrome. *Neuropsy-chology* 1998;12(1):146-53.

[6]   Kodituwakku PW. Defining the behavioral phenotype in children with fetal alcohol spectrum disorders: A review. *Neurosci Biobehav Rev.* 2007;31(2):192-201.

[7]   Kelly SJ, Day N, Streissguth AP. Effects of prenatal alcohol exposure on social behavior in humans and other species. *Neurotoxicol. Teratol.* 2000;22(2):143-9.

[8]   Kupersmidt JB, DeRosier ME. How peer problems lead to negative outcomes: An integrative mediational model. In: Kupersmidt JB, Dodge KA, eds. *Children's Peer Relations: From Development to Intervention*. Washington, D.C.: American Psychological Association, 2004:119-38.

[9]   Streissguth AP, Sampson PD, Barr HM, Book-stein FL, Olson HC. The effects of prenatal exposure to alcohol and tobacco: Contributions from the Seattle Longitudinal Prospective Study and implications for public policy. In: Needleman HL, Bellinger D, eds. *Prenatal Exposure to Toxicants: Developmental Consequences*. Baltimore, MD: The Johns Hopkins University Press, 1994:148-83.

[10]   Jacobson JL, Jacobson SW. Methodological considerations in behavioral toxicology in infants and children. *Dev. Psychol.* 1996;32(3):390-403.

[11]   Jacobson SW, Chiodo LM, Sokol RJ, Jacobson JL. Validity of maternal report of prenatal alcohol, cocaine, and smoking in relation to neurobehavioral outcome. *Pediatrics* 2002;109(5):815-25.

[12]   Sattler JM. *Assessment of children.* San Diego, CA: Jerome M. Sattler, 2001.

[13]   Sparrow SS, Bella DA, Cicchetti DV. *A Manual for the Vineland.* Circle Pines, MN: American Guidance Services, 1984.

[14]   Streissguth AP, Aase JM, Clarren SK, Randels SP, LaDue RA, Smith DF. Fetal alcohol syndrome in adolescents and adults. *J. Am. Med. Assoc* 1991; 265(15):1961-7.

[15]   Thomas SE, Kelly SJ, Mattson SN, Riley EP. Comparison of social abilities of children with fetal alcohol syndrome to those of children with similar IQ scores and normal controls. *Alcohol Clin. Exp. Res.* 1998;22(2):528-33.

[16] Whaley SE, O'Connor MJ, Gunderson B. Comparison of the adaptive functioning of children prenatally exposed to alcohol to a nonexposed clinical sample. *Alcohol Clin. Exp. Res.* 2001; 25(7):1018-24.

[17] Coggins TE, Friet T, Morgan T. Analyzing narrative productions in older school-age children and adolescents with fetal alcohol syndrome: An experimental tool for clinical applications. *Clin. Linguist Phon.* 1998;12(3):221-36.

[18] Schonfeld AM, Paley B, Frankel F, O'Connor MJ. Executive functioning predicts social skills following prenatal alcohol exposure. *Child Neuropsychol.* 2006;12(6):439-52.

[19] Coles CD, Brown RT, Smith IE, Platzman KA, Erickson S, Falek A. Effects of prenatal alcohol exposure at school age. I. Physical and cognitive development. *Neurotoxicol Teratol* 1991;13(4): 357-67.

[20] Streissguth AP, Barr HM, Kogan J, Bookstein FL. *Final Report: Understanding the Occurrence of Secondary Disabilities in Clients with Fetal Alcohol Syndrome (FAS) and Fetal Alcohol Effects (FAE).* Seattle, WA: University of Washington Publication Services, 1996.

[21] Adolphs R. Investigating the cognitive neuroscience of social behavior. *Neuropsychologia* 2003; 41(2):119-26.

[22] Lugo JN, Jr., Wilson MA, Kelly SJ. Perinatal ethanol exposure alters met-enkephalin levels of male and female rats. *Neurotoxicol Teratol* 2006; 28(2):238-44.

[23] Spadoni AD, McGee CL, Fryer SL, Riley EP. Neuroimaging and fetal alcohol spectrum disorders. *Neurosci. Biobehav Rev.* 2007;31(2):239-45.

[24] Achenbach TM. *Manual for the Child Behavior Checklist/4-18 and 1991 Profile.* Burlington: Univ Vermont Dept Psychiatry, 1991.

[25] Achenbach TM. *Manual for the Teacher's Report Form and 1991 Profile.* Burlington: Univ Vermont, 1991.

[26] Mattson SN, Riley EP. Parent ratings of behavior in children with heavy prenatal alcohol exposure and IQ-matched controls. *Alcohol Clin. Exp. Res.* 2000;24(2):226-31.

[27] Steinhausen HC, Spohr HL. Long-term outcome of children with fetal alcohol syndrome: Psychopathology, behavior and intelligence. *Alcohol Clin. Exp. Res.* 1998;22(2):334-8.

[28] Spohr HL, Willms J, Steinhausen HC. Fetal alcohol spectrum disorders in young adulthood. *J. Pediatr.* 2007;150(2):175-9.

[29] Carmichael Olson H, Streissguth AP, Sampson PD, Barr HM, Bookstein FL, Thiede K. Association of prenatal alcohol exposure with behavioral and learning problems in early adolescence. *J. Am. Acad. Child Adolesc. Psychiatry* 1997;36(9):1187-94.

[30] Sood B, Delaney-Black V, Covington C, Nordstrom-Klee B, Ager JW, Jr., Templin T, et al. Prenatal alcohol exposure and childhood behavior at age 6 to 7 years: I. Dose-response effect. *Pediatrics* 2001; 108(2):34-42.

[31] Brown RT, Coles CD, Smith IE, Platzman KA, Silverstein J, Erickson S, et al. Effects of prenatal alcohol exposure at school age. II. Attention and behavior. *Neurotoxicol. Teratol.* 1991;13(4):369-76.

[32] Coles CD, Platzman KA, Raskind-Hood CL, Brown RT, Falek A, Smith IE. A comparison of children affected by prenatal alcohol exposure and attention deficit, hyperactivity disorder. *Alcohol Clin. Exp. Res.* 1997;21(1):150-61.

[33] Nanson JL, Hiscock M. Attention deficits in children exposed to alcohol prenatally. *Alcohol Clin. Exp. Res.* 1990;14(5):656-61.

[34] Nash K, Rovet J, Greenbaum R, Fantus E, Nulman I, Koren G. Identifying the behavioural phenotype in fetal alcohol spectrum disorder: Sensitivity, specificity and screening potential. *Arch. Womens Ment Health* 2006;9:181-6.

[35] Steinhausen HC, Willms J, Metzke CW, Spohr HL. Behavioural phenotype in foetal alcohol syndrome and foetal alcohol effects. *Dev. Med. Child Neurol.* 2003;45(3):179-82.

[36] Roebuck TM, Mattson SN, Riley EP. Behavioral and psychosocial profiles of alcohol-exposed children. *Alcohol Clin. Exp. Res.* 1999;23(6):1070-6.

[37] Schneider ML, Moore CF, Kraemer GW. Moderate level alcohol during pregnancy, prenatal stress, or both and limbic-hypothalamic-pituitary-adrenocortical axis response to stress in rhesus monkeys. *Child Dev.* 2004;75(1):96-109.

[38] Burd L, Klug MG, Martsolf JT, Kerbeshian J. Fetal alcohol syndrome: Neuropsychiatric phenomics. *Neurotoxicol. Teratol.* 2003;25(6):697-705.

[39] Fryer SL, McGee CL, Matt GE, Riley EP, Mattson SN. Evaluation of psychopathological conditions in children with heavy prenatal alcohol exposure. *Pediatrics* 2007;119:e733-41.

[40] Famy C, Streissguth AP, Unis AS. Mental illness in adults with fetal alcohol syndrome or fetal alcohol effects. *Am. J. Psychiatry* 1998;155(4):552-4.

[41] Barr HM, Bookstein FL, O'Malley KD, Connor PD, Huggins JE, Streissguth AP. Binge drinking during pregnancy as a predictor of psychiatric disorders on the structured clinical interview for DSM-IV in young adult offspring. *Am. J. Psychiatry* 2006;163(6):1061-5.

[42] Hill SY, Lowers L, Locke-Wellman J, Shen S. Maternal smoking and drinking during pregnancy and the risk for child and adolescent psychiatric disorders. *J. Stud. Alcohol* 2000;61(5):661-8.

[43] Lowe J, Handmaker N, Aragón C. Impact of mother interactive style on infant affect among babies exposed to alcohol in utero. *Infant Ment. Health J.* 2006;27(4):371-82.

[44] O'Connor MJ, Kasari C. Prenatal alcohol exposure and depressive features in children. *Alcohol Clin. Exp. Res.* 2000;24(7):1084-92.

[45] O'Connor MJ. Prenatal alcohol exposure and infant negative affect as precursors of depressive features in children. *Infant Ment Health J.* 2001; 22(3):291-9.

[46] O'Connor MJ, Kogan N, Findlay R. Prenatal alcohol exposure and attachment behavior in children. *Alcohol Clin. Exp. Res.* 2002;26(10):1592-602.

[47] O'Connor MJ, Paley B. The relationship of prenatal alcohol exposure and the postnatal environment to child depressive symptoms. *J. Pediatr. Psychol.* 2006;31(1):50-64.

[48] O'Malley K, Huggins J. Suicidality in adolescents and adults with fetal alcohol spectrum disorders. *Can. J. Psychiatry* 2005;50(2):125.

[49] Sher L. Prenatal alcohol exposure, circadian rhythm, and serotonin. Med Hypotheses 2004; 63(6):1081.

[50] Sakata-Haga H, Dominguez HD, Sei H, Fukui Y, Riley EP, Thomas JD. Alterations in circadian rhythm phase shifting ability in rats following ethanol exposure during the third trimester brain growth spurt. *Alcohol Clin. Exp. Res.* 2006;30(5): 899-907.

[51] Wilcoxon JS, Kuo AG, Disterhoft JF, Redei EE. Behavioral deficits associated with fetal alcohol exposure are reversed by prenatal thyroid hormone treatment: A role for maternal thyroid hormone deficiency in FAE. *Mol. Psychiatry* 2005; 10(10):961-71.

[52] Fast DK, Conry J, Loock CA. Identifying fetal alcohol syndrome among youth in the criminal justice system. *J. Dev. Behav. Pediatr.* 1999;20(5): 370-2.

[53] Schonfeld AM, Mattson SN, Riley EP. Moral maturity and delinquency after prenatal alcohol exposure. *J. Stud. Alcohol.* 2005;66(4):545-55.

[54] Lynch ME, Coles CD, Corley T, Falek A. Examining delinquency in adolescents differentially prenatally exposed to alcohol: The role of proximal and distal risk factors. *J. Stud. Alcohol.* 2003;64:678-86.

[55] Yates WR, Cadoret RJ, Troughton EP, Stewart M, Giunta TS. Effect of fetal alcohol exposure on adult symptoms of nicotine, alcohol, and drug dependence. *Alcohol Clin. Exp. Res.* 1998;22(4): 914-20.

[56] Enoch MA, Goldman D. Genetics of alcoholism and substance abuse. *Psychiatr. Clin. North Am.* 1999;22(2):289-99.

[57] Baer JS, Barr HM, Bookstein FL, Sampson PD, Streissguth AP. Prenatal alcohol exposure and family history of alcoholism in the etiology of adolescent alcohol problems. *J. Stud. Alcohol* 1998;59(5):533-43.

[58] Baer JS, Sampson PD, Barr HM, Connor PD, Streissguth AP. 21-year longitudinal analysis of the effects of prenatal alcohol exposure on young adult drinking. *Arch. Gen. Psychiatry* 2003;60(4): 377-85.

[59] Alati R, Al Mamun A, Williams GM, O'Callaghan M, Najman JM, Bor W. In utero alcohol exposure and prediction of alcohol disorders in early adulthood: A birth cohort study. *Arch. Gen. Psychiatry* 2006;63(9):1009-16.

[60] Grant T, Huggins J, Connor P, Streissguth A. Quality of life and psychosocial profile among young women with fetal alcohol spectrum disorders. *Ment. Health Aspects Dev. Disabil* 2005;8(2):33-9.

[61] Paley B, O'Connor MJ, Kogan N, Findlay R. Prenatal alcohol exposure, child externalizing behavior, and maternal stress. *Par Science Prac.* 2005;5(1):29-56.

[62] Paley B, J. OCM, Frankel F, Marquardt R. Predictors of stress in parents of children with fetal alcohol spectrum disorders. *J. Dev. Behav. Pediatr.* 2006;27(5):396-404.

[63] Kalberg WO, Buckley D. FASD: What types of intervention and rehabilitation are useful? *Neurosci. Biobehav. Rev.* 2007;31:278-85.

[64] O'Connor MJ, Frankel F, Paley B, Schonfeld AM, Carpenter E, Laugeson EA, et al. A controlled social skills training for children with fetal alcohol spectrum disorders. *J. Consult Clin. Psychol.* 2006; 74(4):639-48.

[65] Frankel F, Paley B, Marquardt R, O'Connor M. Stimulants, neuroleptics, and children's friendship training for children with fetal alcohol spectrum disorders. *J. Child Adolesc. Psychopharmacol.* 2006;16(6):777-89.

[66] Grant T, Huggins J, Connor P, Pedersen JY, Whitney N, Streissguth A. A pilot community intervention for young women with fetal alcohol spectrum disorders. *Community Ment. Health J.* 2004;40(6): 499-511.

[67] Coe J, Sidders J, Riley K, Waltermire J, Hagerman R. A survey of medication responses in children and adolescents with fetal alcohol syndrome. *Ment Health Aspects Dev. Disabil.* 2001; 4(4):148-55.

[68] O'Malley KD, Koplin B, Dohner VA. Psychostimulant clinical response in fetal alcohol syndrome. *Can. J. Psychiatry* 2000;45(1):90-1.

[69] Oesterheld JR, Kofoed L, Tervo R, Fogas B, Wilson A, Fiechtner H. Effectiveness of methylphenidate in Native American children with fetal alcohol syndrome and attention

deficit/hyperactivity disorder: A controlled pilot study. *J. Child Adolesc. Psychopharmacol.* 1998;8(1):39-48.

In: Alcohol-Related Cognitive Disorders   ISBN: 978-1-60741-730-9

Editors: L. Sher, I. Kandel, J. Merrick pp. 111-123   © 2009 Nova Science Publishers, Inc.

Chapter 6

MENTAL HEALTH DISORDERS COMORBID WITH FETAL ALCOHOL SPECTRUM DISORDERS

Larry Burd, Christine Carlson and Jacob Kerbeshian

ABSTRACT

This chapter will discuss relevant issues in the diagnosis of mental disorders comorbid with fetal alcohol spectrum disorders (FASD). We present a theoretical model of the effect of prenatal alcohol exposure on neurobehavioral development and a systematic review of published data on the mental disorders in subjects with an FASD. We have found that prenatal alcohol exposure is associated with high rates of mental disorders, 48 papers reporting on 3,343 subjects. The most common mental disorder comorbid with FASD is attention deficit - hyperactivity disorder occurring in 48% of subjects with FASD. Cognitive impairment is also very common. It appears that prenatal alcohol exposure have differential effects on outcomes leading to large increases in rates of some, but apparently not most mental disorders. We discuss strategies to improve the diagnosis of mental disorders in FASD and the multiplicity of uses for this important data.

INTRODUCTION

Of the four million annual pregnancies in the United States (US), about 40% of women drink some alcohol during pregnancy and about 3% to 5% of women drink heavily throughout pregnancy [1]. The prevalence of alcohol use by women during their childbearing years in the US was 54.6% in 2001 [1]. Frequent alcohol use was reported by 12.5% and third trimester drinking by 4.6% of pregnant women in 2001. For the four million pregnancies each year in the US, these rates translate to 500,000 pregnant women drinking at least weekly and about 80,000 with high levels of persistent exposure throughout pregnancy. Thus, the cumulative number of prenatally exposed infants, children, and adolescents alone would be in the millions.

Recent epidemiologic and clinical evidence suggest a wide range of adverse outcomes from prenatal alcohol exposure (PAE) [2]. The adverse outcomes include the four categorical diagnoses of fetal alcohol syndrome, partial FAS, alcohol-related neurodevelopmental disorders (ARND), and alcohol related birth defects (ARBD). The umbrella term for these syndromal categories is fetal alcohol spectrum disorders (FASD), which technically is not a diagnosis. The boundaries for diagnosis and clinical differentiation among these categorical entities are still emerging.

Current prevalence estimates for FASD range from a conservative rate of 0.5 (FAS only) to 9.1 cases per 1,000 live births for all FASD [3,4]. This estimate suggests that the number of affected pregnancies in the annual birth cohort in the US would range from 2,000 (4 million pregnancies x rate of 0.5 per 1,000 live births) to 36,400 (4 million pregnancies x rate of 9.1 per 1,000 live births) [3,4]. If the mother continues to drink during subsequent pregnancies, the recurrence rate for FASD could be as high as 75% [5,6]. The mortality risk for people with FASD is more than doubled. The mortality risk for siblings is increased 530%, and the maternal mortality rate in the 10-year period after the birth of the child with FASD is about 4.5% [7]. The societal implications of PAE are substantial. The annual cost of care for affected people is estimated to be $3.6 billion dollars in the US and the lifetime cost of care for FAS is $2.9 million dollars per case [8].

Prenatal alcohol exposure is a worldwide public health problem. In South Africa, some areas have a rate of FASD in live-born infants of 4% or higher [9]. The prevalence rates are also very high in Russia (10). Not surprisingly, PAE rates appear to be increased in populations having other risks associated with poor outcomes, including poverty, poor diet, smoking, and limited access to prenatal care and advanced obstetric facilities.

Maternal alcohol use is a frequent method of fetal exposure to a common xenobiotic and is widely accepted as an important causal factor in adverse outcomes, including birth defects, developmental disabilities, and mental illness. In figure 1, we demonstrate the entry of ethanol into the fetal environment. The exposed fetus has blood alcohol levels (BAL) nearly equivalent to maternal BAL as levels increase and peak. Fetal alcohol exposure is then prolonged since the primary mechanism for metabolizing fetal BAL is the reab-sorption of ethanol into the maternal blood stream. The fetus, even near term, has a very modest capacity for ethanol metabolism (Burd et al in press).

The effects of PAE are typically accompanied by the effects of smoking, poor diet, and other substance use in a mother who herself may have been exposed to these same adversities during her gestation. One would not be surprised to find that exposure to these other risk factors coupled with multiple episodes of maternal intoxication (e.g., if the woman drinks heavily two times a week the infant has 80 periods of intoxication before a term birth) would result in long term neurobehavioral abnormalities.

The mechanism of neurocognitive damage from PAE is conceptualized as a continuum from decreased neuronal populations, individual and regional neuronal damage, focal damage to the developing brain (migration abnormalities), and generalized dysmorphology of the fetal brain (microcephaly). However, even in the absence of easily demonstrable neurological damage, high rates of developmental delays, mental illness, and signs of developmentally inappropriate behavior are frequently seen in PAE infants and children [11].

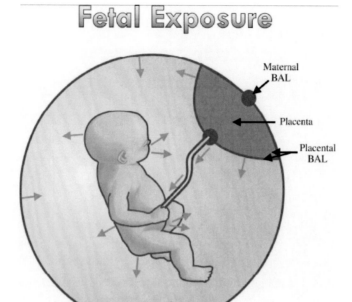

Figure 1. Schematic of alcohol entering the fetal environment and amniotic fluid. Alcohol is cleared from the amniotic fluid at a reduced rate compared to the fetus. BAL = blood alcohol level.

Prenatal alcohol exposure results in a highly variable pattern of adverse outcomes, wherein the primary outcomes are an increased frequency of birth defects and multiple neuropsychiatric impairments. The severity of negative outcome depends on the dose and the timing of PAE during fetal development, the additional exposure to other environmental teratogens that often accompany PAE (smoking, poor diet, other drug use), and other fetal and maternal genetic /epi-genetic factors that modify the susceptibility to adversity (figure 2). The three broad pathways to adverse out-comes comprise the following:

1. causal outcomes wherein PAE is a prepotent cause of an adverse outcome (mental retardation is one example);
2. a decreased threshold of expression for adverse outcomes wherein a subthreshold genetic liability and/or an environmentally induced pre-disposition for mental disorder are expressed as a result of PAE (depression may be a useful example); and
3. PAE increases the severity of discrete neuropsychiatric disorders that might have emerged in any case due to significant other vulnerabilities (ADHD would be an example).

Much of the increased severity of negative outcome in individuals with FASD appears to be the result of the numbers of comorbidities expressed.

The mechanisms of brain damage or dysfunction in individuals with a history of PAE have been based primarily on the association of central nervous system neuropathology and neurobehavioral deficits (e.g., epilepsy, development delays, mental illness) [12-14].

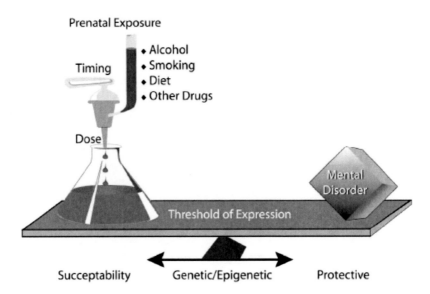

Figure 2. Graphic presentation of prenatal alcohol exposure and other factors that modify outcomes.

In figure 3, we present a theoretical model of the neuropsychiatric manifestations of PAE. We have drawn on the work of Muller [15] and Goodlett [16] to expand our view of the mechanisms of PAE resulting in damage or dysfunction to the central nervous system during fetal and postnatal development. Four principles will be used to refine the model we have presented in figure 3.

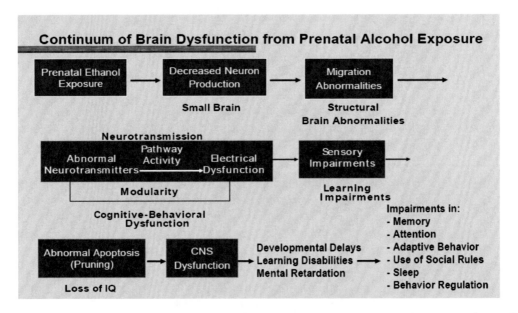

Figure 3. A schematic of neurocognitive deficits from PAE emphasizing the progressive and cumulative impairments from prolonged prenatal alcohol exposure (PAE).

1. Prenatal alcohol exposure produces a distributed (generalized) perturbation of central nervous system function that can be viewed as a disruption of neural networks. This disruption is manifested as an intermediate localized neuropathology(ies) or as a discrete pathophysiology(ies). Thus, in PAE, brain abnormalities and dysfunctions are reciprocally as likely to be the result of adverse outcomes as the cause. The effect of these brain abnormalities and dysfunctions on normal neuro-development leads to a feedback loop in which the altered neurodevelop-mental factors further modify the effects of brain abnormalities and dysfunctions. This transactional model leads to a more parsimonious and dynamic understanding of outcomes in FASD. Thus, PAE results in an abnormal experiential environment during crucial developmental periods, which has a role equally important to that of fetal alcohol exposure.

2. The abnormal experiential effects on development, brain growth, and function have influences that last long after the period of fetal exposure to alcohol. These can be conceptualized as both biologic and psychosocial epigenetic processes. The outcomes in PAE can as well be seen as the child's response to continuing biopsychosocial adversity as to a more or less static biologic effect resulting from exposure of brain to alcohol during fetal development [17]. These have important implications for the child's development and should influence secondary and tertiary prevention or interventions provided to the child after PAE. In this model, the effects of experience and the environment (lack of nurturance, deviant experience, abuse, multiple foster home placements, impaired social skills, mental retardation, speech and language disorders, temperament, vision or hearing loss, etc.) all contribute to brain development and function.

3. Related to #2 above, we have described the complexity principle, which can be summarized as having one abnormal event increasing the risk for a second [11]. Having two abnormal events in life increases the risk for a third and so on. This principle has been very useful in understanding the role of adversity on future development. As most experienced clinicians realize, the long term outlook for children is increasingly compromised when they are exposed to an increasing number of adversities in their life and the duration of exposure to the adversities lengthens.

4. Lastly, we need a more critical examination of the timing and dosing of developmental interventions. Many infants and children with PAE or FASD have multiple tactical habilitative interventions early in life that are the developmental equivalent of non-targeted polypharmacy. A global intervention strategy is often lacking. Many and likely most of the habilitative developmental interventions provided to infants and children can have unintended adverse consequences for the child. For example, placement in foster care might protect the already precariously attached infant or child from abuse or neglect, but at the same time, suddenly expose that infant or child to a new and stressful environment that further increases attachment stress. One hour per day of special education may improve reading but places the child in an atypical school environment for the equivalent of 31 school days per year (1 hour each day x 186 school days = 31 6-hour school days). Prescribing larger doses of intervention may decrease the time for family interaction and play time, resulting in a great deal of additional family stress from meetings and financial burden. The negative consequences of these tactical, but not strategic,

developmental interventions are greatly underappreciated by clinicians or systems of care who see in them the opportunity for enhancing developmental potential. The possibility for harm from such interventions is often underestimated, especially over the long term. This appraisal of developmental interventions is not meant to suggest that they are not useful but rather that they must be planned with far more deliberation and with a greater appreciation of the unintended effects they may have on development. Because the negative effects resulting from most developmental interventions have never been studied, possibly, many will be found to be neutral in efficacy when harm and benefit are compared, and hence cost ineffective. The need for a careful risk versus benefit analysis for specific developmental interventions is even more important when such interventions are provided to infants and children who already have multiple ongoing developmental challenges. This is clearly a much neglected area of research and seems to remain a low priority for funding.

Although the sequelae of PAE include a wide range of neurocognitive impairments and birth defects, the outcome for most affected individuals is influenced primarily by the number, severity, and duration of their developmental impairments and mental disorders. In this paper, we use a systematic review of published literature on PAE and the prevalence of mental disorders to examine what is currently known about that relationship. Our review focuses on mental disorders and does not duplicate a recent comprehensive review of neuro-cognitive impairments [18]. We then discuss PAE as a naturalistic model for population and individual research on neurodevelopmental disorders and mental disorders. We conclude with a policy recommendation dealing with inclusion of FASD in the Diagnostic and Statistical Manual of Mental Disorders (DSM) and the development of a unique code for the FASDs in the International Classification of Diseases (ICD).

SEARCH STRATEGY AND FINDINGS

We developed a search strategy to locate published papers on PAE and mental illness using the MeSH terms: prenatal alcohol exposure, fetal alcohol syndrome, mental disorders, case reports, epidemiology, and prevalence. The search covered the years 1970 to the present. PubMed and the MeSH terms and references from other articles were used to expand our search. We then hand searched the reference lists of papers we located for additional publications.

We located each paper and reviewed the abstract to determine if the paper met our inclusion criteria. We included papers that discussed diagnosed FASD and the related categorical diagnoses and mental illness in humans. For papers in which the abstract did not support inclusion, we reviewed the methods section before any final exclusion. We also included studies on ethanol and mental retardation.

We excluded papers that did not examine the effects of ethanol on the development of mental illness, papers not in English, papers on animal studies and papers without an FASD or related diagnosis.

We found 48 papers meeting our inclusion criteria. We grouped these papers and summarized the largest similar studies. Mental retardation (MR) in subjects with an FASD was reported in 72 people (20 with borderline/mild MR, 18 with moderate MR and 10 with severe/profound MR).

Attention deficit-hyperactivity disorder (ADHD) has been reported to be a common outcome in FASD. The summary of the data from 3,178 cases of FASD indicated that 1,523 subjects (47.9%) had a diagnosis of ADHD. Nine cases of autism were reported in subjects with FASD. We found single case reports of Tourette syndrome [19], schizophrenia [20] and Rett syndrome [21].

DISCUSSION

About 40% of pregnant women in the US have some alcohol exposure, usually before the pregnancy is confirmed. In nearly 4% to 6% of pregnancies, the exposure is heavy (more than four drinks per occasion and drinking 2-7 days per week) and continuing throughout pregnancy. For many women, this exposure occurs in the context of a family history of, and hence a genetic liability for, substance abuse. A genetic risk for substance abuse carries with it a risk for a wide range of mental disorders. A model of this multivariate interaction of risk factors and modifiers is presented in figure 2.

Thus, PAE should be viewed as both a neurological and behavioral dermatogen. In addition to prenatal exposure to neurobehavioral dermatogens accompanied by an increased genetic risk for alcoholism and other mental disorders, the infant and child with PAE is also exposed to an environment which is abnormal and very likely negatively influences infant and child behavior. For many infants, the exposure to environmental adversity is prolonged and for some, may intensify when the infant's demands on caretakers are unmet. This prolonged period of exposure to adversity acts to greatly increase the risk for expression of a developmental disability and or a mental disorder.

Fetal Alcohol Spectrum Disorders and Psychiatric Comorbidity

As noted above, in our clinical experience a critical factor in the outcome for infants and children after PAE is the number, severity, and duration of the developmental adversities to which they are exposed, although there are occasional exceptions to this dictum. The treatment of the comorbid conditions then offers the best hope for the reduction in the number, severity and duration of these adversities, especially sensory impairments, speech and language disorders, and behavior disorders. Whereas birth defects, if severe, can have a life-defining role for infants or children, this is usually not the primary cause of impairment in FASD. Many of the abnormal somatic phenotypic signs used to increase specificity in the diagnosis of FASD have little impact on developmental outcome. Certainly, few children have life-altering adversity from a thin upper lip, flattened philtrum, or decreased palpebral fissure length. For most children, adolescents, and especially for adults, the less specific findings in FASD have the greatest impact on outcomes. Depression, mental retardation, ADHD, oppositional defiant disorder, or even the ubiquitous sleep disorders have far more potent roles in outcomes than do the physical features of FASD. The issue of how to append these common mental disorders or developmental disorders to PAE or to one of the FASD is complex. We will grapple with this issue.

The advent of DSM-III (Diagnostic and Statistical Manual of Mental Disorders) heralded a sea of change in the conceptualization of mental disorders. Subsequent versions of the DSM have carried on the basic paradigm of diagnostic entities being defined by a probabilistic clustering of specific symptoms, which, upon crossing a statistical threshold, rise to a level of acceptable certainty to make a diagnosis. In their very titles, the DSM notes that they are manuals for diagnosing mental disorder, namely a departure from normal order, rather than diagnosing mental disease or mental illness. The DSM is primarily a vehicle for making categorical diagnoses, i.e., taking a symptomatic cross-section of an individual over a limited period of time and to determine whether diagnostic thresholds are reached. Even inherently dimensional conditions such as ADHD are diagnosed using a categorical symptomatic framework. In the case of ADHD, the symptom specific criteria serve as a proxy for the intensity of neuropsychiatric constructs along a distribution curve encompassing normality at one end and severe neuropsychiatric developmental pathology at the other.

In the DSM, the symptom criteria are based primarily on subjective and observable behavioral data. Such features as severity of disorder are either inferred or addressed in terms of psychosocial dysfunction, which to an extent may be environmentally mediated. The course of the disorder is addressed in one of two manners. The first is that of symptom duration, which is often critical in crossing the threshold to diagnosis. The course of disorder is otherwise addressed by elements of acuity, subchronicity, chronicity, or a residual state. The framers of the DSM attempted to address some of the deficiencies of the manual through the promulgation of the multiaxial framework. Behavioral syndromal conditions are addressed on axes I and II. Physical conditions, which may or may not be directly relevant to axes I and II, are listed on axis III. Axis IV addresses psychological and social stressors that might be relevant to the condition. Axis V attempts to capture impairment severity.

The multiaxial framework of DSM does allow for the incorporation of a biopsychosocial backdrop for individual case analysis (individual phenotype) and for the study of associated other factors across groups of individuals with a specific mental disorder (population derived phenotypes). However, it may artificially excise such factors from being critical features of making a specific diagnosis. In the DSM schema, FASD would be an Axis III condition and thus in a different frame of reference than Axis I or Axis II conditions with which it might be comorbid.

In light of the above, Rett disorder is interesting, because of its departure from the prominent template of features of other DSM diagnoses. The case of Rett disorder may have relevance to defining a diagnosis of FAS or FASD in future iterations of the DSM. All eight DSM criteria must be met to qualify for the diagnosis. There are no alternative constellations of symptoms, which in various combinations would reach a threshold for diagnosis. A physical finding is included in the symptom list, namely normal head circumference at birth, and deceleration of head growth thereafter. Developmental course over time is specifically addressed rather than being inferred or represented by the proxy of a categorical symptom. A specific bio-marker for the condition—namely an abnormality at the genetic locus that codes for the MECP2 protein—is not incorporated into the schema, but this may be reflective of the state of knowledge of Rett's syndrome at the time of deliberations regarding DSM-IV. Sunderland et al [22] have made a case for including biomarkers as specifiers for diagnoses in future iterations of the DSM. However, inclusion of a genetic biomarker as a not-necessary diagnostic criterion for Rett disorder could result in a complex diagnostic situation, wherein one child might have a DSM diagnosis of Rett's disorder with a negative MECP2 genetic finding and another child might have a positive MECP2 study but not meet the other DSM criteria for Rett's disorder. Making the inclusion of a positive MECP2 genetic finding a necessary criterion for a diagnosis of Rett disorder would exclude those patients with the Rett syndrome phenotype who are negative for the genotype. These issues concerning the inclusion of Rett's disorder in the DSM serve as a parallel to the inclusion of the specific FASD disorders in the manual.

How can one incorporate the biomarkers, physical findings, environmental teratogens, and clinical course in what is predominantly a categorical crosssectional behavioral diagnostic scheme? The problem of incorpor-ating environmental exposure in DSM diagnostic criteria echoes that of inclusion a specific genetic abnormality. Phenotype variability, severity and complexity are often not adequately captured by DSM or by any other comprehensive nosology. A useful example is environmental lead exposure. The parallel with PAE should be apparent. The neurocognitive phenotype from environmental lead exposure has a wide range, including cognitive impairment, ADHD, and learning disabilities. The outcomes have crude but identifiable dose-dependent risk, wherein increasing lead levels lead to decreasing IQ. Yet, most cases of lead exposure do not have DSM-diagnosable mental retardation because most exposed and affected children have subthreshold cognitive impairments [23-25]. Many cases, however, have a DSM constellation of comorbidities, such as various and sundry learning disorders and ADHD, none of which is specific for or unique to lead toxicity [23-25].

The degree of diagnostic specificity for the four FASD categorical diagnoses is currently problematic. Currently, no nomenclature has been identified that has demonstrated the necessary diagnostic performance criteria for the delineation of the four categorical conditions in FASD. As currently conceptualized, FASD is a dimensional spectrum diagnosis that is roughly equivalent to the DSM's broad category level of nonspecificity for pervasive developmental disorders or anxiety disorders. When seeking the holy grail of a behavioral phenotype for FASD, we are currently limited to looking for associations between relatively specific DSM diagnoses, such as ADHD or panic disorder and a relatively nonspecific FASD diagnosis. We are undermined by a system shift in which we append factors of greater specificity to those of lesser specificity.

Although we have described a number of reasons how including a diagnosis of FASD or of one or more of its component diagnoses in a future iteration of the DSM would be problematic, we believe the prospect is well worth pursuing. Fetal alcohol spectrum disorder is a significant public health problem. Significant neuropsychiatric impairment and morbidity is found in individuals with FASD. The research agenda for FASD would be strengthened with agreed upon diagnostic criteria. In facilitating this goal, we might use the case of criteria for Rett's disorder as a template. For this project, we would recommend conflating specific diagnostic elements from FAS through ARND, including PAE; physical criteria (PAE, microcephaly, growth retardation); neurological symptoms; cognitive symptoms; and specific behavioral symptoms. From this list of criteria, one would develop a hierarchy of necessary symptoms and other symptoms that would allow for the achievement of sufficiency of symptoms for a diagnosis. Category A for a necessary symptom might be "convincing likelihood of prenatal alcohol exposure". Category B could include a sufficient number of physical, cognitive, behavioral, and emotional symptoms. The result would be a concurrent symptomatic probability grid. One might then define a cut point in the list either sequentially or numerically above which one would define the behavioral phenotype. These symptoms would be drawn from available research and would clearly be refined by future research.

A useful interim step may well be the inclusion of unique ICD codes for FASD, using the categories of FAS, partial FAS and perhaps ARND, if acceptable criteria can be developed. This approach would improve the data for prevalence studies using billing codes and identify other currently underappreciated comorbid conditions which may result in increased costs to quality of life, to society, and to the economy.

Lastly, a number of other crucial but as yet unanswered questions remain regarding FASD and mental illness.

- To what degree and how does a noxious abnormal psychosocial environment result in the modification of an individual's neurobehavioral phenotype after PAE?
- To what degree is that phenotype entrenched and to what degree is it modifiable?
- What are the most efficacious strategies to prevent further developmental disruption and what habilitative interventions might improve outcomes for infants, children, adolescents and adults after PAE?
- What does FASD look like in the elderly? PAE is not a new problem. Roughly half the population of the United States has been prenatally exposed to alcohol, at least to a minor degree. There must be innumerable cases unaccounted for. Where are they?

ACKNOWLEDGMENTS

This paper has been supported by the following grants: (1) Northern Plains Prenatal and Infant Health Consor-tium, Department of Health and Human Services (HHS) from National Institutes of Health/National Institute of Child Health and Human Development #5 U01 HD045935-04 (NIH); (2) Fetal Alcohol Syndrome Prevention, Department of Health and Human Services (HHS) from Centers for Disease Control and Prevention (CDC) #U24/CCU823298-04; (3) Consortium on Fetal Alcohol Syndrome, Center for Substance Abuse Pre-vention (CSAP) from Substance Abuse and Mental Health Services Administration (SAMHSA) 4 H79 SO12843-01-1, and (4) Early Predictators of Adverse Neurobehavioral Outcomes, National Institute of Health (NIH) National Institute of Child Health and Human Development (NICHD) #P20 MD001631-02.

REFERENCES

[1]   Floyd RL, Sidhu JS. Monitoring prenatal alcohol exposure. *Am. J. Med. Genet C Semin Med. Genet.* 2004;127(1):3-9.
[2]   Stratton KR, Howe CJ, Battaglia FC, Institute of Medicine. *Fetal alcohol syndrome-diagnosis, epi-demiology, prevention, and treatment.* Washington, DC: Nat Acad Press, 1996.

[3]   Sampson PD, Streissguth AP, Bookstein FL, Little RE, Clarren SK, Dehaene P et al. Incidence of fetal alcohol syndrome and prevalence of alcohol-related neurodevelopmental disorder. *Teratology* 1997;56(5):317-26.

[4]   Abel EL. *Fetal alcohol abuse syndrome*. New York: Plenum Press, 1998.

[5]   Burd L, Martsolf J, Kerbeshian J. Diagnosis of FAS: A comparison of the fetal alcohol syndrome diagnostic checklist and the Institute of Medicine criteria for fetal alcohol syndrome. *Neurotoxicol Teratol* 2003;25(6):719-24.

[6]   Abel EL. Fetal alcohol syndrome in families. *Neurotoxicol Teratol* 1988;10(1):1-2.

[7]   Burd L, Klug MG, Martsolf J. Increased sibling mortality in children with fetal alcohol syndrome. *Addict Biol.* 2004;9(2):179-86.

[8]   Lupton C, Burd L, Harwood R. The cost of fetal alcohol spectrum disorders. *Am. J. Med. Genet C Semin. Med. Genet* 2004;127C(1):42-50.

[9]   May PA, Gossage JP, White-Country M, Good-hart K, Decoteau S, Trujillo PM et al. Alcohol consumption and other maternal risk factors for fetal alcohol syndrome among three distinct samples of women before, during, and after pregnancy: the risk is relative. *Am. J. Med. Genet C Semin Med. Genet* 2004;127(1):10-20.

[10]   Warren KR, Calhoun FJ, May PA, Viljoen DL, Li TK, Tanaka H et al. Fetal alcohol syndrome: An international perspective. *Alcohol Clin. Exp. Res.* 2001;25(5 Suppl):202S-6S.

[11]   Burd L, Cotsonas-Hassler T, Martsolf J, Kerbeshian J. Recognition and management of fetal alcohol syndrome. *Neurotoxicol. Teratol.* 2003; 25(6):681-8.

[12]   Streissguth AP, Aase JM, Clarren SK, Randels SP, LaDue RA, Smith DF. Fetal alcohol syndrome in adolescents and adults. *JAMA* 1991;265(15): 1961-7.

[13]   Spadoni AD, McGee CL, Fryer SL, Riley EP. Neuroimaging and fetal alcohol spectrum disorders. *Neurosci. Biobehav Rev.* 2007; 31(2):239-45.

[14]   Sowell ER, Mattson SN, Kan E, Thompson PM, Riley EP, Toga AW. Abnormal cortical thickness and brain-behavior correlation patterns in indi-viduals with heavy prenatal alcohol exposure. *Cereb Cortex* 2007 Apr 18 [Epub ahead of print].

[15]   Muller RA. The study of autism as a distributed disorder. *Ment. Retard Dev. Disabil Res. Rev* 2007; 13(1):85-95.

[16]   Goodlett CR, Horn KH. Mechanisms of alcohol-induced damage to the developing nervous system. *Alcohol Res. Health* 2001; 25(3):175-84.

[17]   Haley DW, Handmaker NS, Lowe J. Infant stress reactivity and prenatal alcohol exposure. *Alcohol Clin. Exp. Res.* 2006;30(12):2055-64.

[18]   Mattson SN, Riley EP. A review of the neurobehavioral deficits in children with fetal alcohol syndrome or prenatal exposure to alcohol. *Alcohol Clin. Exp. Res.* 1998;22(2):279-94.

[19]   von Gontard A, Deget F. Gilles de la Tourette's syndrome in a girl with fetal alcohol syndrome. *J. Stud. Alcohol.* 1996;57(2):219-20.

[20]   Slavney PR, Grau JG. Fetal alcohol damage and schizophrenia. *J. Clin. Psychiatry* 1978;39(10):782-3.

[21]   Zoll B, Huppke P, Wessel A, Bartels I, Laccone F. Fetal alcohol syndrome in association with Rett syndrome. *Genet Couns* 2004; 15(2):207-12.

[22]   Sunderland T, Hampel H, Takeda M, Putnam KT, Cohen RM. Biomarkers in the diagnosis of Alz-heimer's disease: are we ready? *J. Geriatr Psychiatry Neurol.* 2006;19(3):172-9.

[23] Spivey A. The weight of lead. Effects add up in adults. *Environ. Health Perspect* 2007;115(1):A30-A36.

[24] Chen A, Cai B, Dietrich KN, Radcliffe J, Rogan WJ. Lead exposure, IQ, and behavior in urban 5- to 7-year-olds: does lead affect behavior only by lowering IQ? *Pediatrics* 2007;119(3):e650-e658.

[25] Lead exposure in children: prevention, detection, and management. *Pediatrics* 2005;116(4):1036-46.

[26] Streissguth AP, Clarren SK, Jones KL. Natural history of the fetal alcohol syndrome: a 10-year follow-up of eleven patients. *Lancet* 1985;2(8446): 85-91.

[27] Iosub S, Fuchs M, Bingol N, Stone RK, Gromisch DS. Long-term follow-up of three siblings with fetal alcohol syndrome. *Alcohol Clin. Exp. Res.* 1981;5(4):523-7.

[28] Nanson JL. Autism in fetal alcohol syndrome: a report of six cases. *Alcohol Clin. Exp. Res.* 1992;16(3):558-65.

[29] Ernhart CB, Greene T, Sokol RJ, Martier S, Boyd TA, Ager J. Neonatal diagnosis of fetal alcohol syndrome: not necessarily a hopeless prognosis. *Alcohol Clin. Exp. Res.* 1995;19(6):1550-7.

[30] Tenbrinck MS, Buchin SY. Fetal alcohol syndrome: Report of a case. *JAMA* 1975;232(11): 1144-7.

[31] Roccella M, Testa D. Fetal alcohol syndrome in developmental age. Neuropsychiatric aspects. *Minerva Pediatr* 2003;55(1):63-74.

[32] Char F. Fetal alcohol syndrome with noonan phenotype. *Birth Defects Orig. Artic. Ser* XII[5]; 81-4,1976.

[33] Gabrielli O, Salvolini U, Coppa GV, Catassi C, Rossi R, Manca A et al. Magnetic resonance imaging in the malformative syndromes with mental retardation. *Pediatr Radiol.* 1990;21(1):16-9.

[34] Miceli LA, Marsh EJ, Jarrett TE. Fetal alcohol syndrome—physical and intellectual manifestations: comparison of two cases. *J. Am. Osteopath Assoc.* 1978;78(2):116-21.

[35] Marcus JC. Neurological findings in the fetal alcohol syndrome. *Neuropediatrics* 1987;18(3):158-60.

[36] Mulvihill JJ, Klimas JT, Stokes DC, Risemberg HM. Fetal alcohol syndrome: seven new cases. *Am. J.Obstet Gynecol.* 1976; 125(7):937-41.

[37] Mattson SN, Riley EP, Jernigan TL, Ehlers CL, Delis DC, Jones KL et al. Fetal alcohol syndrome: a case report of neuropsychological, MRI and EEG assessment of two children. *Alcohol Clin. Exp. Res.* 1992;16(5):1001-3.

[38] Usowicz AG, Golabi M, Curry C. Upper airway obstruction in infants with fetal alcohol syndrome. *Am. J. Dis. Child* 1986; 140(10):1039-41.

[39] Neidengard L, Carter TE, Smith DW. Klippel-Feil malformation complex in fetal alcohol syndrome. *Am. J. Dis. Child* 1978; 132(9):929-30.

[40] Root AW, Reiter EO, Andriola M, Duckett G. Hypothalamic-pituitary function in the fetal alcohol syndrome. *J. Pediatr.* 1975; 87(4):585-8.

[41] Qazi Q, Masakawa A, Milman D, McGann B, Chua A, Haller J. Renal anomalies in fetal alcohol syndrome. *Pediatrics* 1979; 63(6):886-9.

[42] LaDue RA, Streissguth AP, Randels SP. Clinical considerations pertaining to adolescents and adults with Fetal Alcohol Syndrome. In: Sonderegger TB, ed. *Perinatal substance abuse: research findings and clinical implications*. Baltimore: Johns Hopkins Univ Press, 1992:104-31.

[43] Harris SR, MacKay LL, Osborn JA. Autistic behaviors in offspring of mothers abusing alcohol and other drugs: a series of case reports. *Alcohol Clin. Exp. Res.* 1995;19(3):660-5.

[44] Qazi QH, Madahar C, Masakawa A, McGann B. Chromosome abnormality in a patient with fetal alcohol syndrome. *Curr. Alcohol.* 1979;5:155-61.

[45] Van Biervliet JP. The foetal alcohol syndrome. *Acta Paediatr. Belg* 1977;30(2):113-6.

[46] Shaywitz SE, Caparulo BK, Hodgson ES. Devel-opmental language disability as a consequence of prenatal exposure to ethanol. *Pediatrics* 1981;68 (6):850-5.

[47] Beattie JO, Day RE, Cockburn F, Garg RA. Alcohol and the fetus in the west of Scotland. *Br.Med. J. (Clin. Res. Ed)* 1983;287(6384):17-20.

[48] Spohr HL, Willms J, Steinhausen HC. Prenatal alcohol exposure and long-term developmental consequences. *Lancet* 1993; 341(8850):907-10.

[49] O'Connor MJ, Shah B, Whaley S, Cronin P, Gunderson B, Graham J. Psychiatric illness in a clinical sample of children with prenatal alcohol exposure. *Am. J. Drug Alcohol Abuse* 2002;28 (4):743-54.

[50] Burd L, Klug M, Martsolf J, Kerbeshian J. Fetal alcohol syndrome: Neuropsychiatric Phenomics. *Neurotoxicol Teratol.* 2003;25(6):697-705.

[51] Bhatara V, Loudenberg R, Ellis R. Association of attention deficit hyperactivity disorder and gesta-tional alcohol exposure: an exploratory study. *J. Atten. Disord* 2006;9(3):515-22.

[52] Steinhausen HC, Willms J, Spohr HL. Long-term psychopathological and cognitive outcome of children with fetal alcohol syndrome. *J. Am. Acad Child Adolesc. Psychiatry* 1993; 32(5):990-4.

[53] Spohr HL, Steinhausen HC. Follow-up studies of children with fetal alcohol syndrome. *Neuropedi-atrics* 1987;18(1):13-7.

[54] Steinhausen HC, Nestler V, Spohr HL. Develop-ment and psychopathology of children with the fetal alcohol syndrome. *J. Dev. Behav. Pediatr.* 1982; 3(2):49-54.

[55] Spohr HL, Willms J, Steinhausen HC. The fetal alcohol syndrome in adolescence. *Acta Paediatr. Suppl.* 1994;404:19-26.

[56] Iosub S, Fuchs M, Bingol N, Gromisch DS. Fetal alcohol syndrome revisited. *Pediatrics* 1981;68(4): 475-9.

[57] Steinhausen HC, Gobel D, Nestler V. Psycho-pathology in the offspring of alcoholic parents. *J. Am. Acad. Child Psychiatry* 1984; 23(4);465-71.

[58] Caruso K, ten Bensel R. Fetal alcohol syndrome and fetal alcohol effects. The University of Minn-esota experience. *Minn. Med.* 1993; 76(4):25-9.

[59] Fryer SL, McGee CL, Matt GE, Riley EP, Mattson SN. Evaluation of psychopathological conditions in children with heavy prenatal alcohol exposure. *Pediatrics* 2007;119(3):e733-e741.

[60] Famy C, Streissguth AP, Unis AS. Mental illness in adults with fetal alcohol syndrome or fetal alcohol effects. *Am. J. Psychiatry* 1998; 155(4): 552-4.

In: Alcohol-Related Cognitive Disorders   ISBN: 978-1-60741-730-9
Editors: L. Sher, I. Kandel, J. Merrick pp. 125-142   © 2009 Nova Science Publishers, Inc.

Chapter 7

ADOLESCENTS WITH PRENATAL ALCOHOL EXPOSURE

Carmen Rasmussen and Katy Wyper

ABSTRACT

Prenatal alcohol exposure can result in life-long primary and secondary disabilities in affected individuals. Adolescents with Fetal Alcohol Spectrum Disorder (FASD) and/or prenatal alcohol exposure display high rates of many risky behaviors. In this chapter, we review the risky behaviors common in adolescents with FASD, including trouble with the law, delinquency, substance abuse, disrupted school experience and dropping out of school, inappropriate sexual behavior, suicidality, psychopathology, and maladaptive behavior. Next, we review factors that are related to high risk behaviors in individuals with FASD, which include executive functioning deficits, impaired decision making, and abnormalities of the prefrontal cortex. Finally, we discuss why adolescence is a period of increased risk taking and poor decision making, and how individuals with FASD are particularly vulnerable during adolescence.

INTRODUCTION

Prenatal alcohol exposure (PAE) can result in life-long primary and secondary disabilities. Fetal Alcohol Spectrum Disorder (FASD) refers to the array of physical, cognitive, behavioral, and/or learning deficits found in children whose mothers consumed alcohol during pregnancy [1]. FASD is an umbrella term used to refer to a set of more specific diagnoses, including fetal alcohol syndrome (FAS), partial fetal alcohol syndrome (pFAS), alcohol related neurodevelopmental disorder (ARND), and fetal alcohol effects (FAE) [1]. Some of the primary disabilities (reflecting CNS dysfunction) associated with FASD include neuropsychological impairments in the areas of executive functioning (EF) [2], memory, attention, visual-spatial abilities, declarative learning, planning, cognitive flexibility, processing speed [3], as well as language and motor delays [4]. Children with FASD are at risk of a lower IQ, poor academic achievement, and learning problems [5], as well as structural and functional brain damage [6]. Secondary disabilities are those that are not present from birth but rather are a consequence of the primary disabilities and limited understanding of effective interventions [6]. In this paper, we first review the high-risk behaviors that are common in adolescents with FASD, and then we discuss factors (e.g., EF deficits, damage to the prefrontal cortex, and other factors that put youth at risk) that contribute to these problematic behaviors.

HIGH RISK BEHAVIORS IN ADOLESCENTS WITH FASD

Secondary Disabilities of FASD

In a large-scale study, Streissguth and colleagues [7-8] investigated the impact of secondary disabilities on the lives of fetal alcohol affected children, adolescents and adults. Using The Life History Interview (LHI), they measured the prevalence of six common secondary disabilities among 415 individuals (ranging in age from 6-51 years) with FAS or FAE. Disrupted school experience was reported in 14% of children and 61% of adolescents/adults. Trouble with the law occurred in 14% of children, and 60% of adolescents and adults. Over 90% of the sample had mental health problems, with no difference in the rate between children and adolescents or adults. Eight percent of children in the study had been confined (for psychiatric purposes only), whereas half (50%) of adolescents and adults had been both hospitalized (for psychiatric reasons and for drug/alcohol treatment) and incarcerated. Alcohol/drug problems were reported by 35% of the subjects who were 12 years or older, with alcohol use being more prevalent than drug use. Finally, 39% of children and 49% of adolescents and adults displayed inappropriate sexual behaviors including promiscuity. Sixty-seven percent of the participants had experienced physical or sexual abuse or had been victims of domestic violence; 50 of the 53 females who reported inappropriate sexual behavior had also been victims of sexual or physical abuse, or had experienced violence toward them selves.

The authors identified five key factors that can protect affected individuals from these negative outcomes, including living in a high quality positive home environment, long-term living arrangements, not being exposed to violence, receiving services for developmental disabilities, and having a diagnosis before age 6 [7-8]. Three variables were identified as increasing the likelihood of secondary disabilities: receiving an FAE diagnosis instead of an FAS diagnosis, having an IQ above 70, and higher scores on the Fetal Alcohol Behavior Scale, which measures behaviors typical of fetal alcohol exposure. An important point to note regarding the results of this study is that the majority (80%) of this sample size was not reared by their biological mother, and many of the participants had been victims to adverse experiences other than being prenatally exposed to alcohol. Psychological tests on the subjects in this study showed that people affected by FASD have specific deficits in adaptive behaviors, which may play a role in risk taking. Interestingly, adaptive behavior scores fell significantly below normative scores of non-FASD individuals with similar IQ [7,8].

Delinquency and FASD

Some of the deficits that often characterize individuals with FASD are problems with judgment, understanding consequences, planning and organization, controlling impulses, and making decisions [6]. Moreover, individuals with PAE have been shown to exhibit maladaptive behaviors such as impulsivity, teasing/bullying, dishonesty (lying, cheating and stealing), avoiding school or work, intentional destruction of property, sexual inappropriateness, physical aggression, and self-injury [9]. FASD has also been linked to behavior problems and delinquency in adolescents, as well as problems with alcohol and drug use [10].

In a study comparing problem behaviors in fetal alcohol-exposed children (aged 6-16) and children with ADHD, Nash et al [11] found that the alcohol-exposed children displayed higher rates of problematic behaviors than did children with ADHD. Of particular concern among the fetal alcohol group was the prevalence of delinquent behaviors, including cruelty, bullying, or meanness to others (48% of children), lying or cheating (90% of children), stealing from home (59% of children) and stealing from outside of the home (45% of children). Furthermore, 97% children with fetal alcohol exposure lacked guilt after misbehaving.

Using a standardized moral maturity questionnaire, Schonfeld et al [12] found a significant association between heavy PAE and higher rates of delinquency, as well as lower overall moral maturity as compared with a control group matched on gender, age, handedness, socioeconomic status (SES) and ethnicity. The authors investigated 27 youth (aged 10-18 years) and found that adolescents prenatally exposed to heavy amounts of alcohol scored higher than did control subjects on the Conduct Disorder Questionnaire, which measures such delinquent behaviors as truancy, stealing, lying, and fighting. Not surprisingly, the home environment was predictive of delinquency in that youth living in biological or foster homes were more likely to engage in delinquent behaviors than youth living in adoptive homes. A deficit in moral reasoning and judgment is one factor that may potentially underlie delinquent behavior. One piece of evidence supporting this association is that both moral immaturity and delinquent behavior become more severe with age. Clearly, individuals with FASD are particularly prone to delinquent behaviors; yet some researchers suggest that this inclination may be due to factors (e.g., family and individual characteristics) other than PAE [13].

FASD in the Criminal Justice System

Adolescents and adults with FASD are at particular risk of ending up in the criminal justice system. Recall that in Streissguth's studies [7,8] 60% of adolescents and adults with FASD had been in trouble with the law and 50% had been confined. Fast et al (14) evaluated the prevalence of FASD in a sample of almost 300 youth who had been remanded for a psychiatric inpatient assessment. The results were alarming: during the time the study was conducted, 23.3% of youth had either full FAS (1%) or FAE (22.3%). This ratio is more than 10 times the incidence in the general population. However, only 3 of the 67 youth identified in this study as being alcohol-exposed had had a previous diagnosis, highlighting the lack of awareness in the general community about the impact of fetal alcohol exposure. A recent

Canadian report indicated that 10% of inmates had an FASD, which is a proportion 10 times higher than that in the general population (15).

FASD and Psychopathology

Streissguth and O'Malley [16] and others have noted poor neuropsychiatric outcomes associated with FASD, particularly in terms of maladaptive behavior, mental illness, and alcohol and drug dependence. In young adults, PAE is also associated with increased psychiatric disorders and traits [17]. O'Connor et al [18] noted very high rates of psychiatric disorders among children with PAE, with 87% of their sample meeting the criteria for a psychiatric disorder; 61% for mood disorders, 35% for bipolar disorder, and 26% for major depressive disorder. Furthermore, PAE has been associated with depressive symptoms among 6-year-old children, particularly for girls [19].

Fryer et al [20] compared psychopathological factors among alcohol-exposed children and non-alcohol-exposed children matched on age, gender, and SES. The authors found that almost all (97.44%) of the alcohol-exposed children were diagnosed with an axis 1 disorder, which is a much larger proportion than the 40% of non-alcohol-exposed control children. Specifically, alcohol-exposed children differed from non-affected children in ADHD, depressive disorders, oppositional defiant disorder (ODD), conduct disorder (CD), and specific phobia, with the greatest difference being in the ADHD category. The prevalence of ODD and CD in individuals with FASD may help to explain the over-representation of these individuals in the justice system.

In a large-scale longitudinal study on the association between prenatal exposure to alcohol in the form of binge drinking and the development of psychiatric disorders, Barr et al [17] assessed 431 participants on 23 different axis I and II disorders from the DSM-IV (e.g. substance abuse, depression, anxiety, psychosis, paranoid personality, antisocial personality, narcissistic personality, etc.). Participants who were prenatally exposed to one or more binges of alcohol were significantly more likely to meet the criteria for six of the disorders: axis I somatoform disorder (odds ratio of 7.21), substance dependence/abuse disorders (odds ratio of 2.56), and axis II paranoid (odds ratio of 3.87), passive-aggressive (odds ratio of 3.27), antisocial (odds ratio of 3.01), and personality disorders (odds ratio of 2.24). In a pilot study on the psychosocial profile of 11 young women with FASD, Grant et al [21] documented significant problems with psychiatric illness, behavioral issues, and a poor quality of life.

FASD and Alcohol/Drug Use

The link between fetal alcohol exposure and the later development of alcohol/drug problems is well-documented [22-26]. For instance, in a longitudinal birth cohort study, Alati et al [24] examined the effect of PAE on the development of alcohol disorders. The authors interviewed over 2500 subjects at 21 years of age and found that 25% of the participants had an alcohol disorder, and 6.1% were classified as alcohol dependent. Individuals born to mothers who had consumed three or more drinks per occasion during pregnancy were more than 2 (2.47 to 2.04) times more likely to have alcohol disorders in early adulthood. Moreover, this effect remained after taking into consideration whether the individual had a father and/or sibling with an alcohol disorder. Prenatal exposure to alcohol in early pregnancy was found to be a stronger predictor of alcohol disorder than was exposure in late pregnancy [23].

In a related view, Yates et al [25] examined the link between PAE and later dependence on nicotine, alcohol, and drugs. The authors used the adoption paradigm in an attempt to separate genetic and environmental in-fluences on substance dependence. Participants (ranging in age from 18 to 45 years) were identified as high-risk adoptees if their biological parent was diagnosed as having an alcohol and/or drug dependency, or antisocial personality. As well, documentation was reviewed from adoption agencies, hospitals, and prisons to determine whether the participants had confirmed PAE. A control group was matched on adoption agency, age, sex, and age of the biological mother at the time of adoption. The results suggest that PAE has a significant influence on the development of nicotine, alcohol, and illicit drug dependence, even when controlling for biological parental alcohol abuse and dependence. However, Yates and colleagues also found that peer influence had a highly significant effect on substance dependence. That is, associating with individuals identified by adoptive parents as "bad friends" influenced greatly the dependence on nicotine, alcohol, and drugs. Thus, whereas biological factors are significant in the development of substance dependency, environmental influences must not be ruled out entirely.

Similarly, Baer et al [22] studied drinking behavior in 433 young adults prenatally exposed to alcohol and found that PAE was significantly related to alcohol problems later in life, even after controlling for factors such as sex, family history of alcohol-related problems, prenatal exposure to nicotine/drugs, and family environment. Specifically, while rates of drinking appear to be unaffected by PAE, alcohol dependency and the negative consequences of heavy drinking (such as passing out, becoming sick, etc.) were significantly correlated with fetal alcohol exposure.

Griesler and Kandel [23] found a significant effect of maternal prenatal drinking on adolescent drinking, even after controlling for potentially influential factors such as maternal current drinking, maternal delinquency in adolescence, closeness to the mother, parental monitoring of the adolescent, prohibition of drinking, and behavior problems in childhood. The daughters of moderate to heavy drinkers were three times more likely to have consumed alcohol during their lifetime than were daughters whose mothers did not drink while pregnant. Moreover, these subjects were six times more likely to have consumed alcohol during the past year than were non-exposed females. Interestingly, this effect was not found in boys whose mothers drank alcohol during pregnancy.

Suicidality in FASD

The rate of suicide and attempted suicide increases significantly in late teens and early adulthood, and this behavior occurs more frequently in rural as opposed to urban communities [27]. Many of the risk factors for suicide, such as mental health problems, disrupted school experience, trouble with the law, confinement, inappropriate sexual behavior, impulsivity, alcohol/drug problems, dependent living, and problems with employment overlap with the disabilities of those affected by FASD. Although sparse, the literature on suicidality in adolescents and adults with FASD establishes that such individuals are at particular risk of suicide and attempted suicide. O'Malley and Huggins [28] carried out a pilot study of 11 individuals affected by FASD. Over half [6] the participants reported attempted suicide, with two being classified as a severe attempt, three as a moderate-risk attempt, and one as a low-risk attempt. This rate of attempted suicide is drastically higher than the general Canadian population rate of 4.6%. While the results are preliminary, they shed light on an issue that clearly deserves attention.

Social Deficits and FASD

Kelly et al [29] suggest that one issue underlying many behavioral problems reported by individuals with FASD is a general social deficit. Children exposed to alcohol tend to have poor social skills [30], and research indicates that the social impairments may become more pronounced with age [31-32]. Streissguth et al [33] found that among adolescents and adults with FASD (mean age 17 years) adaptive functioning skills were at the level of a 7-year-old, with deficits being most pronounced on socialization skills. Such children also tended to have difficulty understanding the consequences of their actions and lacked initiative, understanding of social cues, and reciprocal friendships. Many adolescents also tended to lie, cheat, steal, lack consideration, and appear unhappy [33].

FACTORS RELATING TO HIGH RISK BEHAVIORS

Executive Functioning Deficits in FASD

One of the core deficits in children with FASD is on measures of EF (executive functioning). The term executive functioning refers to higher-order cognitive processes involved in thought and action under conscious control [34], usually to achieve a goal [35-36], and involves such abilities as planning, monitoring, switching, inhibiting, and energization [37]. Executive functioning is thought to be mediated by the frontal cortex [38-39].

Mattson et al [40] found that, relative to typically developing children, children (aged 8 to 15 years) with heavy PAE had significant difficulty on EF tests of planning ability (a tower test), cognitive flexibility, inhibition, concept formation, and reasoning. Children with PAE are also impaired on EF tests measuring verbal and non-verbal fluency [41]. Similarly, Kodituwakku et al [42] found that children with FASD display deficits on measures of planning and strategy use (tower test), attention, and some measures of fluency. Many researchers have found children and adolescents with FASD to be impaired on the Wisconsin Card Sorting Test (WCST), which involves inhibition, set-shifting, and use of feedback [3,36,42-43].

In a recent study, we found that children and adolescents (aged 8 to 16 years) with FASD had difficulty on many tests of EF, including measures of cognitive flexibility, inhibition, some measures of verbal fluency, abstract thinking, deductive reasoning, hypothesis testing, problem solving, and concept formation [44]. Furthermore, older children showed more difficulty relative to the norm than did younger children on tests measuring verbal fluency, inhibition, deductive reasoning and verbal abstract thinking, suggesting that some EF deficits may become more pronounced during adolescence. Finally, adults with FASD are impaired on a variety of EF tasks [45-46].

The bulk of this previous research has been on cognition-based or 'cool' EF tests, which are thought to be mediated by the dorsolateral prefrontal cortex [34,36]. In contrast, emotion-related or 'hot' executive functions are associated with the orbitofrontal cortex (including orbital/ventral and medial regions), which is involved in the regulation of motivated and emotional behavior, processing affective and non-affective stimuli, response to reward and punishment stimuli, and decision making [34,36,47].

Kodituwakku et al [48] compared children and adolescents (aged 7 to 19 years) with PAE, with and without FAS (n = 20), with control children on an emotional-related learning task (visual discrimination reversal task), and a conceptual set-shifting task (WCST). On the visual discrimination reversal task, participants were shown two images, one of which was previously randomly chosen to be rewarding (emotional aspect). The participant had to figure out which was the rewarding and non-rewarding image by receiving feedback and gaining points for correct responses. After the participant reached the learning criterion, the reinforcement contingencies changed. An extinction condition was also included in which both images were non-rewarding. The alcohol-exposed children were slower to reach the learning criterion, completed fewer reversals, and had more variability in extinction as compared with the control group. Group differences on reversal learning were still significant after controlling for performance on the WCST (conceptual set-shifting) and intelligence. Thus, Kodituwakku et al [48] concluded that conceptual and emotional set-shifting could be independent functions in FASD, although the children displayed deficits in both areas.

Recently, Rasmussen et al [49] found that children with FASD displayed deficits on a parental behavioral rating scale of EF; the Behavioral Rating Inventory of Executive Functioning (BRIEF). The mean scores on all scales were in the clinically significance range, with children showing most difficulty on inhibition (particularly for females), working memory, and initiation. Similarly, Kodituwakku et al [48] found that relative to control subjects, children and adolescents with FASD showed deficits on the Children's Executive Functioning Scale, a behavioral measure of social appropriateness, inhibition, problem solving, initiative, and motor planning.

Executive Function Deficits and Risk Behavior

The significant EF deficits in individuals with FASD likely contribute to the numerous high risk behaviors common during adolescence. Specifically, impairments in EF skills such as planning, organizing, cause-effect reasoning, learning from past mistakes, and the lack of social adaptability may be factors related to why youth with FASD are overrepresented in the justice system [50]. The connection between poor EF and juvenile delinquency has been well-documented in other populations. For example, juvenile offenders are impaired on many tests of neuropsychological functioning, including cognitive ability, inhibition and set-shifting, visuospatial functioning, planning, and verbal memory-language functioning [51]. Adolescent and adult offenders demonstrate EF deficits in the areas of social competency, judgment, foresight, perspective taking, impulsivity, immaturity, and aggression.

Inhibition appears to be one aspect of EF that is strongly related to delinquency and high-risk behaviors. Inhibition deficits predict future violent offences [52] and later delinquency among male adolescents [53-54]. The relation between impaired inhibition and delinquency is strongest among early-onset offenders [55]; inhibition is also related to moral maturity [12] and juvenile psychopathy [56-57]. The substantial inhibition deficits common in alcohol-affected individuals (particularly during adolescence) likely places such individuals at increased risk for problematic behaviors that result from an inability to control one's behavior. Finally, the inappropriate sexual behaviors common in individuals with FASD may also be related to underlying EF deficits, as previous research shows that sex offenders are impaired on tests of attention and EF [58].

Frontal Lobe Functions

Given the host of EF deficits common in individuals with FASD, a better understanding of frontal lobe pathology and development is necessary. In short, the prefrontal cortex is divided into three zones: the medial frontal cortex, which is involved in motivated behavior and apathy (motor, cognitive, and affective); the orbitofrontal cortex, which is involved in more socially based functions and decision making; and the dorsolateral cortex, which is involved in more cognitive executive functions [38]. The frontal lobe is involved in EF, planning, reasoning, and impulse control [59]. In particular, the dorsolateral cortex is involved in inhibition and thinking ahead, and the ventromedial cortex in emotion regulation, learning from experience, and weighing risks and rewards [59].

Decision Making and Prefrontal Cortex

The orbitofrontal cortex and specifically the ventromedial areas of the prefrontal cortex have both been implicated in decision making [60]. Individuals with damage to the ventromedial prefrontal cortex (VMPF) are notoriously poor at making decisions in real life and perform poorly on tests of decision making [61]. An example of the latter is the Gambling Task [62], which involves real-life decision making, with rewards and punishments. On this task, the participants are given $2,000 in fake money to start and are told to choose cards one at a time from any of four decks. After the card is selected, the game indicates whether the participant wins or loses money (or both), and the goal is to gain as much money as possible (the games lasts for 100 trials). Unknown to the participants from the outset, two of the decks are advantageous and two are disadvantageous. The advantageous decks allow the participants to gain more money in the long run because these cards have fewer losses, but they also have lower immediate rewards. The two disadvantageous decks yield less money in the long run because they have more losses, but they also have higher immediate rewards. Participants with VMPF damage consistently choose more often from the disadvantageous decks, whereas normal and brain-damaged controls choose more often from the advantageous decks. Bechara et al [62] concluded that individuals with VMPF damage are insensitive to punishment and consequences and are driven by immediate rewards, and these findings have been reinforced in other studies [63].

Studies of individuals with damage to the VMPF have indicated that such individuals display unique personality and behavioral characteristics, similar to those of sociopaths. In fact, some researchers use the term 'acquired sociopathology' to refer to these patients [61].

The characteristics include the following: (1) low and inappropriate emotion expression; (2) poor emotional control (frustration, irritability); (3) impaired decision making, particularly in social contexts (deficits in judgment, flexibility, social appropriateness and empathy); (4) poor goal-directed behavior (difficulty with planning, initiation, and diligence); and (5) lack of recognition of these personality and behavior changes [61]. Interestingly these behavioral characteristics are strikingly similar to those of individuals with FASD and PAE.

Case studies [61] of individuals with early damage to the prefrontal cortex (in particular the VMPF) yield even more similarities to individuals with FASD. The first case review by Tranel [61] is of a girl who had sustained damage to her frontal lobe at 15 months of age (but had been normally developing until the incident). As she grew up, she was characterized as not responding to punishment, displaying problematic behaviors in school, running away from home, stealing, lying, and cheating. She was sent to treatment facilities, but was released because she ran away, did not follow the rules, and did not make improvements. She was sexually active at a young age, had a baby at 18 years of age, and had difficulty caring for this baby as she was apathetic and did not meet the baby's needs. She became dependent on external supports and could not keep a job, because she skipped work, was not dependable, and did not follow rules. She did not show regret or guilt and was indifferent toward her problematic behaviors [61].

The second case was of a boy who had a tumor in his frontal lobe at age 3 years [61]. In school, he displayed poor attention and impulsivity and had difficulty interacting with other children, adapting to new situations, and handing in assignments on time. Later, he demonstrated poor judgment, difficulty in keeping a job and managing money, and poor hygiene. He stole, lied, and could not keep friends. He fathered a child at a young age and was irresponsible in caring for the child. He had difficulty thinking ahead and planning, and he too showed little guilt or remorse. On subsequent testing, both patients had difficulty on certain cognitive EF tests, the Gambling Task, as well as tests of social and moral reasoning [61].

Both individuals described above sustained very specific damage to the frontal cortex (the VMPF) and as a result, they present with a host of social, moral, and decision making deficits that are very similar to those experienced by individuals with FASD. Given these similarities, one may hypothesize that individuals with FASD may also have damage to the prefrontal cortex, which would help explain some of their high risk behaviors and poor decision making.

Frontal Cortex and FASD

Considerable evidence has shown that prenatal exposure to alcohol has a negative effect on the frontal cortex. Children and adolescents with PAE show a smaller brain size and abnormal brain shape, specifically in the frontal lobe and left hemisphere [64]. Prenatal alcohol exposure is associated with reduced brain growth in the frontal lobe [65-66]. Wass et al [67] found that among fetuses of pregnant women, alcohol exposure was specifically related to a decreased size of the frontal cortex, with many of the fetuses having heavy alcohol exposure being below the 10th percentile in frontal cortex size. Mihalick et al [68] examined behavior as well as neuron numbers in the medial prefrontal cortex (mPFC) in rats prenatally exposed to alcohol. The rats had a significant decrease in the number of neurons in the mPFC and had difficulty with reversal learning, inhibition, and transfer of learning.

Adolescents and adults with FASD show altered brain metabolism in the frontal areas [69]. In rats, PAE reduces the level of complexin proteins in the frontal cortex, which are thought to be involved in neuro-transmission, synaptic plasticity, and cognition [70]. Further, individuals with PAE show significant cortical thickness in the right frontal regions [71]. Thus, PAE appears to have a unique negative effect on the development of the frontal cortex, but more research is needed in this area to substantiate these claims and to better understand the mechanisms involved.

Prefrontal Cortex Development during Adolescence

Clearly, damage to the prefrontal cortex leads to unique behavioral and social deficits, and the prefrontal cortex is especially susceptible to PAE. We also know that adolescence is a period when individuals are particularly vulnerable to risk taking behaviors, and this too is related to the development of the prefrontal cortex. The frontal lobe area of the brain continues to develop well into adolescence and even into the mid-twenties [59] and the prefrontal cortex is one of the last brain areas to mature [72]. In particular, the brain areas involved in inhibition, response to rewards and risks, and emotional regulation show significant changes during adolescence [73]. Performance on the Gambling Task improves throughout adolescence, suggesting that the VMPF cortex and its connections are developing at this time [74].

Steinberg [73] suggests that adolescents are particularly vulnerable because their behavioral and cognitive systems are developing at a different rate than their brains. The requirement to regulate behavior and affect also increases during adolescence. Steinberg [73] theorizes that during early adolescence, pubertal changes result in sensation-seeking, emotional arousal, and reward orientation, yet the frontal systems of the brain continue to mature until late adolescence, and this disjunction results in adolescents being particularly vulnerable to risky behaviors and difficulty regulating their behavior and affect. The disparity between adolescent brain development and behavior is particularly disconcerting for adolescents with FASD who are known to have abnormalities of the prefrontal cortex, which likely creates an even larger gap between their behavioral and cognitive capabilities, making them especially vulnerable to high risk behaviors.

Adolescent Decision Making and Risk Taking

Risky behavior during adolescence is very concerning because it is related to poor adult outcomes, and, in general, the earlier the risky behavior occurs the poorer the adult outcome [75]. Risky Behaviors from the National Youth Risk Behavior Survey [76] are defined as substance use (alcohol, drugs, tobacco, smoking), sexual intercourse and lack of protection, fighting, carrying weapons, driving risks (drinking, not wearing seatbelt), suicide attempts, lack of exercise, and being overweight.

Risk taking may be related to a number of factors during adolescence: sensation-seeking, impulsivity, thrill-seeking, depression, and individual differences. Adolescent goals are more for immediate gratification, and adolescents may also view some risky behaviors as rational [59]. Adolescents and adults differ on many aspects of behavior. Adolescents have more difficulty with delay of gratification, inhibition, thinking ahead, and planning. Compared with adults, adolescents are less able to recognize and learn from consequences and view the consequences as less harmful [59]. These behavioral differences may be related to immature brain development during adolescence [59].

Studies indicate that adolescents are aware of the risks and negative outcomes of their behaviors, but that they change their thinking patterns to accommodate the incongruities between their behaviors and the associated risks [77]. Interestingly, when looking at perception of hypothetical risks, few differences are found between adolescents and adults, but in real life, adolescents are more likely than adults to take risks [73]. Steinberg [73] suggests that adolescents do not rationally weigh the risks and consequences of their behaviors and that they may be more influenced by social and emotional factors, such as peer pressure and impulse control and differences in self regulation, resulting in poorer decisions and more risky behaviors.

Peer groups also influence risky behavior. One study of adolescents (13-16 years), youth (18-22 years), and adults (24 and older) found that younger individuals were more likely to take risks than were older individuals, and risky behavior was related to peers [78]. When the participants were in a group of peers, they demonstrated more risky behavior and focused more on the pros than on the cons of the risks than when alone. The adolescent and youth groups were the most influenced by peers. The social skills deficits in children with FASD can result in such children having difficulty making and keeping friends, and thus many turn to delinquent peers for acceptance. These peers, who display many problematic behaviors, will have a negative effect on a child with FASD, who is easily influenced, vulnerable, and naïve.

Adolescents are, in principle, able to make rational decisions but in reality, their decisions are highly influenced by (a) the context in which they are situated, (b) peers, (c) unfamiliar events, (d) spur of the moment and passionate situations, and (e) how they weigh the risks and benefits of their decisions [59].

At-Risk Youth

Other groups of youth are particularly at risk for problematic and risk taking behaviors. Rosser et al [79] examined EF between two groups of youth: a substance and criminally involved group and a resilient group who were not substance or criminally involved but who came from similar demographics. Both groups were tested on the Tower of Hanoi test (a measure of fontal lobe functioning), in which the participant must move disks across a pegboard while following various rules, that is thought to involve inhibition and planning. The substance and criminally involved youth made more moves in less time, indicative of impulsive responding, as compared with the resilient youth who made fewer moves and spent more time doing them. The authors suggest that the behavior of the substance and criminally involved youth is consistent with difficulty with inhibition, which is associated with a less developed prefrontal cortex [76].

Interestingly, evidence has suggested that perceived intelligence is related to risk outcomes. Jaccard et al [80] found that adolescents who perceived themselves as being more intelligent were less likely to display adverse risk outcomes, regardless of their actual IQ. Furthermore, children who are maltreated are at risk for many adolescent risk behaviors [81]. Maltreated youth and youth in foster care display elevated rates of risky behavior (e.g., sexual, delinquent, and violent behaviors; substance use; see [82] for a review). These factors put youth with FASD at even more risk because such individuals may perceive themselves as less intelligent and are often maltreated and placed in foster care.

Children with externalizing behavioral disorders are also vulnerable to risk taking behaviors. Ernst et al [83] suggest that children with externalizing behavior disorders (e.g., ADHD, conduct) may have deficits in decision making because they are impulsive, prefer immediate rewards, and have a tendency to take risks. The authors found that adolescents with externalizing behavior problems had difficulty on a decision making task (the Gambling Task).

Children with ADHD and learning disorders (LD) are at particular risk for antisocial behavior [84]. Specific individual factors that put children at risk for delinquent behavior include "impulsivity; the inability to adopt a future time perspective or to grasp future consequences of behavior; the inability to delay gratification; the inability to self-regulate emotions, especially temper; the need for stimulation and excitement; low harm avoidance; low frustration tolerance; central nervous system dysfunction; low cortical arousal; a predisposition to aggressive behavior; low general aptitude or intelligence; exposure to violence and abuse (as either a victim or a witness); alienation; rebelliousness; association with deviant peers; favorable attitudes toward deviant behavior; peer rejection; alcohol and drug abuse; and early onset of aggressive or problem behavior" [84]. The authors also review family, community and societal factors, including limited resources as a result of deprivation and unemployment, parental antisocial behavior and alcoholism, harsh and inconsistent discipline, poor supervision, low maternal education, family conflict, inconsistency in caregivers and living situations, poor attachment with family, exposure to violence, as well as many community variables such as community disorganization, violence and illegal activities, and isolation [84]. Finally, school-related factors included poor academic achievement, low motivation, peer rejection and interacting with antisocial peers, placement in special education classes, school disorganization, and poor supervision of students. Academic failure may lead to low self esteem and feelings of incompetence and hopelessness [84]. Many of the individual and family factors that put children at risk for antisocial behaviors are common in the life of a child with FASD, again making them even more vulnerable to delinquency.

Children with ADHD have difficulty with self control, inhibition, and regulation of attention, emotions, and behavior, and tend to seek novelty and stimulation, which can make them more susceptible to risky behaviors [85].

Further, co-morbid externalizing and internalizing conditions, as well as EF deficits put these children at increased risk. The risky behaviors common in adolescents with ADHD include difficulties in school, dangerous and distracted driving, sexual activity, substance use, and delinquent behaviors [86]. Children with FASD also tend to have deficits in attention [87] and have a high co-morbidity of ADHD, which could contribute to their behavioral problems.

CONCLUSIONS

Children with FASD display a high rate of risky behaviors, including trouble with the law, delinquency, substance abuse, disrupted school experience and dropping out of school, inappropriate sexual behavior, and suicidality. Such individuals are also prone to psychopathology, particularly in terms of maladaptive behavior and mental illness. The risky behaviors in adolescents with FASD likely result in part from poor decision making and EF deficits, as evidenced by a poorly developed prefrontal cortex. The prefrontal cortex, which is directly implicated in decision making, is negatively affected by PAE, thus putting individuals with FASD at increased risk for engaging in problematic behaviors. Risk taking increases during adolescence because adolescents tend to be more sensation-seeking and reward-driven but have a prefrontal cortex that is still developing. In individuals with FASD, adolescence is a time of heightened vulnerability as these individuals have even more of a gap between their brain/cognitive development and their behaviors. The decision making and EF deficits common in FASD combined with other factors known to increase risky behaviors (ADHD, LD, being maltreated or in foster care, poor environment) predispose adolescents with FASD to risk taking behaviors. An emphasis on improving the cognitive capabilities of individuals with FASD, particularly in terms of EF and decision making, is essential to reduce risky behaviors and to improve the quality of life among individuals with FASD. Furthermore, efforts to ameliorate the environmental factors that make these children even more vulnerable are crucial.

REFERENCES

[1]   Chudley AE, Conry J, Cook JL, Loock C, Rosales T, LeBlanc N. Fetal Alcohol Spectrum Disorder: Canadian guidelines for diagnosis. *Can. Med. Assoc. J.* 2005;172:S1-21.

[2]   Rasmussen C. Executive functioning and working memory in Fetal Alcohol Spectrum Disorder. *Alcohol Clin. Exp. Res.* 2005;29:1359-67.

[3]   Carmichael Olson H, Feldman J, Streissguth AP, Sampson PD, Bookstein FL. Neuropsychological deficits in adolescents with fetal alcohol syndrome: Clinical findings. *Alcohol Clin. Exp. Res.* 1998;22:1998-2012.

[4]   Mattson SN, Riley EP. A review of the neurobehavioral deficits in children with Fetal Alcohol Syndrome or prenatal exposure to alcohol. *Alcohol Clin. Exp. Res.* 1998;22(2):279-94.

[5]   Streissguth AP, Barr HM, Sampson PD, Bookstein FL. Prenatal alcohol and offspring development: The first fourteen years. *Drug Alcohol Depend* 1994;36:89-99.

[6]   Streissguth AP. *Fetal Alcohol Syndrome: A guide for families and communities.* Baltimore, MD: Paul H Brookes, 1997.

[7]   Streissguth AP, Bookstein FL, Barr HM, Sampson PD, O'Malley K, Young JK. Risk factors for adverse life outcomes in fetal alcohol syndrome and fetal alcohol effects. *J. Dev. Behav. Pediatr.* 2004;25(4):228-38.

[8]   Streissguth AP, Barr HM, Kogan J, Bookstein FL. Understanding the occurrence of secondary disabilities in clients with fetal alcohol syndrome (FAS) and fetal alcohol

effects (FAE): *Final report to the Centers for Disease Control and Prevention*. Seattle: Univ Washington, Fetal Alcohol Drug Unit, 1996.

[9]   LaDue RA, Streissguth AP, Randels SP. *Clinical considerations pertaining to adolescents and adults with fetal alcohol syndrome*. Baltimore, MD: Johns Hopkins Univ Press, 1992.

[10]   Carmichael Olson H, Streissguth AP, Sampson PD, Barr H, Bookstein FL, Thiede K. Association of prenatal alcohol exposure with behavioral and learning problems in early adolescence. *J. Am. Acad. Child Adolesc. Psychiatry* 1997;36(9):1187-94.

[11]   Nash K, Rovet J, Greenbaum R, Fantus E, Nulman I, Koren G. Identifying the behavioural phenotype in Fetal Alcohol Spectrum Disorder: Sensitivity, specificity and screening potential. *Arch. Women Ment. Health* 2006;9:181-6.

[12]   Schonfeld AM, Mattson SN, Riley EP. Moral maturity and delinquency after prenatal alcohol exposure. J. *Stud. Alcohol* 2005;66:545-54.

[13]   Lynch ME, Coles CD, Corley T, Falek A. Examining delinquency in adolescents differentially prenatally exposed to alcohol: The role of proximal and distal risk factors. *J. Stud. Alcohol.* 2003;64: 678-86.

[14]   Fast D, Conry J, Loock C. Identifying fetal alcohol syndrome among youth in the criminal justice system. *J. Dev. Behav. Pediatr.* 1999;20:370-2.

[15]   Sanders C. Ten percent of inmates victims of Fetal Alcohol. *Winnipeg Free Press.* 2007.

[16]   Streissguth AP, O'Malley K. Neuropsychiatric implications and long-term consequences of Fetal Alcohol Spectrum Disorders. *Semin. Clin. Neuropsychia*try 2000;5:177-90.

[17]   Barr HM, Bookstein FL, O'Malley KD, Connor PD, Huggins JE, Streissguth AP. Binge drinking during pregnancy as a predictor of psychiatric disorders on the Structured Clinical Interview for DSM-IV in young adult offspring. *Am. J. Psychiatry* 2006;163(6):1061-5.

[18]   O'Connor MJ, Shah B, Whaley S, Cronin P, Gunderson B, Graham J. Psychiatric illness in a clinical sample of children with prenatal alcohol exposure. *Am. J. Drug Alcohol Abuse* 2002;28(4): 743-54.

[19]   O'Connor MJ. Prenatal alcohol exposure and infant negative affect as precursors of depressive features in children. *Infant Ment. Health J.* 2001; 22(3):291-9.

[20]   Fryer S, McGee C, Matt G, Riley E, Mattson S. Evaluation of psychopathological conditions in children with heavy prenatal alcohol exposure. *Pediatrics* 2007;119(3):e733-41.

[21]   Grant T, Huggins J, Connor P, Streissguth A. Quality of life and psychosocial profile among young women with Fetal Alcohol Spectrum Disorders. *Ment Health Aspects Dev. Disabil.* 2005;8(2):33-9.

[22]   Baer J, Sampson PD, Barr H, Connor PD, Streissguth AP. A 21-year longitudinal analysis of the effects of prenatal alcohol exposure on young adult drinking. *Arch. Gen. Psychiatry* 2003;60:377-85.

[23]   Griesler PC, Kandel DB. The impact of maternal drinking during and after pregnancy on the drinking adolescent offspring. *J. Stud. Alcohol* 1998;59(3):292-304.

[24]   Alati R, Mamun AA, Williams GM, O'Callaghan M, Najman JM, Bor W. In utero alcohol exposure and prediction of alcohol disorders in early adulthood: A birth cohort study. *Arch. Gen. Psychiat* 2006;63(9):1009-15.

[25] Yates WR, Cadoret RJ, Troughton EP, Stewart M, Giunta TS. Effect of fetal alcohol exposure on adult symptoms of nicotine, alcohol, and drug dependence. *Alcohol Clin. Exp. Res*. 1998;22(4): 914-20.

[26] Spear NE, Molina JC. Fetal or infantile exposure to ethanol promotes ethanol ingestion in adolescence and adulthood: A theoretical review. *Alcohol Clin. Exp. Res*. 2005;29(6):909-29.

[27] Baldwin M. Fetal Alcohol Spectrum Disorders and suicidality. *Int. Conf. Fetal Alcohol Spectrum Disord*. Victoria, BC: March 2007.

[28] O'Malley K, Huggins J. Suicidality in adolescents and adults with Fetal Alcohol Spectrum Disorders. *Can. J. Psychiat* 2005;50(2):125.

[29] Kelly SJ, Day N, Streissguth AP. Effects of prenatal alcohol exposure on social behavior in humans and other species. *Neurotoxicol. Teratol*. 2000;22(2):143-9.

[30] Roebuck T, Mattson S, Riley E. Behavioral and psychosocial profiles of alcohol-exposed children. *Alcohol Clin. Exp. Res*. 1999;23:1070-6.

[31] Whaley S, O'Connor M, Gunderson B. Comparison of the adaptive functioning of children prenatally exposed to alcohol to a nonexposed clinical sample. *Alcohol Clin. Exp. Res*. 2001; 25:1018-24.

[32] Thomas S, Kelly S, Mattson SN, Riley EP. Comparison of social abilities of children with fetal alcohol syndrome to those of children with similar IQ scores and normal controls. *Alcohol Clin. Exp. Res*. 1998;22:528-33.

[33] Streissguth AP, Aase J, Clarren S, Randels SP, LaDue R, Smith DF. Fetal alcohol syndrome in adolescents and adults. *J. Amer. Med. Assoc*. 1991; 265:1961-7.

[34] Zelazo PD, Mueller U. Executive function in typical and atypical development. In: Goswami U, ed. *Blackwell handbook of childhood cognitive development*. Malden, MA: Blackwell, 2002:445-69.

[35] Welsh MC, Pennington BF, Grossier DB. A normative-developmental study of executive function: A window of prefrontal function in children. Dev Neuropsychol 1991;7:131-49.

[36] Kodituwakku PW, Kalberg W, May PA. The effects of prenatal alcohol exposure on executive functioning. *Alcohol Res. Health* 2001;25(3):192-8.

[37] Stuss D. New approaches to prefrontal lobe testing. In: Miller BL, Cummings JL, eds. *The human frontal lobes*. 2nd ed. New York, NY: Guilford, 2007:292-305.

[38] Stuss DT, Knight RT, eds. *Principles of frontal lobe function*. New York, NY: Oxford Univ Press, 2002.

[39] Miller BL, Cummings JL, eds. *The human frontal lobes: Functions and disorders*. New York, NY: Guilford, 2007.

[40] Mattson SN, Goodman AM, Caine C, Delis DC, Riley EP. Executive functioning in children with heavy prenatal alcohol exposure. *Alcohol Clin. Exp. Res*. 1999;23(11):1808-15.

[41] Schonfeld AM, Mattson SN, Lang A, Delis DC, Riley EP. Verbal and nonverbal fluency in children with heavy prenatal alcohol exposure. *J. Stud. Alcohol*. 2001;62(2):239-46.

[42] Kodituwakku PW, Handmaker NS, Cutler SK, Weathersby EK, Handmaker SD. Specific impairments in self-regulation in children exposed to alcohol prenatally. *Alcohol Clin. Exp. Res*. 1995; 19:1558-64.

[43] Coles CD, Platzman KA, Raskind-Hood CL, Brown RT, Falek A, Smith IE. A comparison of children affected by prenatal alcohol exposure and attention deficit, hyperactivity disorder. *Alcohol Clin. Exp. Res.* 1997;21(1):150-61.

[44] Rasmussen C, Bisanz J. Executive functioning in children with Fetal Alcohol Spectrum Disorder. *Poster presented at the Cognitive Development Society (CDS).* San Diego, CA; 2005 Oct.

[45] Connor PD, Sampson PD, Bookstein FL, Barr HM, Streissguth AP. Direct and indirect effects of prenatal alcohol damage on executive function. *Dev. Neuropsychol.* 2000;18(3):331-54.

[46] Kerns KA, Audrey D, Mateer CA, Streissguth AP. Cognitive deficits in nonretarded adults with fetal alcohol syndrome. *J. Learn Disabil.* 1997;30(6):685-93.

[47] Ogar J, Gorno-Tempini M. The orbitofrontal cortex and the insula. In: Miller BL, Cummings JL, eds. *The human frontal lobes.* 2nd ed. New York: Guilford, 2007:59-67.

[48] Kodituwakku PW, May PA, Clericuzio CL, Weers D. Emotion-related learning in individuals prenatally exposed to alcohol: An investigation of the relation between set shifting, extinction of responses, and behavior. *Neuropsychologia* 2001; 39(7):699-708.

[49] Rasmussen C, McAuley R, Andrew G. Parental ratings of children with Fetal Alcohol Spectrum Disorder on the Behavior Rating Inventory of Executive Function (BRIEF) *J. FAS Int.* 2007; 5(2):1-8.

[50] Moore T, Green M. Fetal Alcohol Spectrum Disorder (FASD): A need for a closer examination by the criminal justice system. *Crim. Rep.* 2004; 19:99-108.

[51] Olvera RL, Semrud-Clikeman M, Pliszka SR, O'Donnell L. Neuropsychological deficits in adolescents with conduct disorder and comorbid bipolar disorder: A pilot study. *Bipolar. Disord* 2005;7(1):57-67.

[52] Parker JS, Morton TL, Lingefelt ME, Johnson KS. Predictors of serious and violent offending by adjudicated male adolescents. *N. Amer J. Psychol.* 2005;7(3):407-17.

[53] Kerr M, Tremblay RE, Pagani L, Vitaro F. Boys' behavioral inhibition and the risk of later delinquency: *Arch. Gen. Psychiat.* 1997;54(9):809-16.

[54] Tremblay RE, Pihl RO, Vitaro F, Dobkin PL. Predicting early onset of male antisocial behavior from preschool behavior: *Arch. Gen. Psychiat* 1994; 51(9):732-9.

[55] Taylor J, Iacono WG, McGue M. Evidence for a genetic etiology of early-onset delinquency: *J. Abnorm. Psychol.* 2000;109(4):634-643.

[56] Roussy S, Toupin J. Behavioral inhibition deficits in juvenile psychopaths: *Aggressive Behav.* 2000; 26(6):413-424.

[57] Lynam DR, Gudonis L. The development of psychopathy: *Annu. Rev. Clin. Psychol.* 2005;1(1): 381-407.

[58] Kelly T, Richardson G, Hunter R, Knapp M. Attention and executive function deficits in adolescent sex offenders: *Child Neuropsychol.* 2002; 8(2):138-43.

[59] Reyna VF, Farley F. Risk and rationality in adolescent decision making: Implications for theory, practice, and public policy. *Psychol. Sci. Public Interest* 2006;7(1):1-44.

[60] Bechara A, Damasio H, Damasio AR. Emotion, decision making and the orbitofrontal cortex: *Cereb Cortex* 2000;10(3):295-307.

[61] Tranel D, ed. Emotion, *decision making, and the ventromedial prefrontal cortex.* New York, NY: Oxford Univ Press, 2002.

[62] Bechara A, Damasio AR, Damasio H, Anderson SW. Insensitivity to future consequences following damage to human prefrontal cortex. *Cognition* 1994;50(1-3):7-15.

[63] Bechara A, Tranel D, Damasio H. Characterization of the decision-making deficit of patients with ventromedial prefrontal cortex lesions. *Brain* 2000;123(11):2189-202.

[64] Sowell ER, Thompson PM, Mattson SN, Tessner KD, Jernigan TL, Riley EP, et al. Regional brain shape abnormalities persist into adolescence after heavy prenatal alcohol exposure. *Cereb Cortex* 2002;12:856-65.

[65] Riley EP, McGee CL, Sowell ER. Teratogenic effects of alcohol: A decade of brain imaging. *Am. J. Med. Genet Part C.* 2004;127C:35-41.

[66] Spadoni AD, McGee CL, Fryer SL, Riley EP. Neuroimaging and Fetal Alcohol Spectrum Disorders. *Neurosci. Biobehav. R* 2007;31(2):239-45.

[67] Wass TS, Persutte WH, Hobbins JC. The impact of prenatal alcohol exposure on frontal cortex development in utero. *Am. J. Obstet. Gynecol.* 2001; 185:737-42.

[68] Mihalick SM, Crandall JE, Langlois JC, Krienke JD, Dube WV. Prenatal ethanol exposure, generalized learning impairment, and medial prefrontal cortical deficits in rats. *Neurotoxicol Teratol* 2001;23:453-62.

[69] Fagerlund A, Heikkinen S, Autti-Ramo I, Korkman M, Timonen M, Kuusi T, et al. Brain metabolic alterations in adolescents and young adults with Fetal Alcohol Spectrum Disorders. *Alcohol Clin. Exp. Res.* 2006;30(12):2097-104.

[70] Barr AM, Hofmann CE, Phillips AG, Weinberg J, Honer WG. Prenatal ethanol exposure in rats decreases levels of complexin proteins in the frontal cortex. *Alcohol Clin. Exp. Res.* 2005;29 (11):1915-20.

[71] Sowell ER, Mattson S, Kan E, Thompson P, Riley EP, Toga A. Abnormal cortical thickness and brain-behavior correlation patterns in individuals with heavy prenatal alcohol exposure. *Cereb Cortex* 2007;12:856-65.

[72] Casey B, Giedd JN, Thomas KM. Structural and functional brain development and its relation to cognitive development. *Bio Psychol.* 2000;54(1-3):241-57.

[73] Steinberg L. Cognitive and affective development in adolescence. *Trends Cog. Sci.* 2005;9(2):69-74.

[74] Hooper CJ, Luciana M, Conklin HM, Yarger RS. Adolescents' performance on the Iowa Gambling Task: Implications for the development of decision making and ventromedial prefrontal cortex. *Dev. Psychol.* 2004;40(6):1148-58.

[75] Pergamit M, Huang L, Lane J. *The long term impact of adolescent risky behaviors and family environment*: Washington, DC: US Dept Health Human Serv, 2001.

[76] The United States Center for Disease Control and Prevention. *National Youth Risk Behavior Survey,* 2005.

[77] Gerrard M, Gibbons FX, Benthin AC, Hessling RM. A longitudinal study of the reciprocal nature of risk behaviors and cognitions in adolescents: What you do shapes what you think, and vice versa. *Health Psychol* 1996;15(5):344-54.

[78] Gardner M, Steinberg L. Peer influence on risk taking, risk preference, and risky decision making in adolescence and adulthood: An experimental study. *Dev. Psychol.* 2005;41(4):625-35.

[79] Rosser R, Stevens S, Ruiz B. Cognitive markers of adolescent risk taking: A correlate of drug abuse in at-risk individuals. *Prison J.* 2005;85(1): 83-96.

[80] Jaccard J, Dodge T, Guilamo-Ramos V. Meta-cognition, risk behavior, and risk outcomes: The role of perceived intelligence and perceived knowledge. *Health Psychol.* 2005;24(2):161-70.

[81] Nickoletti P, Taussig HN. Outcome expectancies and risk behaviors in maltreated adolescents. *J. Res. Adolescence* 2006;16(2):217-28.

[82] Taussig HN. Risk behaviors in maltreated youth placed in foster care: A longitudinal study of protective and vulnerability factors. *Child Abuse Negl.* 2002;26(11):1179-99.

[83] Ernst M, Grant SJ, London ED, Contoreggi CS, Kimes AS, Spurgeon L. Decision making in adolescents with behavior disorders and adults with substance abuse. *Am. J. Psychiat* 2003;160 (1):33-42.

[84] Appalachia Educational Laboratory. Preventing antisocial behavior in disabled and at-risk. http:// www.ldonline.org/article/5973. Accessed January 9, 2007.

[85] Goldstein S. AD/HD and adolescence: A formula for risk and vulnerability. http://www.schwab learning.org/articles.aspx?r=736andf=allart. Accessed January 9, 2007.

[86] Goldstein S. Risky behavior in teens with AD/HD. http://www.schwablearning.org/ articles.aspx?r=737. Accessed January 9, 2007.

[87] Jacobson JL, Jacobson SW. Effects of prenatal alcohol exposure on child development: Alcohol Res Health 2002;26(4):282-6.

In: Alcohol-Related Cognitive Disorders   ISBN: 978-1-60741-730-9
Editors: L. Sher, I. Kandel, J. Merrick pp. 143-156   © 2009 Nova Science Publishers, Inc.

Chapter 8

FETAL ALCOHOL SPECTRUM DISORDER: CURRENT ISSUES AND FUTURE DIRECTIONS

Kelly Nash, Erin Sheard, Joanne Rovet and Gideon Koren

ABSTRACT

Fetal Alcohol Spectrum Disorders (FASDs) currently represent the leading cause of mental retardation in North America, ahead of Downs syndrome and cerebral palsy. The damaging effects of alcohol on the developing brain have a cascading impact on the social and neurocognitive profiles of affected individuals. Researchers investigating the profiles of children with FASD have found impairments in learning and memory, executive functioning, and language, as well as hyperactivity, impulsivity, poor communication skills, difficulties with social and moral reasoning, and psychopathology. The primary goal of this chapter is to examine current issues pertaining to the identification of a behavioural phenotype in FASD, as well as addressing related screening and diagnostic concerns. We conclude that future research initiatives comparing children with FASD to non-alcohol exposed children with similar cognitive and socioemotional profiles should aid in uncovering the unique behavioural phenotype for FASD.

INTRODUCTION

After decades of research, the damaging effects of prenatal alcohol exposure have been well documented. Historically, suggestions that prenatal alcohol exposure may lead to neurodevelopmental impairments were dismissed for explanations en vogue at the time, such as heredity, leaving the teratogenic effects of prenatal alcohol exposure (PAE) unrecognized until the late 1960s. At this time consistent results emerged in France and the United States [1], drawing similar conclusions regarding the appearance and behaviour of alcohol-exposed offspring. By 1973 the constellation of symptoms resulting from prenatal alcohol exposure was named Fetal Alcohol Syndrome [2]. It is now widely recognized that PAE may lead to fetal alcohol spectrum disorder (FASD), a term which encompasses both full-blown fetal alcohol syndrome (FAS), as well as fetal alcohol effects (FAE) or alcohol-related neurodevelopment disorder (ARND), which present as behavioural or cognitive abnormalities in the absence of dysmorphology [3] Even at low doses, PAE has been associated with long-term cognitive difficulties [4] and there is no known safe ingestion limit [5]. To date, researchers are still working to fully understand the scope and mechanisms of prenatal alcohol effects.

Early research appeared to indicate that PAE represented a continuum of severity of effects, with FAS being the most severe form [6]. However, recent research has demonstrated that this is not the case; individuals with FAS, partial FAS, and ARND exhibit equivalent impairments [7] and qualitatively similar cognitive profiles (8, 9). Although the pattern of primary disabilities is similar in FAS and ARND (7,10), ARND may, in fact, be even more susceptible to negative long term outcomes than FAS (11). Due to the presence of characteristic facial dysmorphology, a child with FAS is more likely to be identified and diagnosed early in life, while diagnosis is often delayed or missed in ARND, even though the deficits are evident by 4 years of age or earlier [11]. Despite years of research highlighting the negative impact of PAE, it is still a leading cause of mental retardation [12] and neurobehavioural deficits in cognitive and socioemotional functioning [13]. In the US, the prevalence of FAS is estimated at 0.5-2 per 1000 and FASD at 10 per 1000 births [14], and comparable estimates of 1 to 6 per 1000 live births have been made in Canada [6], with variations within and between countries [15]. Despite a number of primary prevention efforts, the rates have remained unchanged over the years.

Screening and Diagnosis

FASD is not a simple clinical diagnosis; rather, it is an umbrella term for wide range of possible consequences of PAE. Our use of the term FASD includes the full spectrum of disorders resulting from PAE. Diagnosis of FAS was first standardized by the Institute of Medicine [16] and is defined by International Classification of Disease (ICD-9 and ICD-10). Under IOM classification, four criteria must be met for a diagnosis of FAS: (i) severe intrauterine or postnatal growth deficiency with height and/or weight at less than 10th percentile, (ii) craniofacial dysmorphology including smooth philtrum, thin vermilion, and small palpebral fissures, (iii) central nervous system damage that is either structural or neurological; although functional impairment is also assessed it is not sufficient for diagnosis, and (iv) prenatal alcohol exposure, which may be confirmed, unknown, or disconfirmed. Diagnostic categories include FAS with or without confirmation of alcohol exposure, partial FAS, ARND, or alcohol-related birth defects (ARBD).

Alternative diagnostic methods include the University of Washington's 4-Digit Diagnostic Code [17], which ranks each of the 4 key features highlighted in the IMO guidelines on a Likert scale to derive a clinical code that differentiates FAS from other categories. The Washington Likert scales offer more precision in describing and measuring the features than the IOM guidelines (1=absence of feature, 4= extreme expression). Given the overlapping criteria, in practice the IOM and Washington guidelines are often integrated in diagnosis. For instance, the Canadian Guidelines blend IOM and Washington criteria in addition to criteria for diagnosing FAS, partial FAS and ARND [6].

Given the time and resources required to diagnosis FASD, screening tools are being developed to identify at-risk individuals who require further assessment. Novel screening tools using biomarkers such as fatty acid ethyl ester levels in meconium or hair are currently being developed in an effort to support the more traditional diagnostic procedures [18]. Also promising are rapid and easy-to-administer screening tools. These screening tools may be especially helpful in accessing populations in remote or rural areas. One example screening tool, developed by Nash and colleagues [19], utilizes 12 items from a standardized tool for assessing behaviour, the Child Behaviour Checklist, shown to reliably differentiate between FASD, attention-deficit hyperactivity disorder (ADHD), and typically developing children. A specific subset of characteristics have been identified as unique to FASD, which includes a lack of guilt, cruelty, acting young, lying or cheating, stealing from home or stealing from outside of the home. In an effort to expedite the diagnostic process, children identified through screening could then be referred for diagnostic evaluation (see table 1).

The importance of early diagnosis must be emphasized. Although the primary and secondary disabilities from PAE are extremely costly, debilitating, and lifelong, they can be mitigated with early intervention [11]. Current research findings show a substantial protective effect of early diagnosis and treatment in alleviating later associated mental health problems [11]. Diagnosis of FAS may also be easier in young children as craniofacial dysmorphology becomes less pronounced over time [20]. The single biggest challenge to early intervention is delayed diagnosis.

Cognitive Profile

An important question in FASD research is whether or not PAE results in a clearly definable and identifiable cognitive-behavioural profile also known as a phenotype. FASD certainly has a complex and varied phenotypical profile, although key cognitive and behavioural features are evident [13].

The resultant primary disabilities reflect the extensive and varied nature of the brain damage caused by PAE. Alcohol acts on the central nervous system through multiple mechanisms and impacts several cognitive domains. In contrast to the dysmorphology, the primary cognitive disabilities do not show age related improvement [21] and persist into adulthood [11]. Although this is not an exhaustive list, primary disabilities in FASD include reduced IQ, learning disabilities and lower achievement scores, language difficulties, attention problems, working memory, executive functioning, learning, and problems in socioemotional functioning.

A more thorough understanding of the cognitive-behavioural phenotype in FASD is necessary for improving diagnosis, particularly as it relates to neuropsychological impairment and to developing effective interventions. Indeed, the severe consequences of PAE on the developing brain demonstrate the need for a diagnostic process that should more strongly emphasize the neuropsychological profile [6, 9].

A comprehensive review of the cognitive deficits associated with FASD is beyond the scope of this chapter; thus, we seek to highlight key areas of impairment and identify the gaps and limitations in our understanding of the cognitive-behavioural outcome in FASD.

Table 1. Screening checklist for FASD behavioral phenotype

Step 1: Identifying behaviour suggestive of FASD

The following questions should be asked of the child's parent/guardian to determine whether the child's behaviour is suggestive of FASD.

1. Does your child act too young for his/her age?
2. Does your child have difficulty concentrating, and can't pay attention for long?
3. Is your child disobedient at home?
4. Does your child lie or cheat?
5. Does your child lack guilt after misbehaving?
6. Does your child act impulsively and without thinking?
7. Does your child have difficulty sitting still/is restless/hyperactive?

If the parent/caregiver answers 'yes' to at least six out of seven items this is suggestive of FASD with 86% sensitivity and 82% specificity. If the child does not exhibit behavior consistent with ADHD (i.e., answer is negative for questions 2, 6, 7), then a score of 3 out of the 4 following questions needs to be positive:

1) Does your child lack guilt after misbehaving?
2) Does your child lie or cheat.
3) Is your child disobedient at home?
4) Does your child act too young for his/her age?

Step 2: Differentiating FASD from ADHD

a) The child needs to exhibit two of the following three items

1. Does your child experience lack guilt after misbehaving?
2. Does your child display acts of cruelty, bullying or meanness to others?
3. Does your child act young for his/her age?

b) OR the child needs to exhibit three of the following six items:

1. Does your child experience lack guilt after misbehaving?
2. Does your child display acts of cruelty, bullying or meanness to others?
3. Does your child act young for his/her age?
4. Does your child steal from home?
5. Does your child steal outside of home?
6. Does your child lie and cheat?

IQ and Academic Achievement

Prenatal alcohol exposure has a deleterious effect on IQ and academic achievement and may result in profound learning disabilities. The earliest work on FASD linked prenatal alcohol exposure to significant impairments in IQ, with the severity of dysmorphology relating to degree of mental deficiency [22]. Indeed, alcohol is widely recognized as the leading cause of preventable mental retardation, occurring more frequently than the other two most common birth defects combined [12] and the deficits are enduring across the lifespan [11].

Streissguth and colleagues (23) reported an almost 7-point decrease in IQ in 7-year old children exposed to an ounce of alcohol per day mid-gestation. Severity of dysmorphogenesis correlates with IQ, with IQ scores ranging from 55 if manifestations are severe to a normal score of 82 with less pronounced manifestation [22]. Average IQ estimates using standardized instruments are typically between 65-70, although variability ranges from about 20 to 105 (normal). For instance, Abel [24] reported an average IQ of 67, with over half scoring below 70, indicating mental retardation. IQ is impaired on both the verbal and performance scales [25], although verbal deficits may become increasingly marked with age [26]. Unlike spelling and reading, a particular deficit in mathematics has been noted, with deficits exceeding those that would be predicted from IQ scores (4). This impaired intellectual function contributes to academic difficulty [4], despite evidence that IQ is not the best predictor of academic achievement [27].

Children and adolescents with FASD report negative academic experiences and parents and teachers report below average academic achievement. Average academic functioning falls at the grade 2-4 level [4], a level of functioning that does not solely reflect IQ and points to other contributing factors like a poor post-natal environment. Children with PAE are at increased risk for learning disabilities and are more likely to be placed in remedial or special educational settings, to be suspended, or to drop-out [28]. In children without full-blown FAS, however, the learning disabilities are sometimes mistakenly attributed to motivational issues rather than brain damage, compounding the problem [29] and limiting access to proper intervention. As the child ages and the academic demands increase, the problems are marked with greater task difficulty, a need for more monitoring and an increasingly negative attitude toward academic work.

Language and Communication

Language problems as indicated on IQ measures have been consistently noted; for example, Streissguth et al [28] noted a discrepancy between verbal IQ and performance IQ, with greater impairment in the verbal realm. Indeed, language problems tend to present early in FASD [30] and may be a trigger for referral. Initial language delays are often exacerbated hearing disorders, as hearing is important in normal language acquisition, reception, and expression [31]. In 3-year olds, Greene and colleagues [32] found no relation between alcohol exposure and language in the absence of craniofacial dysmorphometry; however, some speech delay and language deficits may reflect a higher-level central auditory processing disorder [31]. Language delays are also evident into the school years, but because individuals with FASD tend to have adequate social speech (33) the language and communication problems may go unnoticed or untreated. A child with FASD may seem to be typically verbal, but there is often a striking contrast between their use of verbal language and the comprehension and understanding.

The most salient impairments are in receptive language [27], resulting in difficulty understanding and interpreting information, whereas expressive language is stronger. That said, both components of language are impaired in FASD, with 82% showing receptive and 76% showing expressive [34] performance greater than one standard deviation below the mean. The severity of language impairment in FASD correlates with socioemotional disturbance [35], emphasizing the critical role of language in social cognition. Language is a significant area of impairment in FASD, but there are few studies with a primary emphasis on language.

Attention

Attentional deficits are a core problem in FASD. However, the precise nature of these deficits, and more specifically the relation between attentional deficits in FASD and Attention Deficit Hyperactivity Disorder (ADHD), is not well understood. Linnet et al. [36] reviewed maternal factors in ADHD risk and found no significant relation between PAE and ADHD, although many others have found a link between PAE and ADHD symptoms (37) and ADHD prevalence may increase with amount of PAE [38].

ADHD is the most commonly reported co-morbid disorder associated with FASD [38], yet some researchers believe that the attentional profile in FASD is unique or presents as an ADHD phenocopy. O'Malley and Nanson [37] reviewed literature on the FASD-ADHD link and concluded that in FASD, ADHD is more likely to be the earlier-onset inattentive subtype. Coles and colleagues (39) reported that children with FAS had more attentional problems in encoding and shifting focus, whereas non-exposed children with ADHD were most impaired in focused and sustained attention. Subtle differences in attentional profiles may help to differentiate ADHD-like symptoms resulting from PAE from ADHD. This point is particularly poignant given that some individuals with FASD may be misdiagnosed as having ADHD as the primary diagnosis, resulting in missed or inappropriate interventions. Furthermore, the aspects of attention most impaired in FASD – encoding and shifting – implicate a more general problem in working memory and executive functioning respectively. Burden et al [40] investigated the effect of PAE on the components of attention and found that working memory was the aspect of attention most adversely affected by PAE. Consistent with Coles et al [39], no association between sustained or focused attention and PAE was found.

Executive Functioning and Working Memory

Executive functioning (EF) refers to a broad spectrum of goal-oriented abilities that include working memory, planning, decision-making, cognitive flexibility, inhibition, reasoning, and problem solving. Global deficits affecting both the verbal and non-verbal domains in multiple aspects of EF have been reported in FASD from childhood to adulthood, independent of facial dysmorphology (9). Although few studies have looked at the role of affect, emotional EF processing also appears to be impaired in FASD [41]. Mattson et al [42] demonstrate that EF impairments are not merely a reflection of component process deficits in basic skills such as reading or motor speed, but are true deficits in higher level executive processes. Rasmussen [9] highlights the sweeping EF impairments as measured on a variety of tasks across the lifespan and independent of FASD diagnosis. Deficits may be particularly evident in high demand settings such as school, as reflected by the fact that teacher ratings indicate greater EF difficulty that parent ratings [26].

Cognitive flexibility, for example, involves dividing and shifting attention. On a task requiring the child to flexibly meet changing criterion, as in the Wisconsin Card Sorting Task, children with FASD will persevere on the wrong category after the criterion has shifted [39]. Planning is similarly impaired, illustrated by poor performance on tasks such as the Tower of Hanoi, which requires the participant to plan ahead to make the minimum number of moves necessary to replicate a pattern [43]. Deficits in inhibitory control have been reported and map onto reported behavioural problems of impulsivity, although inhibitory deficits may be task specific. For example, Mattson et al [42] reported impairments in response-inhibition on a Stroop task requiring participants to inhibit one response (word naming) in lieu of the correct response (colour naming), although this deficit has not been consistently found [43].

Working memory (WM) is a central feature of EF processes and is thought by some to be the core deficit in FASD (43). Deficits in the maintenance and manipulation of information are observed on measures such as forward and backward digit span [23], trigram recall with rehearsal prevention (44), and the n-Back task [45]. These WM deficits are thought to underlie the extensive EF deficits in FASD [43] and may exceed impairment predicted by overall IQ (44, but see also reference 9 for deficits mediated by IQ). Although WM and EF deficits in FASD are widely acknowledged, Rasmussen [9] highlights the paucity of interventions and treatments designed to target EF impairments; the undertaking of such important initiatives should serve to reduce the prevalence of secondary disabilities such as academic failure, socio-behavioural disturbance, and societal difficulty.

Learning and Memory

In FASD, learning and memory impairments are particularly evident in spatial memory and associative learning and are primarily linked to acquisition rather than storage and retrieval of information [46]. The affected memory processes are mediated by the hippocampus and not coincidentally, the hippocampus is thought to be particularly vulnerable to the effects of PAE [47]. Animal models support the hypothesis of vulnerability in spatial learning suggestive of hippocampal impairment; alcohol exposed rats are impaired at the Morris water maze, T-mazes and radial arm mazes [48]. There is evidence that children and adolescents exposed to alcohol prenatally have similar visuo-spatial memory deficits. Comparable deficits in Morris water maze learning is evident [49] and Uecker and Nadel [50] found particular problems with object location and only subtle weaknesses in object memory, although others have found spatial deficits to be confounded with impaired verbal memory [51]. Indeed, verbal memory may not be spared and deficits are reported [25].

Memory impairment has a variety of forms, and encompasses recall omission, intrusions, perseverations and poor recognition discrimination [46]. Impairments in recall are more consistently reported than deficits in recognition [52] and impairments may affect explicit tasks more so than implicit [53]. Even in infants, recognition memory may be relatively spared [54]. Furthermore, verbal learning is impaired, but there does appear to be normal long-term retention of previously learned visual and verbal material. For example, difficulty learning a word list is not related to difficulty in retaining the list once learned [55]. Priming also seems to be effective and there are typical benefits of previous exposure in FASD relative to controls [53]. Memory impairment in FASD is complex; both visual and verbal recall is affected, but recognition, long-term retention, implicit memory and specific sub-types of memory (e.g. facial memory; 50), may be spared.

Socioemotional Functioning

Socioemotional functioning, defined as the interplay between affective processing and social behaviour, is not well understood in FASD. As typical development of language and executive functioning may be critical for the development of social cognition, impairments may have a cascading impact on socioemotional development [35,56]. Indeed, degree of cognitive dysfunction reliably predicts behaviour problems in FASD [41]. The problems in socioemotional behaviour also exceed what would be expected based on IQ alone and seem to reflect an arrest, rather than a delay, in function [57].

Key problems in atypical attachment and difficulty regulating state [58] begin in early infancy with irritability, disturbed sleep patterns, and feeding problems. In early life, the children may present as talkative, rambling, and overly inquisitive, therefore overshadowing behaviour problems [29]. At approximately school age, children with FASD show an arrest in socioemotional development [59] with problems typically presenting around 6 years of age [60]. Steinhausen [61] reports that in childhood, severe deficits in the social domain are seen, highlighted by characteristic reports of impulsivity, aggression, and mood lability.

More subtle deficits in the ability to infer from another's perspective (theory of mind), in the reading of social cues, and in social withdrawal negatively impacts social interaction. Parents report that the children are highly prone to hyperactivity, disruptivity, impulsivity, and delinquency [62, 63] and teachers report less social competency and greater aggression in the classroom [64]. The negative behaviour is accompanied by a lack of guilt, an inability to learn from past mistakes and deficits in moral judgments as they pertain to relationships with others [19, 65]. Parent ratings suggest that the most salient deficit may be improper socialization as it relates to responding to social cues, considering consequences of actions, and interpersonal skills [66].

The socioemotional defects evident in infancy do not attenuate over time, but rather increase with age [57] and may actually set the stage for disrupted socioemotional function across the lifespan [58]. Similarly, maladaptive social behaviours may have a more detrimental impact with age, as behaviours that seem cute or endearing at a young age become increasingly inappropriate. For instance, excessive friendliness and affection [67] raise concerns about safety and appropriate social interaction [29]. The long-term consequences of socioemotional impairment are distressing.

Psychopathology

Socioemotional deficits may precede the onset of psychopathology or other secondary disabilities which include mental health disorders (90%), drug and alcohol abuse (50%), trouble with the law (50%), trouble at school (60%), and employment problems (70%) to name a few [29], often putting individuals at risk for developing psychopathology. In a recent attempt to address this issue, Fryer et al [68] examined psychopathological conditions (secondary disabilities) in a community sample of children with FASD. Results revealed that 97% of the FASD sample met criteria for a DSM-IV axis I disorder. Compared to controls, children with FASD were more likely to meet criteria for ADHD, depressive disorders, Oppositional Defiant Disorder (ODD), Conduct Disorder (CD), and specific phobia. Perhaps most notable from their findings is that there were substantially more co-morbid diagnoses in the alcohol exposed group (71%) than the control group, particularly among the disruptive disorders. This finding is especially important as many of the social and emotional problems reported by parents and teachers of children with FASD are disruptive in nature [19, 35].

One aspect of psychopathology that has received little attention in adolescents with FASD is moral maturity. Using Kohlberg's stages of moral development, Schonfeld and colleagues [56] were the first to examine this issue; compared to controls, children with FASD were focused on reducing negative consequences on the self (stage 2), whereas controls demonstrated concern for others and social norms (stage 3). Additionally, children with FASD were found to have poor social judgment, trouble learning from experience, failure to consider the consequences of their actions, and demonstrated difficulty communicating in social contexts. Most notable from this study is the finding that underdeveloped levels of moral maturity in children with FASD were related to elevated levels of delinquency, particularly stealing and conduct problems. Interestingly, similar results were found by Nash et al [19] using individual items from the Child Behaviour Checklist.

Recently, efforts have been made to elucidate the early manifestations and specific underpinnings of the social and emotional disturbances seen in FASD. However, what remains striking is that the majority of research efforts continue to focus heavily on the cognitive deficits, whereas secondary disabilities and their precursors remain largely ignored in individuals with FASD.

CONCLUSIONS

Research examining the FASD profile has evolved tremendously since FAS was first introduced into the medical literature in the 1960s. It is clear that early intervention and a positive rearing environment provides the best chance of circumventing the devastating secondary disabilities for individuals with FASD. However, research also indicates that we are far from understanding the full spectrum of strengths and weaknesses that typify individuals with FASD, thus impeding our ability to identify a specific neurobehavioural phenotype.

Identifying the phenotype is further complicated by the fact that many children with FASD also share profiles or co-morbid diagnoses of children with other clinical conditions, such as ADHD, Oppositional-Defiant Disorder, and Conduct Disorder. Therefore, it will be especially important for future research to delineate the FASD profile from these other childhood disorders.

Until then, developing interventions that specifically target FASD will be difficult. On a societal level, with the cost estimated to be up to 1.4 million dollars in intervention across the lifespan of an individual with FASD (4), FASD remains a critical public health concern and can only be alleviated with early intervention initiatives. In both economic and individual terms, the costs of the impact of the disorder on the families of individuals with FASD are immeasurable, consequently, in so far as it is possible, the primary goal of research efforts should be to provide hope for individuals with FASD and their families.

REFERENCES

[1]   Lemoine P, Harousseau II, Borteyru JP, Menuet JC. Les enfants de parents alcooliques: anomalies observees a propos de 127 cas. *Ouest Med* 1968;21: 476-82.

[2]   Jones KL, Smith DW, Ulleland CN, Streissguth AP. Pattern of malformation in offspring of chronic alcoholic mothers. *Lancet* 1973;1(7815):1267-71.

[3]   Clarren SK, Smith DW. The fetal alcohol syndrome. Lancet 1978;35(10):4-7.

[4]   Streissguth AP, Aase JM, Clarren SK, Randels SP, LaDue RA, Smith DF. Fetal alcohol syndrome in adolescents and adults. *JAMA* 1991;265(15):1961-7.

[5]   Koren G, Caprara D, Jacobson S, Chan D, Porter K. Is it all right to drink a little during pregnancy? *Can. Fam Physician* 2004;50:1643-44.

[6]   Chudley AE, Conry J, Cook JL, Loock C, Rosales T, LeBlanc N et al. Fetal alcohol spectrum disorder: Canadian guidelines for diagnosis. *CMAJ* 2005;172(5 Suppl):S1-S21.

[7]   Mattson SN, Riley EP, Gramling L, Delis DC, Jones KL. Neuropsychological comparison of alcohol-exposed children with or without physical features of fetal alcohol syndrome. *Neuropsychology* 1998;12(1):146-53.

[8]   Mattson SN, Riley EP. A review of the neurobehavioral deficits in children with fetal alcohol syndrome or prenatal exposure to alcohol. *Alcohol Clin. Exp. Res.* 1998;22(2):279-94.

[9]   Rasmussen C. Executive functioning and working memory in fetal alcohol spectrum disorder. *Alcohol Clin. Exp. Res.* 2005;29(8):1359-67.

[10] Steinhausen HC, Spohr HL. Long-term outcome of children with fetal alcohol syndrome: psychopathology, behavior, and intelligence. *Alcohol Clin. Exp. Res.* 1998;22(2):334-8.

[11] Streissguth AP, Bookstein FL, Barr HM, Sampson PD, O'Malley K, Young JK. Risk factors for adverse life outcomes in fetal alcohol syndrome and fetal alcohol effects. *J. Dev. Behav. Pediatr.* 2004;25(4):228-38.

[12] Abel EL, Sokol RJ. Maternal and fetal characteristics affecting alcohol's teratogenicity. *Neurobehav Toxicol Teratol* 1986; 8(4):329-34.

[13] Kodituwakku PW. Defining the behavioral phenotype in children with fetal alcohol spectrum disorders: a review. *Neurosci. Biobehav. Rev.* 2007;31(2):192-201.

[14] May PA, Gossage JP. Estimating the prevalence of fetal alcohol syndrome: a summary. *Alcohol. Res. Health* 2001;25(3):159-67.

[15] Nulman I, O'Hayon B, Gladstone J, Koren G. The effects of alcohol on the fetal brain: the nervous system tragedy. In Slikker W, Chang LW, editors. *Handbook of Developmental Neurotoxicology*. San Diego, CA: Acad Press, 1998:567-86.

[16] Institute of Medicine of the National Academy of Sciences Committee to Study Fetal Alcohol Syndrome . In: Stratton K, Howe C, Battaglia F, eds. *Fetal alcohol syndrome. Diagnosis, epidemiology, prevention and treatment*. Washington, DC: Nat Acad Press, 1996:17-32..

[17] Astley SJ, Clarren SK. A fetal alcohol syndrome screening tool. *Alcohol Clin. Exp. Res.* 1995;19(6):1565-71.

[18] Caprara DL, Nash K, Greenbaum R, Rovet J, Koren G. Novel approaches to the diagnosis of fetal alcohol spectrum disorder. *Neurosci. Biobehav. Rev.* 2007;31(2):254-60.

[19] Nash K, Rovet J, Greenbaum R, Fantus E, Nulman I, Koren G. Identifying the behavioural phenotype in Fetal Alcohol Spectrum Disorder: sensitivity, specificity and screening potential. *Arch. Womens Ment Health* 2006; 9(4):181-6.

[20] Spohr HL, Steinhausen HC. Follow-up studies of children with fetal alcohol syndrome. *Neuropediatrics* 1987;18(1):13-7.

[21] Steinhausen HC, Willms J, Spohr HL. Long-term psychopathological and cognitive outcome of children with fetal alcohol syndrome. *J. Am. Acad Child Adolesc. Psychiatry* 1993;32(5):990-4.

[22] Streissguth AP, Herman CS, Smith DW. Intelligence, behavior, and dysmorphogenesis in the fetal alcohol syndrome: a report on 20 patients. *J. Pediatr.* 1978;92(3):363-7.

[23] Streissguth AP, Barr HM, Sampson PD. Moderate prenatal alcohol exposure: effects on child IQ and learning problems at age 7 ½ years. *Alcohol Clin. Exp. Res.* 1990;14(5):662-9.

[24] Abel EL. *Fetal Alcohol Syndrome*. Oradell, NJ: Med Economics, 1990.

[25] Mattson SN, Riley EP, Gramling L, Delis DC, Jones KL. Heavy prenatal alcohol exposure with or without physical features of fetal alcohol syndrome leads to IQ deficits. *J. Pediatr.* 1997;131(5):718-21.

[26] Rasmussen C, Horne K, Witol A. Neurobehavioral functioning in children with fetal alcohol spectrum disorder. *Child Neuropsychol.* 2006;12(6):453-68.

[27] LaDue RA, Streissguth AP, Randels SP. Clinical considerations pertaining to adolescents and adults with fetal alcohol syndrome. In: Sonderegger TB, ed. *Perinatal substance abuse: Research findings and clinical implications*. Baltimore, MD: Johns Hopkins Univ Press, 1992:104-33.

[28] Streissguth AP, Barr HM, Kogan J, Bookstein FL. Final report: understanding the occurrence of secondary disabilities in clients with fetal alcohol syndrome (FAS) and fetal alcohol effects (FAE). Seattle, WA: Univ Washington Publ Serv, 1996.

[29] Niccols A. Fetal alcohol syndrome and the developing socio-emotional brain. *Brain Cogn.* 2007;65(1):135-42.

[30] Coles CD, Kable JA, Drews-Botsch C, Falek A. Early identification of risk for effects of prenatal alcohol exposure. *J. Stud. Alcohol* 2000;61(4):607-16.

[31] Church MW, Kaltenbach JA. Hearing, speech, language, and vestibular disorders in the fetal alcohol syndrome: a literature review. *Alcohol Clin. Exp. Res.* 1997;21(3):495-512.

[32] Greene T, Ernhart CB, Martier S, Sokol R, Ager J. Prenatal alcohol exposure and language development. *Alcohol Clin. Exp. Res.* 1990;14(6):937-45.

[33] Weinberg NZ. Cognitive and behavioral deficits associated with parental alcohol use. *J. Am. Acad. Child Adolesc Psychiatry* 1997; 36(9):1177-86.

[34] Church MW, Eldis F, Blakley BW, Bawle EV. Hearing, language, speech, vestibular, and dentofacial disorders in fetal alcohol syndrome. *Alcohol Clin. Exp. Res.* 1997;21(2):227-37.

[35] Greenbaum R. Socioemotional functioning and language impairment in children with prenatal alcohol exposure: a comparison with attention deficit hyperactivity disorder. *Doctoral thesis.* Toronto, ON: Univ Toronto, 2004.

[36] Linnet KM, Dalsgaard S, Obel C, Wisborg K, Henriksen TB, Rodriguez A, Kotimaa A, Moilanen I, Thomsen PH, Olsen J, Jarvelin MR. Maternal lifestyle factors in pregnancy risk of attention deficit hyperactivity disorder and associated behaviors: review of the current evidence. *Am. J. Psychiatry* 2003;160(6):1028-40.

[37] O'Malley KD, Nanson J. Clinical implications of a link between fetal alcohol spectrum disorder and attention-deficit hyperactivity disorder. *Can. J. Psychiatry* 2002;47(4):349-54.

[38] Bhatara V, Loudenberg R, Ellis R. Association of attention deficit hyperactivity disorder and gestational alcohol exposure: an exploratory study. *J. Atten. Disord.* 2006;9(3):512-22.

[39] Coles CD, Platzman KA, Raskind-Hood CL, Brown RT, Falek A, Smith IE. A comparison of children affected by prenatal alcohol exposure and attention deficit hyperactivity disorder. *Alcohol Clin. Exp. Res.* 1997;21(1):150-61.

[40] Burden MJ, Jacobson SW, Sokol RJ, Jacobson JL. Effects of prenatal alcohol exposure on attention and working memory at 7.5 years of age. *Alcohol Clin. Exp. Res.* 2005;29(3):443-52.

[41] Kodituwakku PW, May PA, Clericuzio CL, Weers D. Emotion-related learning in individuals prenatally exposed to alcohol: an investigation of the relation between set-shifting, extinction of responses, and behavior. *Neuropsychologia* 2001;39(7):699-708.

[42] Mattson SN, Goodman AM, Caine C, Delis DC, Riley EP. Executive functioning in children with heavy prenatal alcohol exposure. *Alcohol Clin. Exp. Res.* 1999;23(11):1808-15.

[43] Kodituwakku PW, Handmaker NS, Cutler SK, Weathersby EK, Handmaker SD. Specific impairments in self-regulation in children exposed to alcohol prenatally. *Alcohol Clin. Exp. Res.* 1995;19(6):1558-64.

[44] Connor PD, Sampson PD, Bookstein FL, Barr HM, Streissguth AP. Direct and indirect effects of prenatal alcohol damage on executive function. *Dev. Neuropsychol.* 2000;18(3):331-54.

[45] Malisza KL, Allman AA, Shiloff D, Jakobson L, Longstaffe S, Chudley AE. Evaluation of spatial working memory function in children and adults with fetal alcohol spectrum disorders: a functional magnetic resonance imaging study. *Pediatr. Res.* 2005;58(6):1150-7.

[46] Mattson SN, Riley EP, Delis DC, Stern C, Jones KL. Verbal learning and memory in children with fetal alcohol syndrome. *Alcohol Clin. Exp. Res.* 1996;20(5):810-6.

[47] Berman RF, Hannigan JH. Effects of prenatal alcohol exposure on the hippocampus: spatial behavior, electrophysiology, and neuroanatomy. *Hippocampus* 2000;10(1):94-110.

[48] Blanchard BA, Riley EP, Hannigan JH. Deficits on a spatial navigation task following prenatal exposure to ethanol. *Neurotoxicol Teratol* 1987;9(3):253-8.

[49] Hamilton DA, Kodituwakku P, Sutherland RJ, Savage DD. Children with fetal alcohol syndrome are impaired at place learning but not cued-navigation in a virtual Morris water task. *Behav Brain Res.* 2003;143(1):85-94.

[50] Uecker A, Nadel L. Spatial locations gone awry: object and spatial memory deficits in children with fetal alcohol syndrome. *Neuropsychologia* 1996;34(3):209-23.

[51] Kaemingk KL, Halverson PT. Spatial memory following prenatal alcohol exposure: more than a material specific memory deficit. *Child Neuropsychol.* 2000;6(2):115-28.

[52] Willford JA, Richardson GA, Leech SL, Day NL. Verbal and visuospatial learning and memory function in children with moderate prenatal alcohol exposure. *Alcohol Clin. Exp. Res.* 2004;28(3):497-507.

[53] Mattson SN, Riley EP. Implicit and explicit memory functioning in children with heavy prenatal alcohol exposure. *J. Int. Neuropsychol. Soc.* 1999;5(5):462-71.

[54] Jacobson SW, Jacobson JL, Sokol RJ, Martier SS, Ager JW. Prenatal alcohol exposure and infant information processing ability. *Child Dev.* 1993;64(6):1706-21.

[55] Kaemingk KL, Mulvaney S, Halverson PT. Learning following prenatal alcohol exposure: performance on verbal and visual multitrial tasks. *Arch. Clin. Neuropsychol.* 2003;18(1):33-47.

[56] Schonfeld AM, Paley B, Frankel F, O'Connor MJ. Executive functioning predicts social skills following prenatal alcohol exposure. *Child Neuropsychol.* 2006;12(6):439-52.

[57] Thomas SE, Kelly SJ, Mattson SN, Riley EP. Comparison of social abilities of children with Fetal Alcohol Syndrome to those of children with similar IQ scores and normal controls. *Alcohol Clin. Exp. Res.* 1998;22(2):528-533.

[58] Kelly SJ, Day N, Streissguth AP. Effects of prenatal alcohol exposure on social behavior in humans and other species. *Neurotoxicol. Teratol.* 2000;22(2):143-9.

[59] Streissguth AP, Randels SP, Smith DF. A test-retest study of intelligence in patients with fetal alcohol syndrome: implications for care. *J. Am. Acad. Child Adolesc. Psychiatry* 1991;30(4):584-7.

[60] Coles CD, Brown RT, Smith IE, Platzman KA, Erickson S, Falek A. Effects of prenatal alcohol exposure at school age: physical and cognitive development. *Neurotoxicol Teratol.* 1991;13(4):357-67.

[61] Steinhausen HC. Psychopathology and cognitive functioning in children with fetal alcohol syndrome. In: Spohr HL, Steinhausen HC, eds. *Alcohol, pregnancy, and the developing child.* New York, NY: Cambridge Univ Press, 1996:227-48.

[62] Mattson SN, Riley EP. Parent ratings of behavior in children with heavy prenatal alcohol exposure and IQ-matched controls. *Alcohol Clin. Exp. Res.* 2000;24(2):226-31.

[63] Roebuck TM, Mattson SN, Riley EP. A review of the neuroanatomical findings in children with fetal alcohol syndrome or prenatal exposure to alcohol. *Alcohol Clin. Exp. Res.* 1998;22(2):339-44.

[64] Jacobson SW, Jacobson JL, Sokol RJ, Chiodo LM. Preliminary evidence of socioemotional deficits in 7-year-olds prenatally exposed to alcohol. *Alcohol Clin. Exp. Res.*1998;22:61A.

[65] Schonfeld AM, Mattson SN, Riley EP. Moral maturity and delinquency after prenatal alcohol exposure. *J. Stud. Alcohol.* 2005;66(4):545-54.

[66] Olson HC, Feldman JJ, Streissguth AP, Gonzales RD. Neuropsychological deficits and life adjustment in adolescents and young adults with fetal alcohol syndrome. *Alcohol Clin. Exp. Res.* 1992;16:380.

[67] Guinta CT, Streissguth AP. Patients with fetal alcohol syndrome and their caretakers. *Social Casework* 1988;69(7):453-9.

[68] Fryer SL, McGee CL, Matt GE, Riley EP, Mattson SN. Evaluation of psychopathological conditions in children with heavy prenatal alcohol exposure. *Pediatrics* 2007;119(3):e733-41.

PART TWO: ACUTE EFFECTS OF ALCOHOL

In: Alcohol-Related Cognitive Disorders   ISBN: 978-1-60741-730-9
Editors: L. Sher, I. Kandel, J. Merrick pp. 159-175   © 2009 Nova Science Publishers, Inc.

Chapter 9

ALCOHOL AND COGNITIVE FUNCTIONS

Mark T. Fillmore

ABSTRACT

Alcohol is arguably the most widely used and studied drug in human history. The acute effects of alcohol in humans have been studied in laboratories for over a century. Much of the interest in alcohol concerns its debilitating effects on human performance. Originally this interest was fueled by well-founded concerns that alcohol could impair the drinker's ability to operate an automobile. Before the advent of breath analysis devices, "road-side" behavioral tests of motor coordination and mental ability were the only means of detecting "impaired drivers". Thus there was much interest in discerning which aspects of human behavior were most disrupted by a given dose of alcohol. This chapter concerns the acute impairing effects of alcohol on cognitive functions in healthy, non-alcohol dependent adults. The chapter begins by describing how different aspects of human performance are not equally sensitive to the impairing effects of alcohol and that the wealth of research on these differences poses unique challenges for summarizing and communicating this large body of evidence. The chapter then discusses speeded and divided attention tasks as methods commonly used to assess the acute cognitive impairing effects of alcohol and the cognitive theories that have been offered to account for the findings based on these tasks. This is followed by a review of more contemporary methods and techniques that focus on how the drug impairs specific cognitive mechanisms that underlie the control and regulation of behavior. The chapter concludes by explaining how acute impairments of such mechanisms might actually contribute to the abuse potential of alcohol for some individuals.

INTRODUCTION

Many early controlled laboratory investigations of alcohol effects examined a broad range of human performance. The aspects of performance that were tested included simple reaction time, visual and auditory acuity, hand-eye coordination, gross body movement (i.e., body sway), short-term memory, and simple arithmetic and mental tasks [1,2]. One of the earliest and longstanding observations from this research is that all aspects of human performance are not equally sensitive to the impairing effects of alcohol. Yet, characterizing these differences has never been an easy task, in large part because of the enormity of the data and the heterogeneity of approaches used to measure the effects of alcohol on behavior in the laboratory [3]. The difficulties in summarizing a growing volume of research characterized by cross-study differences in methods, doses, and subjects were recognized even as far back as 1940 in a review by Elvin Morton Jellinek (1890-1963) [2].

To cope with this problem, several reviewers employed the concept of a threshold or effective blood alcohol concentration (BAC) to characterize differences in the sensitivities of the various aspects of human performance to the impairing effects of alcohol. The threshold referred to a specific BAC at which the majority of subjects in a given study displayed statistically reliable impairment on a task. The threshold concept was also applied at the meta-analytic level, in which the threshold referred to the BAC at which at least 50% of the studies reported a reliable impairment for a given task [4,5]. Threshold BACs have considerable heuristic appeal, because they provide a simple quanti-tative indication of the degree to which a given aspect of performance is sensitive to the impairing effects of alcohol. The lower the threshold BAC for a task, the more sensitive the behavior is to the impairing effects of alcohol. Using this approach, reviews reported that most behaviors tested in laboratories do indeed have threshold BACs below 0.08%, which is the current "legal limit" for driving an automobile in the United States.

Reviewers also attempted to organize the findings by grouping various tasks and measures together based on common attributes to identify patterns of reliable differences in alcohol sensitivity among broader domains of human functioning [4-6]. Many different grouping criteria have been employed over the years. These have included distinguishing tasks based on complexity [1], relevance to driving performance [5,7,8], cognitive-versus-motor performance, and the degree to which the skill requires controlled, effortful processing rather than being an over-learned or automatic action [6]. The heuristic value of these categorizations for understanding differences in alcohol sensitivity among various types of behaviors has become well recognized among researchers. For example, it is now generally accepted that the BAC threshold for impairment is lower for tasks that are complex or require controlled effortful attention on the part of the drinker [4]. Higher-order cognitive functions, such as decision-making, judgement, and memory have a reliable BAC threshold of impairment of 0.06% [4-8]. The threshold is even lower (0.05%) for the more complex, divided-attention tasks that emphasize the ability to perform two or more activities simultaneously [4-8]. By contrast, the performance of simple tasks is relatively resistant to the effects of alcohol at BACs under 0.08%. For example, reaction time to a simple visual signal is not reliably impaired below a threshold of 0.08%.

EARLY APPROACHES

Speeded Tasks

Among the acute debilitating effects of alcohol, one of the earliest and long standing assumptions is that alcohol disrupts behavior because the drug slows the drinkers' ability to process information. Some of the earliest support for this assumption came from simple reaction-time tasks that showed drinkers were slower to make a behavioral response (e.g., a button press) to a stimulus, such as a light or an auditory signal (9). However, such observations of slowed reactions in these situations could not distinguish between a slowing of some central information processing or slowing of the peripheral motor response itself. More specific tests of slowed information processing followed.

One of the earliest tools to demonstrate that alcohol slows the processing of information was the critical flicker-fusion task. The task presents a strobe-like flashing light to the subject with an increasing "flicker" frequency until it gives the perception of a continuous beam of light, thus changing in appearance from a flicker to a fusion. The subject reports when the light appears continuous and the flicker frequency coinciding with this report is recorded as the "flicker-fusion frequency". Early studies reported by Goldberg (1) found that alcohol lowered the flicker-fusion frequency. Thus, under alcohol, subjects perceived the light as being continuous at slower frequencies than they did when sober. This effect was attributed to a slowing of neural processing of visual information somewhere along the visual pathway between retina and visual cortex.

Other early tasks that implicated an alcohol-induced slowing of information processing were the speeded tasks, in which the subject is required to perform a series of mental operations as quickly as possible. Two of the earliest speeded tasks were the Subtraction Task and the Bourdon Task. The Subtraction task required subjects to count backwards from one hundred by sevens. Performance was usually measured as the time required to reach zero and by the number of subtraction errors made. Alcohol reliably increased the time needed to complete the task and increased errors. The Bourdon Task requires subjects to scan a random list of letters and pencil out each instance of a target letter that is randomly distributed throughout the list. Speed of performance is measured by the number of letters scanned during an interval and errors are measured by the number of target letters missed. Early studies showed that alcohol increased errors on the task and reduced the number of letters that could be scanned in a given time period [1].

The Letter Cancellation Task and Digit Symbol Substitution Task (DSST) are modifications of the Bourdon Task that are commonly used today to evaluate acute drug effects on information processing speed. Also recent are self-paced, interactive forms of these tasks that provide rate-based measures of information processing. One example is the Rapid Information Processing task, which adjusts the rate with which numbers are presented on a computer display as a function of the subject's ability to encode and respond to the numbers [10]. Correct responding increases the presentation rate, and errors slow the presentation rate. Thus, the presentation of information is adjusted to a rate at which the individual can accurately encode and respond. The average rate obtained during a test estimates the subject's rate of information processing. Several studies have showed that alcohol reliably slows information processing on this task [11].

Much evidence for the impairing effects of alcohol in speeded tasks has been interpreted within the framework of stage theories of information processing [12]. These theories postulate a sequence of distinct processes or stages, which operate between the presentation of some stimulus and the resulting response to the stimulus. For example, a common three-stage model asserts that information processing involves three independent components; a perceptual, a central, and a motor process [13]. Each process governs a particular activity that is required by a task. The perceptual process governs the attention to stimuli. The central process interprets and stores the information, and the motor process governs overt behavioral reactions required by a task. Because each component activity is assumed to represent an independent process, each activity should uniquely contribute to the overall measure of task performance. Although evidence for which processing stages are most impaired by alcohol can depend on the nature of the task, it is commonly concluded that early, perceptual stages are comparatively unaffected by alcohol whereas more central stages involving working memory and response selection are most sensitive to the disruptive effects of the drug [8,15].

A limitation of speeded tasks as an indicator of alcohol-induced slowing of information processing is that the tasks can be subject to speed-accuracy trade-off effects [8]. In a speed-accuracy trade-off the intoxicated individual appears to purposely slow performance in an effort to maintain some level of accuracy. Purposely slowing task performance to maintain accuracy might suggest that the slowing effect is a compensatory strategy evoked by the drinker to cope with a disruption of some central stage process, such as response selection, which might represent the primary impairing effect of the drug. This poses difficulties in identifying exactly which stage or stages of information processing are directly disrupted by the drug. Methods of quantifying speed-accuracy trade-offs have been used in alcohol research [15] and there has been research interest in the types of task attributes and drinker characteristics that might be associated with the occurrence of speed-accuracy trade-offs under the drug [16].

Divided Attention Tasks

Trade-off problems involving performance speed are generally avoided by the use of divided attention tasks. These tasks assess the ability to perform two or more activities at once. For example, a divided attention task may require a subject to manually track a rotating target (e.g., perform a pursuit task), while performing some auditory discrimination task (e.g., detecting differences among tones). Thus the subject must maintain a precise level of hand-eye coordination while accurately discrim-inating the pitch of various tones. Performance in these situations is considered to be highly vulnerable to the disruptive influence of alcohol. Reviews of alcohol studies report some of the lowest threshold BACs (e.g., 0.05%) for impairment on tasks involving divided attention [4]. Moreover, it is often found that when the individual tasks are performed in isolation, no impairing effect of alcohol is evident. It is only when the tasks are performed together that impairment is observed. Thus even simple activities that, individually, are entirely unaffected by moderate alcohol doses can demonstrate substantial impairment to those same doses in the divided attention situation [17].

Like speeded tasks, divided attention tasks can be affected by performance trade-offs. But unlike speeded tasks where an individual sacrifices one aspect of performance (i.e., speed) for another (i.e., accuracy,) in the divided attention situation the individual sacrifices one task for another. For example, upon perceiving the intoxicating effects of alcohol an individual might choose to shift attention or effort toward the task that is deemed most important to maintain proficiency, and this shift often occurs at the expense of the other task. To some degree this strategic shifting of attention between tasks invalidates the divided attention model, which is intended to tap the limits of the individual's information processing capacity by forcing the simultaneous performance of multiple activities. Yet, in spite of this limitation, divided attention tasks offer greater ecological validity as models of day-to-day performance of activities outside the laboratory where our attention is routinely divided among multiple demands. For example, common tasks performed outside the laboratory, such as driving, are inherently multi-task in nature and can be further complicated by voluntarily adding additional tasks to them, such as talking on a cellular telephone while driving. Indeed, outside the laboratory, such dual-task activities may be the norm rather than the exception.

Much of the evidence for the impairing effects of alcohol in divided attention scenarios has been interpreted within the framework of capacity theories of information processing [18]. Capacity theories focus on the limitations on information processing. In general, these theories assert that information processing is constrained much like a "bottleneck" in which only one process can be completed at any one time. Capacity limitations on information processing can be revealed when an individual performs two activities at once (i.e., a dual-task situation). For example, performance is degraded in situations that require an individual to respond to each of two stimuli (task 1 and task 2), presented in close temporal proximity [18]. This type of degradation is evident by a slowing of response time to the second stimulus (task 2). The delayed response time is often attributed to a "psychological refractory period", and is assumed to reflect a limitation of information processing in which the response to task 2 must be delayed until processing of task 1 is complete. Fillmore and Van Selst [17] have argued that much of the behaviorally disruptive effects of alcohol are the direct result of an increased constraint on processing information that is directly produced by the drug. In fact, the disruptive effects of alcohol closely resemble the impairing effects of task-related constraints on information processing, such as those produced by dual-task performance, or by conditions that require divided attention among multiple activities.

In sum, the widespread use of speeded and divided attention tasks in alcohol research has been useful in identifying aspects and conditions of performance that demonstrate robust impairments in response to alcohol, as well as the situations in which impairments are likely to be exacerbated (e.g., dual-task/divided attention). The research also adds to our understanding of the under-lying nature of these impairments by implicating a slowing or capacity-reducing effect of alcohol on the drinker's ability to process information. This finding is important because it suggests two fundamental ways in which alcohol might impair information processing, from which many other cognitive and behavioral impairments observed in response to the drug might actually arise.

CONTEMPORARY APPROACHES

Neuropsychological Techniques

During the 1980s and 1990s, alcohol research saw the growing application of traditional neuropsychological tests for studying its acute behavioral effects [19]. This innovation coincided with the popular use of the exec-utive functioning concept. The latter term describes a collection of higher-order cognitive abilities, such as decision-making, sequencing, planning, and organizing behavior. Traditional neuropsychological tests were re-labeled as executive functioning tasks and used to study acute alcohol effects on a host of behaviors. Some tasks commonly used in this regard were the Trails Task, the Wisconsin Card Sorting Test, and the Porteous Maze, Test.

One advantage of using neuropsychological assess-ments is that such tasks have well-established validity, allowing performance deficits to be associated with specific brain regions that might underlie the impaired functions (e.g., frontal lobe vs. temporal lobe function). Thus, acute impairments in response to alcohol on these types of tasks could offer certain insights into the associated brain areas likely being disrupted by the drug. In fact, evidence based on neuropsychological tests of hemispheric functioning suggests that the right hemisphere is more affected by alcohol than the left, which could account for why functions like spatial information processing appear particularly vulnerable to the disruptive effects of alcohol [8,14].

However, many neuropsychological tasks also proved to be poorly suited to measure the acute behavioral effects of alcohol or other drugs. For example, many neuropsychological tasks can be performed only once by a subject, after which any repeated testing would be invalid owing to substantial learning effects on performance. This phenomenon is particularly true of tasks that assess planning and problem solving. Consequently such tasks could not be used to evaluate alcohol effects in within-subjects designs involving repeating testing, such as dose-response studies that require repeated administrations of the test to the same subjects under various doses of the drug.

Another major problem with the neuropsycho-logical tasks in alcohol research is that many of them proved to be rather insensitive to the impairing effects of alcohol at BACs below 0.10%. In hindsight, this finding is not surprising given that many neuropsycho-logical tasks were originally designed to detect severe and debilitating cognitive impairments as symptomatic of neurological disorders or brain injuries. Actually, it is in this respect that neuropsychological tasks have been quite useful in addiction research. Neuropsychological assessments have been integral in demonstrating cognitive deficits that result from long-term, heavy alcohol use, such as memory impairments among Korsakoff's patients [20]. Moreover, such assessments are proving to be sensitive indicators of the potential amelioration of dysfunction that can result from prolonged abstinence from the alcohol.

COGNITIVE TECHNIQUES

Although characterizing the impairing effects of alcohol at a level of complex function is important, identifying specific mechanisms by which the drug might produce such disruptions in complex cognitive operations is also needed. This need is met by the theoretically based approach to task development that typifies the field of cognitive psychology. During the past two decades, alcohol research has seen a growing shift away from descriptive assessments that are based on neuro-psychological tasks to more theoretically driven assessments that examine specific "mechanisms" of behavior. Unlike neuro-psychological approaches that assess complex cognitive operations, this cognitive approach breaks down complex operations to study their component mechanisms. Thus the cognitive approach to studying alcohol impairment is aimed at identifying disturbances in the basic "building blocks" of behavior and, in this sense, is antithetical to the neuro-psychological approach. The next few sections review several cognitive models that focus on inhibitory mechanisms of behavior and describe their current use in the study of alcohol effects.

INHIBITION AND THE CONTROL OF BEHAVIOR

Several theories argue that behavioral control can be reduced to two sets of conflicting mechanisms: inhibitory and activational [21-25]. Considerable research in cognitive neuroscience has focused on inhibitory mechanisms of behavioral control. The ability to withhold or to terminate a behavioral response is considered to reflect an inhibitory cognitive mechanism of behavioral control [23]. The inhibition of behavior is an important function that sets the occasion for many other activities requiring self-restraint and regulation of behavior [26]. Inhibitory mechanisms also have been implicated in self-control disorders. Aggressive and impulsive behaviors that characterize disorders, such as anti-social personality, obsessive-compulsive, and attention deficit/hyperactivity disorders (ADHD), have been attributed to impaired inhibitory mechanisms [26,27].

In recent years, several studies have examined the acute effects of alcohol using theoretically based tasks that model the joint contribution of inhibitory and activational mechanisms in the control of behavior [28-30]. Two of these tasks are the stop-signal and the cued go/no-go task [31,32].

The tasks model behavioral control using a reaction-time scenario that measures the countervailing influences of inhibitory and activational mechanisms. Individuals are required to activate a response to a go-signal quickly and to inhibit a response when a stop-signal occasionally occurs. Activation is typically measured as the speed of responding to go-signals, and inhibition to stop-signals is assessed by the probability of suppressing the response or by the time needed to suppress the response. In these models, inhibition of a response is usually required in a context in which there is a strong tendency to respond to a stimulus (i.e., a pre-potency), thus making inhibition difficult. The validity of these models is well-documented. The models are sensitive to inhibitory deficits characteristic of brain injury [33,34], trait-based impulsivity [35], and self-control disorders, such as ADHD [27,36,37].

Several recent studies using these tasks have provided consistent evidence that moderate doses of alcohol selectively reduce the drinker's ability to inhibit behavior at doses that leave the ability to activate behavior relatively unaffected [29,38]. For example, Fillmore and Weafer [39] used a cued go no-go task to test the impairing effect of alcohol on drinkers' inhibitory control over their behavioral impulses. The cued go no-go task presented go and no-targets to which subjects had to execute a response (go) or to inhibit a response (no-go). The subjects' inhibitory control was tested on two occasions: following a placebo and following an active dose that was sufficient to raise a drinker's BAC to 0.08%. Figure 1 illustrates the results of the study. The figure shows that, compared with placebo, alcohol impaired inhibitory control by increasing the likelihood that drinkers would fail to inhibit responses to no-go targets. By contrast, no effect of alcohol at this dose was observed on the ability of drinkers to execute the responses to go targets as measured by their speed of responding.

What is particularly remarkable about findings such these is the robust impairment that is evident despite the relatively simple nature of the inhibitory response tested. Typically, the sensitivity to alcohol-induced impairment increases as a function of dose and task complexity [40]. However, the impairing effects of alcohol on the ability to inhibit behavior are often observed at BACs at or below 0.08% [41].

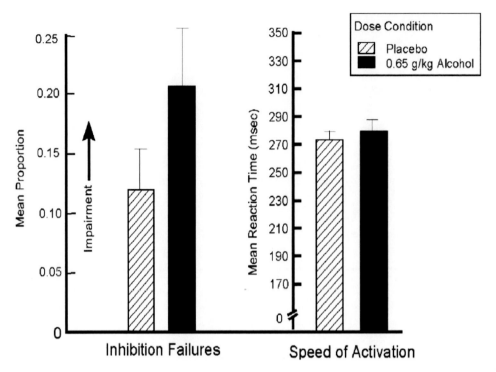

Figure 1. Effect of 0.65 g/kg alcohol and placebo on inhibitory failures to no-go targets and speed of response activation to go targets in a cued go/no-go model .

The findings suggest that activities requiring a quick suppression of actions might be particularly vulnerable to the disruptive influences of alcohol. In addition, alcohol-induced impairment of inhibitory mechanisms might actually exert considerable disruptive influence on higher-order, executive cognitive functions. Many fundamental cognitive and perceptual processes, such as inhibitory mechanisms, are considered to operate in a "bottom-up" fashion to exert increasing influence at each stage of higher-order attentional and cognitive functions.

Thus, the alcohol-induced disturbance of basic control mechanisms, such as inhibitory processes, might actually result in much more pronounced impairments of the higher cognitive operations for which they serve (e.g., decision-making, planning, goal maintenance, etc.).

The findings might also provide some account for the long-standing observation that alcohol intoxication is often characterized by increased impulsivity and aggression. Using the same types of tasks as those described here, deficits of inhibitory control have been identified in individuals with disorders characterized by aggressive or impulsive behaviors, such as attention deficit/hyperactivity disorder (ADHD) and anti-social personality [26,27].

In fact, the acute impairments of inhibitory control that are produced by alcohol closely resemble those inhibitory deficits that are assumed to be symptomatic of externalizing disorders [30]. This raises an intriguing possibility that alcohol temporarily disrupts cognitive functioning in a manner similar to the enduring cognitive disturbances that are characteristic of disorders like ADHD.

INHIBITION AND CONTROL OF ATTENTION

Inhibitory mechanisms are also suspected to facilitate control over attention [42-45]. Distraction from irrelevant stimuli might be reduced by active inhibitory mechanisms, which direct attentional resources away from irrelevant stimuli in the environment [46]. In theory, irrelevant information is internalized as neural representations associated with an active inhibitory gating mechanism, and this inhibition of irrelevant information allows relevant information to be processed free from interference. The influence of these inhibitory mechanisms on attention has been measured using negative priming, anti-saccade, and the inhibition of return tasks [46-48]. In brief, these are reaction time techniques demonstrating that individuals take longer to respond to a stimulus that was recently ignored as being irrelevant compared with a stimulus that was not ignored. The increased response time is attributed to residual inhibition toward the recently ignored stimulus that delays the individual's response to it when it becomes a relevant target and focus of attention. The models support distinct inhibitory mechanisms in the selection of attention and their validity is well-established. Studies show that individuals characterized by poor attention (e.g., schizophrenics, head-injury patients, and those with ADHD) demonstrate reduced inhibitory control against irrelevant stimulus input [49-52].

Recent studies of alcohol using these types of tasks show that the drug reduces the time-cost normally associated with responding to recently ignored stimuli, suggesting that alcohol impairs the normal inhibitory mechanism that directs attention away from irrelevant information [53-55]. For example, Fillmore et al. [54,55] used a negative priming model in which subjects had to respond to the relevant attribute of Stroop color words (i.e., the color of the letters) while ignoring the distracting, irrelevant attribute of the Stroop words (the spelling of the letters). Negative priming is demonstrated as an increased response time to name the attribute of a Stroop word that was just ignored as being irrelevant on the previous trial. The increased response time reflects the additional time needed to overcome residual inhibition that directed attention away from the previously ignored attribute. Fillmore et al [54,55] showed that moderate doses of alcohol (0.56 g/kg) suppressed negative priming effects, suggesting that the drug impairs normal inhibitory or gating processes that control attention.

Alcohol also appears to impair inhibitory processes that aid in visual searches [53]. When scanning a visual environment, attention is directed over different locations until a stimulus of interest is detected. Once attention has been directed away from a location for a sufficient period, the time required for attention to return to that location actually increases relative to the time required to direct attention to a new, previously unattended location. This phenomenon is referred to as inhibition of return (IOR) and appears to reflect the operation of a reactive inhibitory effect that enhances the efficiency of searches by biasing attention toward new information in unexplored locations and away from redundant, old information contained in previously searched locations [48,56]. Abroms and Fillmore [53] examined the IOR effect in response to two doses of alcohol: 0.65 g/kg and 0.45 g/kg. The task briefly presented a visual cue in a peripheral location of a computer display. Following the cue, a simple target stimulus was presented at either the same or a different location, and the subject had to detect the target as quickly as possible by pressing a computer key. The IOR is evident by prolonged detection times for targets that appear at the same location as the cue (same cue-target condition). Abroms and Fillmore found that, compared with placebo, both active alcohol doses reduced the normal IOR effect by shortening its duration. The finding suggests that alcohol impairs an inhibitory mechanism that normally aids in visual search.

The effects of alcohol on inhibitory mechanisms of attention have also been studied by directly examining how the drug alters eye movements (i.e., saccades) toward relevant and irrelevant stimuli. One task used is the delayed ocular response (DOR) task [52,57]. The task requires subjects to focus on a fixation point in the center of the screen while a stimulus in the periphery is suddenly presented to elicit a reflexive saccade toward it. The subjects are instructed, however, to delay (i.e., inhibit) looking at the stimulus for a brief wait interval. The primary measure of task performance is inhibitory failures, which occur when the subject makes a "pre-mature" saccade to the stimulus before the wait interval expires. Studies of individuals with disorders that are characterized by poor inhibitory control and attentional-deficits (i.e., ADHD and schizophrenia) find increased inhibitory failures compared with healthy controls, thus demonstrating the validity of the DOR task as a sensitive measure of inhibitory impairments of attention [52,57].

Abroms, Gottlob, and Fillmore (58) used the DOR task to examine the acute impairing effects of alcohol on the ability to inhibit saccades and found that alcohol increases premature saccades. Figure 2 shows that compared with the placebo, the number of premature saccades increased markedly in response to alcohol. In accord with an inhibition-based account, the evidence suggests that alcohol impairs the drinker's ability to inhibit a reflexive saccade elicited by the sudden onset of the target. In other words, alcohol impairs the drinker's ability to ignore a sudden distraction that competes for attention. Furthermore, the inhibitory mechanism appeared quite sensitive to the disruptive effects of alcohol. The number of premature saccades under the highest dose (0.65 g/kg) was nearly three times greater than that in response to placebo. Also, impairment was evident even in response to the lower dose (0.45 g/kg) that did not produce BACs above 0.065%.

Identifying a suppressing effect of alcohol on inhibitory mechanisms that normally serve to guide attention is important for a number of reasons. Selective impairment of inhibitory mechanisms of attention could provide some account for the general observation that alcohol slows information processing in many situations. For example, the finding by Abroms and Fillmore [53] that alcohol reduces inhibitory mechanisms involved in visual search suggests that redundant searching of previously explored locations might be more likely to occur under the influence of the drug. Unnecessary re-acquisition of visual information would slow the rate at which new information could be obtained and subse-quently processed. This redundancy could dramatically reduce the efficiency of visual search under the drug. Also, high doses of alcohol were not required to produce these impairing effects. The low-dose effects observed support the general notion that inhibitory processes of visual attention might be especially vulnerable to the disruptive effects of this drug. Finally, the evidence that alcohol impairs inhibitory mechanisms of attention is consistent with evidence that the drug also impairs inhibitory mechanisms that control behavioral impulses, as measured by go no-go and stop-signal models [28-30]. Little is known about potential relationships between inhibitory processes involved in attention and those that control suppression of prepotent behavioral responses. Evidence for some interdepen-dence among these mechanisms would contribute much to our understanding about the role of inhibitory mechanisms in the control of attention and behavior [31]. Although the specific nature of inhibitory mechanisms implicated in the control of attention likely differs from those involved in inhibiting prepotent behavioral responses, the consistency of findings con-cerning alcohol effects suggests that activities depending heavily on inhibitory influences might be particularly susceptible to the impairing effects of the drug.

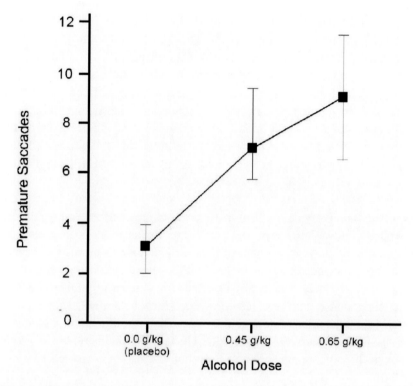

Figure 2. Mean number of premature saccades during DOR task performance in response to 0.0 g/kg, 0.45 g/kg, and 0.65 g/kg alcohol.

ACUTE COGNITIVE IMPAIRMENT AND ALCOHOL ABUSE

The reductionist approach of these contemporary cognitive models has allowed for a better understanding of the general 'disinhibiting' effects of alcohol in terms of the impairments of specific control mechanisms that normally suppress inappropriate actions and gate influence from distracting stimuli. In addition, evidence for the vulnerability of inhibitory mechanisms to alcohol effects could offer important new insights into the development and maintenance of alcohol abuse. Alcohol abuse is an individual difference problem in that whereas most adults are exposed to alcohol, only a few individuals develop abuse-related problems. A long-standing hypothesis is that individuals who develop abuse problems do so, because they experience abnormal reactions to alcohol, such as heightened or dampened responses to the drug. For instance, commonly assumed is that excessive consumption or binge drinking can occur because for certain drinkers, the initial drink itself reinforces or 'primes' continued alcohol intake in the situation [59,60]. Alcohol priming has been demonstrated in alcoholics and social drinkers [59,61-63]. The typical priming procedure in these studies involves the administration of a mild dose of alcohol or placebo followed by measures that assess the priming effect. Such measures typically include increased self-reports of the euphorigenic effects, such as "liking" and "wanting to drink more", as well as behavioral measures of drug reinforcement, such as increased self-administration of alcohol and work output to acquire subsequent doses. Evidence of such priming effects traditionally has been attributed to alcohol's action on brain mechanisms of reward, whereby incentive properties of a small dose reinforce the consumption of greater amounts [64-67].

Although there is little dispute that reward mechanisms play an important role in abuse potential, the acute cognitive impairing effects alcohol might also contribute to abuse by compromising mechanisms involved in the regulation and self-control of behavior and attention [41]. As mentioned earlier, subtle impairments in the operation of inhibitory mechanisms can have a substantial impact on functioning in situations that require control of complex behaviors, including drinking behavior. In particular, inhibitory mechanisms likely play an important role in terminating alcohol use during an episode [19,41,68]. Many drinkers report intentions to limit their alcohol use to one or two drinks only to fail and instead drink excessively [69]. Such accounts have fueled the notion that alcohol reduces control over consumption in certain individuals. Terminating a drinking episode requires the inhibition of ongoing alcohol-administration behaviors and the reallocation of attention away from alcohol-related stimuli. Any impairment of normal inhibitory mechanisms resulting from an initial dose of alcohol could compromise the ability to stop additional alcohol administrations in a drinking situation. Thus, acute alcohol-induced impairment of inhibitory processes could represent an important cognitive mechanism by which an initial alcohol dose promotes subsequent self-administration. Although only speculative at this point, the degree to which alcohol impairs inhibitory control might contribute to the likelihood of self-administration independently of the euphorigenic effects of alcohol that are also experienced by the drinker. Figure 3 illustrates this general working hypothesis by showing how alcohol-induced impairment of cognitive inhibitory processes and its rewarding effects might both operate as independent mechanisms to determine its abuse potential for a given individual.

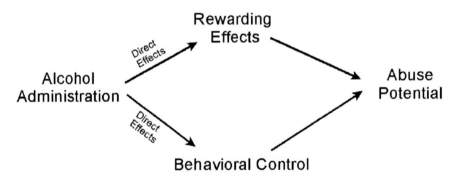

Figure 3. Model illustrating how alcohol promotes abuse potential via two independent mechanisms: increased subjective reward and decreased behavioral control.

CONCLUSIONS

Over the past century, a wealth of information has been gathered concerning the acute effects of alcohol on human behavior. From a historical perspective, many of the methods and techniques used to study alcohol effects have been adopted from those used in behavioral research fields, such as experimental psychology, clinical psychology, and neuropsychology. As such, our knowledge about how alcohol affects human behavior has benefited greatly from advances and developments in those fields. At present, much is being learned about how alcohol alters specific mechanisms of behavioral control and the selection of attention, and this can be credited in large part to significant developments in model-based measurement of cognitive and behavioral functions.

Furthermore, a common interest in such mechanisms is now shared among researchers from many different fields like developmental psychology and behavioral pharmacology. As a result, common methodologies have emerged among research areas that previously differed markedly in the methods and techniques used to evaluate behavior. For example, stop-signal models of inhibitory control have been used for studying behavioral deficits associated with the acute intoxicating effects of alcohol [30] and for studying problematic behavioral symptoms associated with ADHD in children [37]. The broad application of these models, including their incorporation into fMRI and other imaging research, could reveal important similarities and differences in the mechanisms underlying behavioral control deficits observed among different populations, behavioral dis-orders, and classes of abused drugs. Finally, noteworthy is that the dearth of information concerning the link between alcohol effects on basic mechanisms of self-control and the drug's potential for abuse represents a serious gap in our understanding of the transition from social drinking to abusive drinking. A more reductionist analysis of basic mechanisms of behavioral control should provide greater insight into the role of these processes as non-motivational mechanisms of alcohol abuse potential.

ACKNOWLEDGMENTS

This work was supported by Grant R01 AA12895 from the National Institute on Alcohol Abuse and Alcoholism and by Grant R21 DA021027 from the National Institute on Drug Abuse. The author is grateful to Emma Wigglesworth for assistance in preparing this chapter.

REFERENCES

[1]   Goldberg L. Quantitative studies on alcohol tolerance in man: The influence of ethyl alcohol on sensory, motor, and psychological functions referred to blood alcohol in normal and habituated individuals. *Acta Physiol. Scand* 1943;5(suppl 16): 1-128.

[2]   Jellinek EM, MacFarland RA. Analysis of psycho-logical experiments on the effects of alcohol. *Q J Stud. Alcohol* 1940;1:272-371.

[3]   Carpenter JA. Effects of alcohol on some psycho-logical processes: a critical review with special reference to automobile driving skill. *Q J Stud Alcohol.* 1962;23:274-314.

[4]   Holloway FA. Low-dose alcohol effects on human behavior and performance. *Alcohol Drugs Driving* 1995;11:39-56.

[5]   Moskowitz H, Robinson C. Driving-related skills impairment at low blood alcohol levels. *Alcohol Drugs Traffic Safety* 1987;T86:79-86.

[6]   Kruger HP. Effects of low alcohol dosages: a review of the literature. In: Utselmann HG, Berghaus G, Kroj G, eds. Alcohol, drugs, and traffic safety: *Proceeding of the 12th*

international conference on alcohol, drugs, and traffic safety. Cologne: Verlag TUV Rheinland, 1992:763-78.

[7] Mitchell MC. Alcohol-induced impairment of central nervous system function: behavioral skills involved in driving. *J. Stud. Alcohol.* 1985;(suppl 10):109-16.

[8] Linnoila M, Stapleton JM, Lister R, Guthrie S, Eckardt M. Effects of alcohol on accident risk. *Pathologist* 1986;40:36-41.

[9] Carpenter JA. The effect of caffeine and alcohol on simple visual reaction time. *J. Comp. Physiol. Psych* 1959;52:491-6.

[10] Hasenfratz M, Bunge A, Dal Pra G, Battig, K. An-tagonistic effects of caffeine and alcohol on mental performance parameters. *Pharmacol. Biochem. Behav.* 1993;46:463-5.

[11] Fillmore MT, Carscadden J, Vogel-Sprott M. Alcohol, cognitive impairment, and expectancies. *J. Stud. Alcohol.* 1998;59:174-9.

[12] Sternberg S. Memory scanning: mental processes revealed by reaction-time experiments. *Am. Sci.* 1969;57:421-57.

[13] Wesnes K, Simpson P, Christmas L. The assess-ment of human information-processing abilities in psychopharmacology. In: Hindmarch I, Stonier PD, eds. *Human psychopharmacology: measures and methods.* Chichester, UK: Wiley, 1987:79-92.

[14] Koelega HS. Alcohol and vigilance performance: a review. *Psychopharmacology* 1995; 118:233-49.

[15] Maylor EA, Rabbitt PM. Effects of alcohol and practice on choice reaction time. *Percept Psychophys.* 1987;42:465-75.

[16] Fillmore MT, Blackburn J. Compensating for alcohol-induced impairment: Alcohol expectancies and behavioral disinhibition. *J. Stud. Alcohol.* 2002; 63:237-46.

[17] Fillmore MT, Van Selst M. Constraints on information processing under alcohol in the context of response execution and response suppression. *Exp. Clin. Psychopharm* 2002; 10:417-24.

[18] Pashler H. Dual-Task interference in simple tasks: Data and theory. *Psychol. Bull* 1994; 116:220-44.

[19] Lyvers M. "Loss of control" in alcoholism and drug addiction: a neuroscientific interpretation. *Exp. Clin. Psychopharm* 2000;8:225-49.

[20] Bates ME, Bowden SC, Barry D. Neurocognitive impairment associated with alcohol use disorders: implications for treatment. *Exp. Clin. Psychopharm.* 2002;10:193-212.

[21] Fowles DC. Application of a behavioral theory of motivation to the concepts of anxiety and impul-sivity. *J. Res. Personality* 1987;21:417-35.

[22] Gray JA. The behavioral inhibition system: a possible substrate for anxiety. In: Feldman MP, Broadhurst, A, eds. *Theoretical and experimental bases of the behavior therapies.* London, UK: Wiley, 1976:3-41.

[23] Logan GD, Cowan WB. On the ability to inhibit thought and action: A theory of an act of control. *Psychol. Rev.* 1984;91:295-327.

[24] Patterson CM, Newman JP. Reflectivity and learning from aversive events: toward a psycho-logical mechanism for the syndromes of disinhibition. *Psychol. Rev.* 1993;100: 716-36.

[25] Quay HC. Inhibition and attention deficit hyper-activity disorder. *J. Abnorm. Child Psychol.* 1997; 25:7-13.

[26] Barkley RA. Behavioral inhibition, sustained attention, and executive functions: constructing a unifying theory of ADHD. *Psychol. Bull* 1997;121: 65-94.

[27] Tannock R. Attention deficit hyperactivity disorder: advances in cognitive, neurobiological, and genetic research. *J. Child Psychol. Psychiat* 1998;39:65-99.

[28] de Wit H, Crean J, Richards, JB. Effects of d-amphetamine and ethanol on a measure of behav-ioral inhibition in humans. *Behav. Neurosci.* 2000; 114:830-7.

[29] Mulvihill LE, Skilling TA, Vogel-Sprott M. Alcohol and the ability to inhibit behavior in men and women. *J. Stud. Alcohol.* 1997;58:600-5.

[30] Fillmore MT, Vogel-Sprott M. An alcohol model of impaired inhibitory control and its treatment in humans. *Exp. Clin. Psychopharm* 1999;7:49-55.

[31] Logan GD. On the ability to inhibit thought and action: A user's guide to the stop-signal paradigm. In: Dagenbach D, Carr TH, eds. *Inhibitory processes in attention, memory, and language.* San Diego, CA, USA: Academic Press, 1994:189-239.

[32] Miller J, Schaffer R, Hackley SA. Effects of pre-liminary information in a go versus no-go task. *Acta Psychologica* 1991;76:241-92.

[33] Cremona-Meteyard SL, Geffen GM. Event-related potential indices of visual attention following moderate to severe closed head injury. *Brain Injury* 1994;8:541-58.

[34] Malloy P, Bihrle A, Duffy J, Cimino C. The orbi-tomedial frontal syndrome. *Arch. Clin. Neuropsych.* 1993;8:185-201.

[35] Logan GD, Schachar RJ, Tannock R. Impulsivity and inhibitory control. *Psychol. Sci* 1997;8:60-4.

[36] Oosterlaan J, Sergeant JA Inhibition in ADHD, aggressive, and anxious children: a biologically based model of child psychopathology. *J. Abnorm. Child Psychol.* 1996;24: 19-37.

[37] Schachar R, Tannock R, Marriott M, Logan G. Deficient inhibitory control in attention deficit hyperactivity disorder. *J. Abnorm. Child Psychol.* 1995;23:411-37.

[38] Marczinski CA, Fillmore MT. Pre-response cues reduce the impairing effects of alcohol on the execution and suppression of responses. *Exp. Clin. Psychopharm* 2003;11:110-7.

[39] Fillmore MT, Weafer J. Alcohol impairment of behavior in men and women. *Addict* 2004;99: 1237-46.

[40] Maylor EA, Rabbitt PM, James GH, Kerr SA. Effects of alcohol, practice, and task complexity on reaction time distributions. *Quart. J. Exp. Psychol. Hum. Exp. Psychol.* 1992; 49(A):119-39.

[41] Fillmore MT. Drug abuse as a problem of impaired control: current approaches and findings. *Behav. Cog. Neurosci. Rev.* 2003;2:179-97.

[42] Fox E. Negative priming from ignored distractors in visual selection: A review. *Psychon. Bull. Rev.* 1995;2:145-73.

[43] Houghton G, Tipper S. A model of inhibitory mechanisms in selective attention. In: Dagenbach D, Carr TH, eds, *Inhibitory processes in attention, memory, and language.* New York, NY, USA: Academic Press, 1994:53-112.

[44] May CP, Kane MJ, Hasher L. Determinants of negative priming. *Psych Bull* 1995;118: 35-54.

[45] Neill WT, Valdes LA. Facilitatory and inhibitory aspects of attention. In: Kramer AF, Coles MGH, Logan GD, eds, Converging operations in the study of visual selective attention. Washington, DC, USA: *Am. Psychol. Assoc.* 1996:77-106.

[46] Tipper SP. The negative priming effect: inhibitory priming by ignored objects. *The Q J Exp. Psychol.* 1985;37(A):571-90.

[47] Everling S, Fischer B. The antisaccade: a review of basic research and clinical studies. *Neuropsycho-logia* 1998;36:885-99.

[48] Klein RM. Inhibition of return. *Trends Cogn. Sci.* 2000;4:138-47.

[49] Beech AR, Powell TJ, McWilliams J, Claridge GS. Evidence of reduced "cognitive inhibition" in schizophrenia. *Br. J. Clin. Psychol.* 1989;28:110-6.

[50] Gaymard B, Ploner CJ, Rivard S, Vermesch AI, Pierrot-Deseilligny C. Cortical control of saccades. *Exp. Brain Res.* 1998;123:159-63.

[51] Hasher L, Stoltzfus ER, Zacks RT, Rypma B. Age and inhibition. *J. Exp. Psychol. Learn Mem. Cogn.* 1991;17:163-9.

[52] Ross RG, Harris JG, Olincy A, Radant A. Eye movement task measures inhibition and spatial working memory in adults with schizophrenia, ADHD, and a normal comparison group. *Psychiat Res.* 2000;95:35-42.

[53] Abroms BD, Fillmore MT. Alcohol-induced im-pairment of inhibitory mechanisms involved in visual search. *Exp. Clin. Psychopharm* 2004;12: 243-50.

[54] Fillmore MT, Dixon MJ, Schweizer TA. Differ-ential effects of alcohol on responses to negatively and positively primed stimuli. *J. Stud. Alcohol* 2000; 61:872-80.

[55] Fillmore MT, Dixon MJ, Schweizer TA. Alcohol affects processing of ignored stimuli in a negative priming paradigm. *J. Stud. Alcohol* 2000;61:571-8.

[56] Klein RM. Inhibitory tagging system facilitates visual search. *Nature* 1988;334:430-1.

[57] Ross RG, Hommer D, Breiger D, Varley C, Radant A. Eye movement task related to frontal lobe functioning in children with attention deficit disorder. *J. Am. Acad. Child Adolesc Psychiatry* 1994;33:869-74.

[58] Abroms BD, Gottlob L, Fillmore MT. Alcohol effects on inhibitory control of attention: distinguishing between intentional and automatic mechanisms. *Psychopharmacology* 2006;188:324-34.

[59] Ludwig AM, Wikler A, Stark LH. The first drink: psychobiological aspects of craving. *Arch. Gen. Psychiat* 1974;30:539-47.

[60] Marlatt GA, Gordon JR Determinants of relapse: implications for the maintenance of behavior change. In: Davidson PO, Davidson SM, eds, *Behavioral medicine: changing health lifestyles*. New York, NY, USA: Brunner-Mazel, 1980:410-52.

[61] Fillmore MT. Cognitive preoccupation with alcohol and binge drinking in college students: Alcohol-induced priming of the motivation to drink. *Psychol. Addict. Behav.* 2001;15:325-32.

[62] Fillmore MT, Rush CR. Alcohol effects on inhibitory and activational response strategies in the acquisition of alcohol and other reinforcers: Priming the motivation to drink. *J. Stud. Alcohol* 2001;62:646-56.

[63] Kirk JM, de Wit H. Individual differences in the priming effect of ethanol in social drinkers. *J. Stud. Alcohol* 2000;61:64-71.

[64] Koob GF, Le Moal M. Drug abuse: Hedonic homeostatic dysregulation. *Science* 1997; 278:52-8.

[65] Robinson TE, Berridge KC. The neural basis of drug craving: An incentive-sensitization theory of addiction. *Brain Res. Rev.* 1993;18:247-91.

[66] Stewart J, de Wit H, Eikelboom R. Role of unconditioned and conditioned drug effects in the self-administration of opiates and stimulants. *Psychol. Rev.* 1984;91;251-68.

[67] Wise RA, Bozarth MA. A psychomotor stimulant theory of addiction. *Psychol. Rev.* 1987; 94:469-92.

[68] Jentsch JD, Taylor JR. Impulsivity resulting from frontostriatal dysfunction in drug abuse: implica-tion for the control of behavior by reward-related stimuli. *Psychopharmacology* 1999;146:373-90.

[69] Collins RL. Drinking restraint and risk for alcohol abuse. *Exp. Clin. Psychopharm.* 1993;1: 44-54.

In: Alcohol-Related Cognitive Disorders
Editors: L. Sher, I. Kandel, J. Merrick pp. 177-189

ISBN: 978-1-60741-730-9
© 2009 Nova Science Publishers, Inc.

Chapter 10

ATTENTIONAL LAPSES DUE TO ALCOHOL INFLUENCE

Frances Finnigan, Daniela Schulze and Jonathan Smallwood

ABSTRACT

In this chapter we examine the influence of acute alcohol on attentional lapses whilst performing a sustained attention task (SART). The sample consisted of 17 male and seven females. A dose of alcohol achieving 80mg/100ml was administered to subjects before completion of the task. Alcohol led participants to make more errors as the session progressed and report a greater incidence of mind wandering. Importantly, alcohol reduced individuals' ability to recover from a lapse in attention. Although the sample size is small, the study did enable us to gain insight into the detrimental effects of acute alcohol ingestion on mind wandering. The authors anticipate that through the use of thought probes in the context of the SART and a larger sample size, we hope to shed further light on this phenomenon.

INTRODUCTION

In many of today's societies, the law prohibits individuals from engaging in tasks such as operating heavy machinery or driving a car while under the acute influence of alcohol. These tasks share a common skill: they require participants to monitor the environment and their own performance continuously to detect, as early as possible, the sequence of events that can lead to accidents. In tasks requiring continuous attentional supervision, it has recently emerged that thoughts that are unconstrained by the task can have serious consequences for task performance [1]. In this chapter, we consider the possibility that the effects of alcohol consumption on a continuous performance are, in part, due to such brief failures to maintain continuous attentional supervision on the necessary features of the larger task environment.

In the literature, shifts in attention away from the task environment have been variously described as stimulus independent thought (SI) [2], task unrelated thought (TUT) [3-7] zone outs [8,9] or more recently, as mind wandering [1,10]. Despite the variations in terminology, these labels emphasize that, periodically, attention leaves the constraints of the task, often focusing instead on information derived from one's own internal world. Recent neuro-imaging work suggests that the so-called default network [11,12]—a network of cortical and subcortical areas—provides the neural substrates for such experiences [11]. The present study aimed to determine whether mind wandering during a sustained vigilance task is influenced by acute alcohol ingestion. Such a finding would be an important step in understanding the consequences of alcohol on safety conscious industries.

INFLUENCE OF ALCOHOL ON PERFORMANCE

Although it is well known that elevated blood alcohol level (BAL) impairs both behavioral and psychomotor performance on a range of tasks [13-19], it is often the case that these effects are subtle and that even small amounts of alcohol impair performance on many common tasks, even when blood alcohol levels are at or below the legal limit for driving [20]. Such acute alcohol induced impairment may be seen on inhibitory control of attention [21] and cognitive executive function [22]. Moreover, performance impairment can persist for at least two hours after drinking [23-26] and perhaps much longer [27]. Despite alcohol impairing performance on a range of tasks, there is a lack of consistent evidence that the acute administration of alcohol can impair sustained attention [28]. For example, although both a Digit Symbol Task and word recall were impaired following the acute administration of alcohol, no difference was observed in a vigilance task [28]. Moreover, wide individual differences have been seen in the effects of alcohol on reaction time, with some individuals showing faster reaction times that did not vary from baseline [29]. This lack of consistent findings of the effects of alcohol on a simple reaction time task, particularly given the notion that alcohol is often described as the most likely cause of impaired driving, suggests that perhaps alcohol has subtle effects that traditional tasks fail to detect [30,31].

PREDICTING ALCOHOL IMPAIRMENT

It has also been shown that performance at a given time is very poorly correlated with blood alcohol when both performance and BAL were recorded over time. Studies that have charted performance across the ascending and descending limbs of the blood-alcohol curve tend to show characteristic patterns, whereby following the ingestion of alcohol, the blood-alcohol level increases to a peak that is generally associated with maximal impairment of performance. Although the BAL then declines, this decrease does not show a parallel reduction in the degree of performance impairment. For example, it has been shown [23] that reaction time was slowed to about 112% of baseline after a dose of about 40 mg% BAL, but this impairment did not improve as BAL decreased over time. By 120 minutes after drinking, performance was still at 115% baseline, whereas BAL had decreased to below 10% mg% from peak. Furthermore, performance could be better predicted from the initial alcohol dose than from the current BAL. These issues make it difficult to determine the extent to which BAL can be indicative of current levels of impairments.

What is perhaps the greatest concern for our ability to prevent the detrimental effects of alcohol, however, is the dissociation between subjective ratings of alcohol intoxication and objective measures of both BAL and performance deficits. In general, subjects subjectively rate themselves most drunk within the first 15 minutes of drinking and progressively rate themselves less intoxicated despite their rising blood alcohol concentrations [29]. Despite this reduction in subjective impairment, the detrimental effects of alcohol on the rate of processing have been shown to be independent of practice or cognitive judgments [32,33]. Similar to BAL, therefore, subjective intoxication does not provide a reliable index of acute alcohol impairment.

Clearly, to date, little evidence has supported impairment due to alcohol on simple tests of sustained attention. Moreover, research to date does not indicate a simple correlation between dose, current BAL, and impairment in both subjective and objective performance. Such null results are surprising, given the emphasis that society places on drunkenness during routine tasks such as driving, and that BAL is the preferred measure of intoxication.

A recently developed task, the Sustained Attention to Response Task [SART], requires participants to respond to a sequence of stimuli presented on a computer screen, responding to frequent non-target stimuli and withholding a response to an infrequent target. The SART requires participants to perform a simple task while paying close attention not just to the task but also to the manner in which they are performing it [34,35]. This combination of a routine task environment with a need to attend to one's behavior therefore mimics in an important manner the nature of many of the task environments from which alcohol is forbidden.

Failing to attend to the SART in a continuous manner leads to error. The SART has been shown to be sensitive to the individual differences in the frequency of attentional lapses [34] as measured by the Cognitive Failures Questionnaire (CFQ) [36]. The task has also been shown to be sensitive to the experience of task disengagement as measured by a thought sampling methodology (37, Experiments 1 and 2) and retrospecttive self report (37, Experiment 3). Recent research using thought sampling techniques has confirmed that periods in which transcribed verbal reports indicate attention has left the task are associated with errors on the SART [37] and co-vary with physiological indices implicated in task disengagement, such as GSR [38].

One advantage of the SART as a measure of sustained attention is that, because the participants are required to respond continuously to the infrequent target, it is possible to derive a number of additional parameters regarding the nature or character of attentional lapses. For example, generally the response time is rapid before a lapse in attention (34,37,39) a phenomenon that is usually interpreted as a lack of careful or controlled processing of the task. Likewise, following a lapse, the response time lengthens as participants re-establish controlled processing of the task environment, the so called 'oops' phenomenon. Consistent with the notion that deceleration in response time indexes awareness and so recovery from an attentional lapse, participants with traumatic brain injury neither lengthen their response times after an error [34] nor show subjective or physiological awareness that their performance lapsed [38].

In our study, participants performed the SART after consuming either alcohol or placebo. We recorded both behavioral (e.g. response inhibition errors) and subjective indicators of the frequency of mind wandering. In addition, we examined the consequences of acute alcohol consumption on three measures of response time during task performance: (i) response time prior to an error, (ii) response time after an error, and (iii) the deceleration following an error.

OUR EXPERIENCE

Seventeen male and seven female volunteers (see table 1 for demographic details) were recruited by local advertising in and around the university. Females were specifically included in this study because data on alcohol and ingestion are seriously lacking in this area. Females were given a pregnancy test (Predictor Pregnancy, Predictor Frameset) to ensure that they were not unknowingly pregnant. All volunteers gave informed consent to participate. Inclusion depended upon satisfactory completion of a health-check questionnaire, a history of moderate social drinking (a score of less than 3 on Short Michigan Alcoholism Screening Questionnaire (SMAST) [40], and absence of current medication. Participants received a £15 disturbance allowance, £5:00 taxi fare and £5:00 food voucher (redeemable by the university refectory) on completion of the study. Participants were free to terminate the study without reason at any time. A between-group design was employed to avoid the asymmetrical transfer of treatment effects that often afflict within-subjects designs [41,42]. Subjects were allocated at random to either to the alcohol (n=12) or control (n=12) condition. Alcohol was administered as vodka (37% v/v/ ethanol). Doses were calculated per liter of body water computed from height, weight, and age, which has been advocated as a more accurate method than body weight alone [43]. The dose was chosen to achieve peak BAL of 80mg/100 ml. The alcohol was mixed with an equal volume of water and diabetic orange juice (Robinsons Orange No Added Sugar). For placebo and alcohol mixtures, 4 ml of vodka was floated on the surface of the drink and the rim of the glass was swabbed with alcohol.

To mask any taste of alcohol [44] all participants first sucked a 5 mg benzocaine 'Tyroset' lozenge and a menthol flavored cough sweet 'Halls Mentholyptus extra strong' before ingesting the mixture. BALs were assessed using a Lion Alcometer, SD 400 series (Lion Laboratories, Cardiff, Wales, UK) which was calibrated at weekly intervals. Participants performed the standard SART [34], which consisted of single digit alpha numeric stimuli (X or Y) presented in the centre of a VDU against a black background. The target stimulus was the digit Y. All stimuli were non-masked and presented on the screen for 1000 ms. The inter-stimulus interval (ISI) was 1000 ms, during which time the screen was blank. The rate of stimuli presentation was comparable with that employed on standard SART tasks (34). In the present study, the duration of each test session on the task was ten minutes. A short practice session was carried out before the first task. Participants also completed the Thinking Content component of the Dundee Stress State Questionnaire (DSSQ) [45], which is a sixteen-item questionnaire considering the content of thinking during a recently completed task. The instrument assesses (i) Task Appraisal (e.g. 'I thought about how I should work more carefully' or 'I thought about my level of ability' and (ii) Task Disengagement (e.g. 'I thought about my personal worries' or 'I thought about something than happened earlier today'). Each item contains eight factors that are measured on a five-point Likert scale ranging from 'Never' to 'Very Often'. Participants also completed a seven-day retrospective drinking diary and a drinking-history questionnaire and subjective mood as assessed by an 11-item Subjective Feelings Question-naire [29].

Participants were required to abstain from alcohol, drugs, and mediation for 24 hours before the test day. To control for stomach content, participants were instructed to refrain from eating or drinking anything except water for 4 hours before the test. Smokers were requested to have their last cigarette one hour before the test.

Upon arrival at the laboratory, participants gave informed consent to participate in the study. They were breathalyzed, first to ensure blood alcohol levels were zero and second to familiarize them with the breatha-lyzing procedure. Females were then asked to take a pregnancy test. Volunteers were then randomly assigned to an alcohol/placebo condition. Demographic details were obtained. The participants then completed a practice session on the SART, consisting of ten non-target and two target stimuli presented in a random order. Pilot studies had shown that such practice provided good performance stability. Following practice, baseline SART performance measures were obtained. Participants consumed the 'Tyrozet' and 'Hall' lozenges during baseline testing and then received their drink, which had to be consumed within 10 min. All drinks were prepared out-with the laboratory. Over the next 10 minutes, participants completed the questionnaires and drinking diaries.

To ensure that our study measured the effects of alcohol over the ascending and descending limbs of the blood alcohol curve (BAC) and at peak, testing commenced and continued every 20 minutes over an 80-minute period (giving five data points for each participant) with BAL and subjective feelings measured before each testing session and the thinking component of the DSSQ assessed at the end of each test session. After the final breath test (2 hours after drinking), participants were debriefed, given tea/coffee, and directed to the university refectory fo a snakc to offset the effects of fasting.

WHAT WE FOUND

Table 1 contains demographic information, physical characteristics and drinking history information. Independent- sample t-test on these variables revealed no significant group differences, p > .05 for all comparisons.

Table 1. Description of the individuals allocated to the control and alcohol conditions

	Control	SD	Alcohol	SD
Age in years	27.83	6.81	29.92	7.86
SMAST	0.50	0.80	0.58	0.67
Weight in kg	70.50	15.62	71.08	13.29
Height in cm	173.67	7.15	171.75	5.53
Years education	16.92	3.60	18.42	3.65
Previous wk drinking in units of alcohol	20.83	19.79	31.54	14.91
Previous wk drinking frequency of drinking sessions	2.67	2.10	3.83	1.34
Age first drink (yrs)	13.17	2.92	13.42	3.94
Age first drunk (yrs)	15.00	2.04	14.92	3.82
Age drinking at current level	18.33	1.72	19.58	3.73
Self-reported quantity consumed during average drinking session (units)	10.33	10.36	8.45	5.52
Self-reported frequency of drinking in drinking sessions	2.44	1.90	3.21	1.67
Family history of drinking problems	0.33	0.49	0.42	0.51

Figure 1 shows BAL over the 80-minute observation period as a function of alcohol dose. As expected, there was no evidence of alcohol ingestion for those who had ingested placebo. A mixed ANOVA indicated that the difference between the two groups was reliable [$F(1,21)$= 520, $p < .001$]. A test session by group interaction was significant, indicating that the BALs for those in the alcohol group decreased systematically over the course of the five test sessions [$F(4,87)$=17.2, $p < .001$].

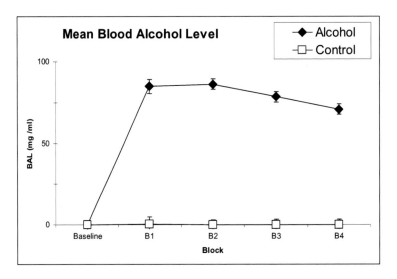

Figure 1. Blood alcohol levels assessed by breath analysis as a function of alcohol dose. Alcohol was administered to approximate blood alcohol level of 80 mg/100 ml (see text).

The frequency with which each group reported 'task appraisal' and 'task disengagement' is presented in figure 2 (A,B). Mixed ANOVA revealed no group differences in the frequency for 'task appraisal' although a general decrease in this measure was observed for both groups over the five test sessions [$F(4,88)$=3.55, $p < .01$]. By contrast, the analysis of 'task disengagement' indicate an increase in this measure over the same test period [$F(4,88)$=5.7, $p < .01$]. In addition, marginally higher levels of 'task disengagement' were reported for those participants in the alcohol condition [$F (1,22)$=2.9, $p = .09$]. Individual ANOVA conducted for each test session of the task over the 80- minute test period of this group revealed that the self-reported higher levels of task disengagement was significant during the first test session only [$F(1,22) = 4.38$, $p < .05$].

The consequences of alcohol ingestion on the probability of making errors on the SART over time are presented in figure 3. One participant allocated to the alcohol condition failed to respond to 202 of the correct targets and was excluded. Mixed ANOVA revealed a reliable interaction between the effects of alcohol and SART errors over time [$F(4, 84) = 2.85$, $p< .05$, Partial Eta Squared=.12]. Post hoc tests constrained to each experimental condition and containing these outlier individuals revealed that participants in the alcohol condition made greater errors across all cells relative to baseline [$p<.01$ for each block]. In the control group the number of errors was only greater at block 3 ($p < .05$). Alcohol, therefore, led to increases in the extent to which SART errors accrued during task performance.

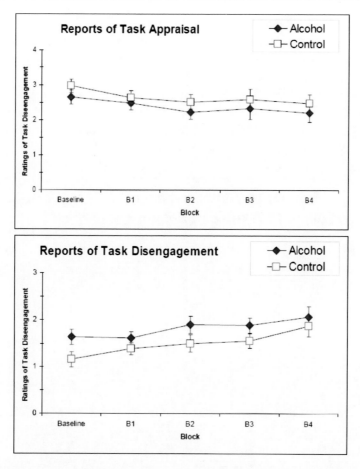

Figure 2. The likelihood of verbal reports of task appraisal (top) and task disengagement (bottom) over the five sessions of the task.

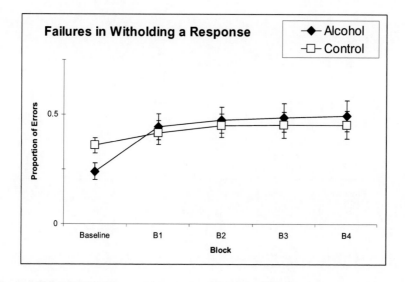

Figure 3. Probability of an error over the course of the experiment.

The study used mixed ANOVA to contrast the effects of alcohol on the RT associated with failures to withhold a response correctly. Alcohol condition was included as a between-participant factor with repeated measures on block. Consideration of the average response time over four stimuli before failing to withhold a response yielded an effect of block only [$F(4,88) = 3.1$, $p < .05$ MSE = 959, Partial Eta Squared = .12] indicating that response time before errors tended to decrease over the course of the testing session, irrespective of alcohol consumption (figure 4, Upper Panel). A comparable pattern was identified when comparing the response time following an error (figure 4, Lower Panel).

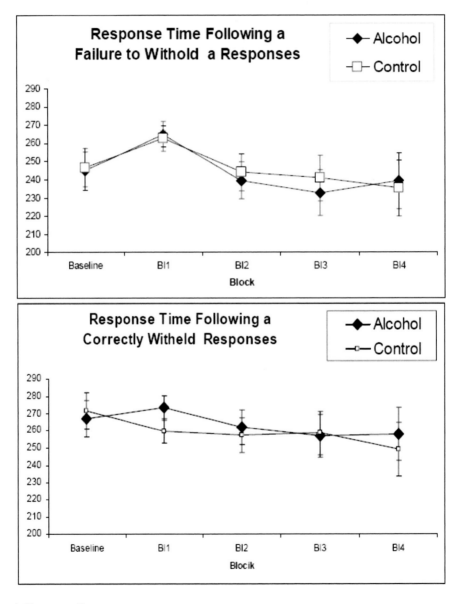

Figure 4. Response times.

Finally, we examined the lengthening in RT following an error. This analysis tended toward a Block X Condition interaction [$F (4, 88) = 2.1$, $p = .07$, MSE = 32, Partial Eta

Squared = .09]. Subsequent contrast analysis indicated that the time course of this interaction fitted a reliable linear trend [F (1,22) = 6.6, p = .17, p < .05 MSE = 17, Partial Eta Squared=.23] indicating that participants in the control condition showed maximal decreases in RT following an error in the early sessions, whereas participants in the alcohol condition showed maximal deceleration in later blocks of the task. Consistent with these different time courses, the decrease in RT was reliably larger in the control condition than the alcohol group in Block 1 [t (22) = 2.4, p = .023].

DISCUSSION

The results of our investigation indicated that acute alcohol ingestion could lead to increases in the extent to which the mind wanders during sustained attention. As can be observed from figure 3, participants in the alcohol condition showed a statistically significant increase in errors across the five test session. Although an increase in errors was also observed for those in the control group, this effect was less consistent. Additional analysis of response time suggested that recovery from an attentional lapse was impaired in the alcohol group early in the session (figure 5). In addition, verbal reports (see figure 2) indicated a higher level of subjective accounts of 'task disengagement' for those in the alcohol condition, however, this effect was significant for the early points in the testing session only. No significant group differences were found for 'task appraisal'.

Although a significant effect of alcohol consumption was observed across several different measures of mind wandering, the specific pattern varied across different sessions of the task.

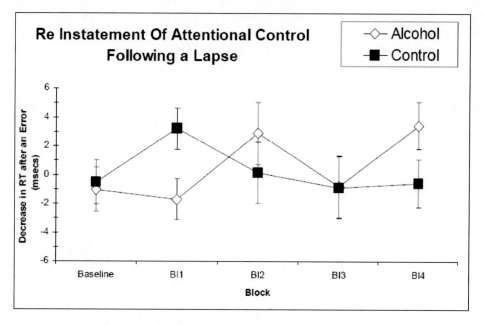

Figure 5. Reinstatement of attentional control following a lapse.

For example, the participants' ability to recover from an attentional lapse and questionnaire measures of 'task disengagement' showed the greatest discrepancy between the alcohol and control conditions in the early blocks of the session (blocks 1 and 2), and so broadly paralleled the BAL curve. On the other hand, the probability of errors on the SART was greater over each of the five test sessions for the alcohol conditions. One explanation for these discrepancies may be that these measures of attentional lapses could be differentially related to the experience of being intoxicated. For example, it has been found [29] that participants rate themselves most drunk within the first 15 minutes of drinking, and progressively rate themselves less intoxicated as time elapses, despite rising blood alcohol concentrations. It is thus possible that the explicit experience of intoxication engenders particularly elaborate mind-wandering from which the participants have difficulty disengaging. As the session progressed, the acute experience of intoxication could decrease and, the resultant alcohol 'come down' could be responsible for the increase in the number of attentional lapses.

A second reason for the partial dissociation between the acute effects of alcohol on the two measures may reflect the nature of awareness of these attentional lapses. For example, the experience of mind wandering has been suggested [1] to be the result of two different cognitive processes—the decoupling of attention from the constraints of the task, and a simultaneous lack of awareness that one has temporarily ceased to monitor ones own performance. Possibly, the acute effects of alcohol on 'task disengagement' are such that they are targeted at the individual's ability to recognize his/her own attentional lapse. Early in the session, alcohol impaired participants' ability to recover from an attentional lapse (block 1), whereas verbal reports of these episodes were higher in block 2. Recent neuro-imaging work indicates that the anterior cingulate is responsible for the detection of failures in both subjective [46] and behavioral lapses [47], and so it could be that our results further underline that acute alcohol ingestion targets frontal brain regions leading attentional lapses to remain unrecognized or uncorrected for longer than when in a sober state [15]. The relative failure for drunken individuals to lengthen their response time following an error is consistent with recent work, suggesting that alcohol may selectively impair the ability of participants to catch their own minds wandering [48].

Taken together, the results of this preliminary study lends support to the suggestion that acute alcohol ingestion leads to an increase in mind wandering whilst performing a task that requires sustained attention. Crucially, acute alcohol ingestion may impair an individual's ability to recover from such lapses, particularly during periods of acute intoxication, a process that could be responsible for some of the consequences of alcohol in safety conscious settings like driving. Our data are consistent with the suggestion in the literature [49] that one reason why detecting the effects of acute alcohol ingestion is difficult is because the tasks employed are not sensitive to the drug's sedative effects.

In routine tasks, which require sustained attention over a prolonged period, the detrimental consequences of alcohol may arise from brief failures in the individual's ability to maintain the necessary and continuous attentional supervision. Finally, an interesting possibility that emerges from our data presented is that if mind wandering is increased by acute intoxication, then this process could underscore some of the pleasurable effects of alcohol consumption. Moderate consumption of alcohol could plausibly reduce the inhibitory processes that normally constrains our thoughts upon the current environment, and by so doing, facilitate a form of mental time travel [10], allowing us to escape from some of the more mundane aspects of daily life.

ACKNOWLEDGMENTS

This study was funded by a grant awarded from the Alcohol Education and Research Council (AERC).

REFERENCES

[1]   Smallwood J, Schooler JW. The restless mind. *Psychol Bull* 2006;132(6):946 -58.
[2]   Antrobus J. Information theory and stimulus inde-pendent thought. Br J Psychol 1968;59:423-30.
[3]   Giambra LM. A laboratory method for investi-gating influences on switching attention to task-unrelated imagery and thought. *Conscious Cogn* 1995;4:1-21.
[4]   Smallwood J, Obonsawin MC, Heim SD. Task Unrelated Thought: the role of distributed processing. *Conscious Cogn.* 2003;12:169-89.
[5]   Smallwood J, Baraciaia SF, Lowe M, Obonsawin MC. Task unrelated thought whilst encoding information. *Conscious Cogn.* 2003;12:452-84.
[6]   Smallwood J, Obonsawin MC, Reid H. The effects of block duration and task demands on the experience of task unrelated thought. *Imaginat Cogn. Pers* 2003;22:13-31.
[7]   Smallwood J, O'Connor RC, Sudberry MV, Ballantyre C. The consequences of encoding information on the maintenance of internally generated images and thoughts: The role of meaning. *Conscious Cogn.* 2004;4:789-820.
[8]   Schooler JW, Reichle ED, Halpern DV. Zoning-out during reading: Evidence for dissociations between experience and meta-consciousness. In: Levin D, ed. *Visual meta-cognition: Thinking about seeing.* Praeger (in press).
[9]   Schooler JW. Representing consciousness: Dissociations between consciousness and meta-consciousness. *Trends Cogn. Sci.* 2002;6:339-44.
[10] Mason MF, Norton MI, Van JD, Wegner DM, Grafton ST, Macrae CN. Wandering minds: the default network and stimulus independent thought. *Science* 2007;315:393-5.
[11] Raichle ME et al. A default mode of brain function. *Proc. Natl. Acad. Sci.* 2001;16:676-82.
[12] Greicius MD, Krasnow B, Reiss AL, Menon V. Functional connectivity in the resting brain: a network analysis of the default mode hypothesis. *Proc. Natl. Acad. Sci.* 2003;100(1):253-8.
[13] Abroms, BD, Fillmore, MT. Alcohol-induced impairment of inhibitory mechanisms involved in visual search. *Exp. Clin. Psychopharmacol.* 2004; 59:234-50.
[14] Verster JC, van Duin D, Volkerts ER, Schreuder AHCML, Verbaten MN. Alcohol hangover effects on memory functioning and vigilance performance after an evening of binge drinking. *Neuropsycho-pharmacology* 2003;28(4):740-6.

[15] Ridderinkhof RE, de Vlugt Y, Bramlage A, Spaan M, Elton M, Snel J et al. Alcohol consumption impairs detection of performance errors in medio-frontal cortex. *Science* 2002;298(5601):2209-11.

[16] Moskowitz H, Fiorentina D. A review of the scientific literature regarding the effects of alcohol on driving-related behavior at blood alcohol concentrations of 80mg/dl and lower. Report HS-809-028. Washington, DC: US Dept Transport Nat Highway Traffic Safety Adm, 2000.

[17] Koelega S. Alcohol and vigilance performance: A review. *Psychopharmacology* 1995;118:233-49.

[18] Holloway FA. Low-dose alcohol effects on human behaviour and performance. *Alcohol Drugs Driving* 1995;11:39-56.

[19] Finnigan F, Hammersley RH. Effects of alcohol on performance. In: Jones DM, Smith AP, eds. *Factors affecting human performance*. London, UK: Academic Press, 1992:73-126.

[20] West R, Wilding J, French D, Kemp R, Irving A. Effects of low and moderate doses of alcohol on driving hazard perception latency and driving speed. *Addiction* 1993;88:527-32.

[21] Abroms, BD, Gottlob, LR, Fillmore, MT. Alcohol effects on inhibitory control of attention: Distin-guishing intentional and automatic mechanisms. *Psychopharmacology* 2006;188(3):324-34.

[22] Weissenborn R, Duka D. Acute alcohol effects on cognitive function in social drinkers: their relation- ship to drinking habits. *Psychopharmacology* 2003; 165(3):306-12.

[23] Millar K, Hammersley RH, Finnigan F. Reduction of alcohol-induced performance impairment by prior ingestion of food. *Br. J. Psychol* 1992;83:261-78.

[24] Finnigan F, Hammersley RH, Millar K. The effects of expectancy and alcohol on cognitive-motor performances. *Addiction* 1995;90:661-72.

[25] Maylor EA, Rabbitt PMA, James GH, Kerr SA. Effects of alcohol and extended practice on divided-attention performance. *Percept Psychophys* 1990;48(5):445-52.

[26] Rohrbaugh JW, Stapleton JM, Parasuraman R Frowein HW, Adinoff B, Varner JL et al. Alcohol intoxication reduces visual sustained attention. *Psychopharmacology* 1988;96:443-6.

[27] Cooper TJ. The effects of alcohol on executive function in social drinkers: Even-related potential correlates of cognitive performance. *Doctoral Thesis*. Glasgow, Scotland, UK: Caledonian University, 2004.

[28] Heishman SJ, Arasteh K, Stitzer ML. Comparative effects of alcohol and marijuana on mood, memory, and performance. *Pharmacol. Biochem. Behav.* 1997;58(1):93-101.

[29] Hammersley RH, Finnigan F, Millar K. Individual differences in the acute response to alcohol. *Pers. Individ. Dif.* 1994;17:497-510.

[30] Leung S, Starmer G. Gap acceptance and risk-taking by young and mature drivers, both sober and alcohol-intoxicated, in a simulated driving task. *Accid. Anal. Prev.* 2005;37(6):1056-65.

[31] Borkenstein RF. Driver Characteristics and Impairment at Various BACs. *J. Stud. Alcohol.* 1985;10:3-12.

[32] Maylor EA, Rabbitt PMA. Effects of practice and alcohol on performance of a perceptual-motor task. *Q J Exp. Psychol.* 1987;39A:777-95.

[33] Maylor EA, Rabbitt PMA, Connolly SAV. Effects of alcohol and extended practice on divided-attention performance. *Percept Psychophys* 1989; 45:431-8.

[34] Robertson IH, Manly T, Andrade j, Baddeley BT, Yiend J. Oops: Performance correlates of everyday attentional failures in traumatic brain injured and normal subjects. *Neurospsychologia* 1997;35(6): 747-58.

[35] Manly T, Robertson IH, Galloway M, Hawkins K. The absent mind: Further investigations of sustained attention to response. *Neuropsychologia* 1999;37:661-70.

[36] Broadbent DE, Cooper PF, Fitzgerald P, Parks KR. The cognitive failures questionnaire (CFQ) and its correlates. *Br. J. Clin. Psychol.* 1982;21(1):1-16.

[37] Smallwood J, Davies JB, Heim D, Finnigan F, Sudberry MV, O'Connor et al. Subjective exper-iences and the attentional lapse. Task engagement and disengagement during sustained attention. *Conscious Cogn* 2004;4:789-820.

[38] O'Keefe F, Dockree P, Robertson IH. Awareness deficits in traumatic brain injury mediated by impaired error processing? Evidence from electro-dermal activity. *J. Cog. Neurosci.* 2004;Suppl 31.

[39] Smallwood J, McSpadden M, Schooler JW. The lights are on but nobodies home. *Psychon. Bull Rev.* (in press).

[40] Selzer ML, Vinocour A, Van Rooijen L. A self-administered Short Michigan Alcohol Screening Test (SMAST). *J. Stud. Alcohol.* 1975;36:117-26.

[41] Armitage P, Hills M. The two-period crossover trial. *Statistician* 1982;31:119-31.

[42] Cotton JW. Interpreting data from two-period crossover design. *Psychol. Bull* 1989;106:503-15.

[43] Watson PE, Watson ID, Batt RD. Prediction of blood alcohol in human subjects. *J. Stud Alcohol* 1981;42:547-56.

[44] Fagan D, Tiplady B, Scott DB. Effects of ethanol on psychomotor performance. *Br. J. Anaesth* 1987; 59:961-5.

[45] Matthews G, Joyner L, Gililand K, Campbell SE, Faulconner S. Validation of a comprehensive stress state questionnaire: Towards a state "Big three"? In: Mervielde I, Deary IJ, De Fruyt F, Ostendorf F, eds. *Handbook of coping: Theory, research and applications*. Tilburg, NL: Tilburg Univ Press 1999:333-50.

[46] Mitchell JP, Heatherton TF, Kelley WM, Wyland CL, Wegner DN, Macrae CN. Separating sustained from transient aspects of cognitive control during thought suppression. *Psychol. Sci.* (in press).

[47] Hester R et al. Neural mechanism involved in error processing: A comparison of errors made with and without awareness. *Neuroimage* 2005; 27:602-8.

[48] Sayette M, Schooler JW, Reichle ED. *The effects of alcohol on self and probe caught episodes of zoning-out*. Unpublished manuscript. Pittsburgh: Univ Pittsburgh, 2006.

[49] Finnigan F, Schulze D, Smallwood J, Helanders S. The effects of self-administered alcohol induced hangover attained in a naturalistic setting on psychomotor and cognitive performance and subjective state. *Addiction* 2005;100(11):1680-9.

In: Alcohol-Related Cognitive Disorders   ISBN: 978-1-60741-730-9
Editors: L. Sher, I. Kandel, J. Merrick pp. 191-197   © 2009 Nova Science Publishers, Inc.

Chapter 11

EFFECT OF ALCOHOL ON INTRUSION ERRORS IN SOCIAL DRINKERS

Suchismita Ray and Marsha E. Bates

ABSTRACT

This chapter is a secondary analysis of acute alcohol effects on intrusion errors in social drinkers in immediate free recall and delayed free recall tasks. Our aim was to examine further the mechanism through which intrusion errors occur in delayed recall. Intrusion errors occur when individuals produce information that is not relevant to the task. Previous research suggests that alcoholics are less able than controls to inhibit intrusions (a reflective cognitive function) under both no-intoxication and acute benzodiazepine Halcion intoxication conditions. We hypothesized that acute alcohol intoxication in social drinkers would cause more intrusion errors reflecting impaired reflective cognitive function in the delayed, compared to the immediate, free recall task. Twenty-two (11 male) volunteers participated in two counterbalanced sessions (alcohol, no-alcohol). In the alcohol session, free recall tasks were completed at blood alcohol concentrations between 80-84 mg/dl. Results showed that participants committed significantly more intrusion errors in a delayed recall task during acute alcohol intoxication compared to their no alcohol performance level. In contrast, in the immediate free recall task, participants' number of intrusion errors did not differ between alcohol and no-alcohol conditions. We suggest that by increasing the susceptibility to interference, acute alcohol intoxication caused more intrusion errors in the delayed, than in the immediate free recall task. Finally, the implications of these results in terms of alcohol prevention and intervention are suggested.

INTRODUCTION

Chronic, heavy alcohol consumption is known to increase the likelihood of memory intrusion errors [1,2]. Such studies showed that groups of otherwise cognitively unimpaired alcoholics were less able to inhibit intrusion errors in a task that tested their ability to track the source of remembered knowledge. Intrusion errors occur when individuals produce information that is not relevant to the task, for example, "remembering" an inaccurate antecedent or for example, when asked to recall words from a particular list, participants erroneously remember words from a different list.

The ability to inhibit intrusion errors in remembering has been conceptualized as a controlled information-processing operation that supports reflective cognition functions involving self-monitoring and self-evaluation of performance [1] and is thought to be governed by the frontal lobe [3]. Thus, distinct from quantitative differences in memory functioning, such as the number of words recalled from a list, intrusion errors represent qualitative aspects of memory performance that are informative about a potential mechanism through which alcohol may disrupt behavior. Weingartner and colleagues [2,4] have argued that reflective cognitive functions may play an important role in maintaining patterns of alcohol abuse. From this perspective, impaired reflective cognitive functions may lead to inaccurate risk perceptions and diminished behavioral inhibition [3], and increase risk for the development of alcohol and other drug abuse and dependence [3,5-7].

In view of the implications of impaired reflective cognitive function for risky decision making by both intoxicated alcoholics and social drinkers, surprisingly little research has been done on acute alcohol effects on intrusion errors in either immediate and delayed memory processing tasks. One study found that alcohol-dependent subjects, compared with non-alcohol-dependent controls, were less able to inhibit intrusion errors after the administration of triazolam (benzodiazepine Halcion) [4], while their performance did not differ from controls in the placebo challenge condition. Given that the drug triazolam mimics the acute effects of alcohol, the results suggest that reflective functions in alcohol-dependent persons may be particularly impaired during episodes of acute intoxication.

Our study was designed as a secondary analysis of intrusion error data from a larger study of the effects of acute alcohol intoxication on a broad range of memory processes in social drinkers. The results of the larger study [8,9] showed that acute alcohol intoxication impaired explicit, but not implicit, memory processing across multiple memory task. The present study further aims to characterize the effects of acute alcohol intoxication on reflective cognitive function as measured by the patterns and characteristics of intrusion errors. We examined intrusion errors in both immediate and delayed free recall tasks. In the larger study, the participants performed tasks in the following sequence: List 1 study, Distractor task 1 (word/non-word decisions); List 2 study, List 2 free recall (Immediate Free Recall task); Distractor tasks 2 (word/non-word decisions, frequency monitoring); List 1 free recall (Delayed Free Recall task).

The aim was also to explore a potential mechanism through which intrusion errors may occur in the delayed free recall by separately examining the occurrence of recalled versus unrecalled List 2 words from the immediate free recall task, on List 2 intrusion errors in the delayed free recall task. In the present study, the time difference between the study and the test phase of the immediate recall task was 1/2 min, whereas the time difference between the study and the test phase of the delayed recall task was approximately 43 min. Based on the results of Weingartner et al [4], we predicted that intrusion errors, signaling impaired reflective cognitive function, would be more likely as time passed between the study and the test phase, providing increased opportunities for interference from intervening tasks. Thus, we hypothesized that acute alcohol intoxication in social drinkers would cause more intrusion errors in the delayed, compared with the immediate, free recall task. Given that alcohol interferes with memory storage of list context [10,11] and increases sensitivity to interference [12], we examined recalled versus unrecalled List 2 words from the immediate free recall task on List 2 intrusion errors in the delayed free recall task to shed light on the underlying mechanism.

OUR EXPERIMENT

Twenty-two (11 male) participants individually took part in two counterbalanced sessions (alcohol and no-alcohol) separated by one week. Participants completed both free recall tasks in each session. Individuals over the age of 21 years were recruited. Males who consumed at least four drinks at least twice per month in the previous year, and women who consumed at least three drinks at least twice per month in the previous year were selected for the study. Exclusion criteria used were medical or psychological risks that contraindicated alcohol consumption, any current use of prescribed medication, past or present history of psychiatric, neurological, medical problems or diseases, weight 20% more or less than ideal for their age [13], first language not English, report of childhood learning disability or special education, parental or participant alcohol or drug related problem including treatment, conviction for driving under the influence, blackouts, morning drinking, others' perception of problem use, and a score of >1 on the Brief Mast questionnaire [14]. All the participants provided written informed consent and were reimbursed $75 for their time.

Delayed Free Recall (DFR) Task. Materials for this task consisted of List 1 that contained 90 items of 30 words selected from Ray and Bly [15]. These words were middle familiarity category exemplars from different categories (e.g., 'fruit', 'sport', 'furniture') [16]. The words were presented in different frequencies: six words were presented once, six words presented twice, six words presented three times, six words presented four times and six words presented five times.

Immediate Free Recall (IFR) Task. Materials for this task consisted of List 2 that contained 90 items of 30 words selected from Tracy and Bates [17]. These words did not come from specific categories (e.g., 'soil', 'green', 'book', 'dollar'). These 30 words were presented in different frequencies as described for the DFR Task. The words were chosen to be high in imagery and frequency in the English language.

Each participant completed two experimental sessions (alcohol challenge, no-alcohol) separated by one week. Equated, but not the same, sets of stimulus materials were used in the two experimental sessions. The order of completion of the sessions was randomized with the constraint that order was counterbalanced across participants. In the alcohol condition, participants performed both study and test phases following an alcohol challenge. In the no-alcohol condition, the participants were told not to expect alcohol to eliminate possible bias due to expectancy. All participants were required to fast for four hours before coming to the lab, and the zero blood alcohol concentration (BAC) was confirmed. The participants consumed a weight-adjusted dose of alcohol that produced a blood alcohol concentration (BAC) of approximately 90 mg/dl. Individual alcohol doses were mixed with orange juice in a ratio of 4 parts mixer to 1 part ethanol; the dose was consumed within a 15-minute interval. When a BAC of approx-imately 70 mg/dl was reached, the experimental session began.

DFR Task

Study: Participants saw List 1 of 90 items presented sequentially in a random manner on the computer screen. Each word stayed on the screen for four seconds and during that time participants were required to give a liking rating on individual words on a 7-point scale. Liking ratings were used to promote semantic or deep encoding of individual words [18]. Participants were asked to be careful in performing this task, as they would be asked about the words later. After the study phase of the DFR task, participants took part in a distractor task wherein they made a lexical decision, that is, word/non-word decisions. Then they took part in the IFR task.

IFR Task

Study: Participants gave liking ratings for 90 items on List 2 presented sequentially in a random manner following the same procedure as mentioned above.

Test: Immediately after the study phase, participants were instructed to recall as many words as possible from the studied list (i.e., List 2) during a 2 min interval. The critical measure in this task was the number of words participants mistakenly reported from List 1 (List 1 intrusion errors). Participants then took part in a task where they reported the frequency with which words appeared in the lists, and a task where, after viewing a string of letters, they decided whether it was a word or a non-word. These served as distractors prior to the test phase of the DFR task.

DFR Task

Test: Participants were instructed to recall as many words as possible from List 1 in 2 min. The critical measure in this task was the number of words the participants mistakenly reported from List 2 (List 2 intrusion errors).

OUR FINDINGS

IFR task. The mean BAC at the beginning and at the end of the task was 80 mg/dl (SD = 6) and 84 mg/dl (SD = 11), respectively. The mean number of List 1 intrusion errors in the alcohol and no-alcohol conditions was 0.73 (SD = 1.20) and 0.59 (SD = 1.00), respectively. A repeated measures ANOVA did not show a significant effect of alcohol ($F_{1, 20} = 1.30$, $p > .05$); Gender ($F_{1, 20} = .62$, $p > .05$); or Gender × Alcohol interaction ($F_{1, 20} = 1.81$, $p > .05$) on the number of intrusion errors. Number of intrusion errors was not significantly affected by word frequency ($F_{4, 80} = 0.57$, $p > .05$), nor by its interaction with alcohol ($F_{4, 80} = 0.44$, $p > .05$).

DFR task. The mean BAC at the beginning and at the end of the task was 86 mg/dl (SD = 8) and 83.5 mg/dl (SD = 9.1), respectively. The mean number of List 2 intrusion errors in the alcohol and no-alcohol conditions were 3.76 (SD = 2.19) and 2.81, (SD = 2.42) respectively. A repeated measures ANOVA performed on the intrusion error data showed a significant effect of alcohol (F_1, 20 = 6.29, p < .05, moderate effect size), but no significant effect of Gender (F_1, 20 = .84, p > .05) or Gender × Alcohol interaction (F_1, 20 = 2.11, p > .05). The number of intrusion errors was not significantly affected by word frequency (F_4, 80 = 0.67, p > .05), nor by its interaction with alcohol (F_4, 80 = 0.86, p > .05).

A paired t-test comparison showed that the alcohol condition compared with the no-alcohol condition caused participants in the DFR task to commit more List 2 intrusion errors from the correctly recalled List 2 words in the IFR task (M = 2.0, SD = 1.77 and M = 1.04, SD = 1.94; t21 = 2.37, p < .05). That is, during acute intoxication participants committed more List 2 intrusion errors from the words that they correctly recalled in the IFR task. Alternatively, a paired t-test comparison of List 2 intrusion errors from the unrecalled List 2 words in the IFR task showed that the unrecalled intrusion errors did not vary significantly in the alcohol and no-alcohol conditions (M = 1.59, SD = 1.68 and M = 1.0, SD = 1.20; p > .05).

DISCUSSION

Chronic, heavy alcohol consumption has been found to increase the likelihood of memory intrusion errors in delayed recall tasks [1,2]; acute triazolam administration decreases the ability of chronic alcoholics to inhibit intrusions errors [4]. The results of the present study provide new evidence for a continuum of acute-to-chronic alcohol effects on this aspect of reflective memory performance by demonstrating that young, apparently healthy social drinkers also commit significantly more intrusion errors in a delayed free recall task during acute alcohol intoxication compared with their no-alcohol performance level. In contrast, in the immediate free recall task, participants' number of List 1 intrusion errors did not differ between alcohol and no-alcohol conditions, supporting the prediction that acute intoxication would cause more intrusion errors in the delayed than in the immediate free recall task in social drinkers.

It has been argued that impairment in reflective cognitive functions may play an important role in maintaining heavy patterns of alcohol abuse (4) and may be an important risk factor for the development of alcoholism [3,5-7]. Weingartner et al [2] showed that cognitively unimpaired alcoholics were less able to inhibit intrusion errors in a task that tested their ability to track the source of remembered knowledge, suggesting an impairment of reflective cognitive function.

In the present analysis, we further examined the mechanism through which intrusion errors may occur in the delayed free recall by separately analyzing DFR intrusion errors that were recalled versus unrecalled List 2 words from the IFR task. The results showed that in the DFR task in the alcohol challenge condition, participants committed more List 2 intrusion errors from the correctly recalled List 2 words in the IFR task, whereas List 2 intrusion errors from the unrecalled List 2 words in the IFR task were equivalent in the alcohol and no alcohol conditions. In view of previous research demonstrating that acute alcohol intoxication diminishes the ability to encode and store list context information in the long-term memory [10,11] we suggest that the second set of distractor tasks likely interferes with memory for the list context information more so in the alcohol than in the no-alcohol session. This suggestion is supported by the finding that List 2 intrusion errors from the unrecalled List 2 words in the IFR task were unaffected by alcohol. Thus, compared with the unrecalled words, the recalled words from the IFR task were more readily accessible during alcohol challenge, yet memory for their list context was interfered with more by the distractor tasks. It appears likely that these two factors—heightened accessibility and diminished memory for context—accounted for the enhanced commission of List 2 intrusion errors in the DFR task during acute alcohol intoxication. Noteworthy is that the word presentation frequency did not diminish intrusion errors in either the immediate or the delayed free recall tasks, suggesting that multiple word presentations do not facilitate encoding and storage of words with respect to list context.

From the perspective of facilitating the efficacy of alcohol-abuse prevention and intervention efforts, strategies that promote efficient context encoding during learning may be useful to help inhibit behavior due to maladaptive reflective functions based on irrelevant or misattributed memories. For example, a intervention training paradigm that involved exhaustive learning of the association between the addiction-related stimuli and their negative consequences could possibly be used to compete with positive alcohol use consequences that may already exist in automatic memory systems. As a result, initiation of drinking may activate the negative consequence automatically for participants in such an intervention, which may help them to inhibit their drinking behavior. As this link would be strong, it may not be easily interfered even under acute alcohol intoxication. The traumatic brain injury literature also suggests that improvements to working memory, attention distribution, and management of executive functions might be useful to improving reflective cognitive functions in addiction treatment samples [19].

ACKNOWLEDGMENT

Financial support for this study was provided by the Alcoholic Beverage Medical Research Foundation and the National Institute on Alcohol Abuse and Alcoholism grants K02 AA 00325 and R01 AA015248. We thank Maria Barbier, Angela Babetski, Ilan Danan, Sheryl Sciarappa, Jaclyn Smith, and Pooja Bendala, undergraduate research assistants for helping with various aspects of this study.

REFERENCES

[1]   Heishman SJ, Weingartner HJ, and Henningfield JE. Selective deficits in reflective cognition of polydrug abusers: Preliminary findings. *Psychol. Addict Behav.* 1999;13: 227-31.

[2]   Weingartner HJ, Andreason PJ, Hommer DW, Sirocco, KY et al. Monitoring the source of memory in detoxified alcoholics. *Biol. Psychiatry* 1996;40(1): 43-53.

[3]   Giancola PR, Peterson JB, Pihl RO. Risk for alcoholism, antisocial behavior, and response preservation. *J. Clin. Psychol* 1993;49(3): 423-8.

[4]   Weingartner HJ, Rawlings R, George DT, Eckardt M. Triazolam-induced changes in alcoholic thought processes. *Psychopharmacoly* 1998;138 (3-4):311-7.

[5]   Begleiter H, Porjesz B. Neuroelectric processes in individuals at risk for alcoholism. *Alcohol Alcoholism* 1990;25(2-3):251-6.

[6]   Cloninger R. Neurogenetic adaptive mechanisms in alcoholism. *JSTOR Science New Series* 1987; 236 (4800):410-5.

[7]   Moss HB, Kirisci L. Aggressivity in adolescent alcohol abusers: Relationship with conduct disorder. *Alcohol Clinl. Exp. Res.* 1995; 19(3):642-7.

[8]   Ray S, Bates ME, Bly BM. Alcohol's dissociation of implicit and explicit memory processes: Implications of a parallel distributed processing model of semantic priming. *Exp. Clin. Psychopharmacol.* 2004;12:118-25.

[9]   Ray S, Bates ME. Acute alcohol effects on repetition priming and word recognition memory with equivalent memory cues. *Brain Cogn.* 2006;60: 118-27.

[10] Hashtroudi S, Parker ES, DeLisi LE, Wyatt RJ. On elaboration and alcohol. *J. Verbal Learn Verbal Behav.* 1983;22:164-73.

[11] Hashtroudi S, Parker ES, DeLisi LE, Wyatt RJ, Mutter SA. Intact retention in acute alcohol amnesia. *J. Exp. Psychol. Learn Mem .Cogn.* 1984; 10(1):156-63.

[12] Weingartner H, Murphy DL. State-dependent storage and retrieval of experience while intoxicated. In: Birnbaum IM, Parker ES, eds. *Alcohol and human memory*. Hillsdale, NJ, USA: Lawrence Erlbaum, 1977:159-73.

[13] Metropolitan Life Insurance Company. *Height-weight tables for men and women,* 1983. www. metlife.com/Lifeadvice/Tools/Heightnweight/

[14] Chan AW, Pristach EA, Welte JW. Detection of alcoholism in three populations by the Brief-Mast. *Alcohol Clin. Exp. Res.* 1994;18(3): 695-701.

[15] Ray S, Bly BM. Two routes for activation in the priming of categorical co-ordinates. *J. Gen. Psychol.* (in press).

[16] Battig WF, Montague WE. Category norms for verbal items in 56 categories: A replication and extension of the Connecticut category norms. *J. Exp. Psychol. Monogr.*1969;80(3):1-43.

[17] Tracy JI, Bates ME. The selective effects of alcohol on automatic and effortful memory processes. *Neuropsychol* 1999;13(2):282-90.

[18] Graf P, Shimamura AP, Squire LR. Priming across modalities and priming across category levels: Extending the domain of preserved function in amnesia. *J. Exp. Psychol. Learn Mem. Cogn.* 1985; 11(2):386-96.

[19] Nolan P. Executive memory dysfunctions following mild traumatic brain injury. *J. Head Trauma Rehab.* 2006;21:68-75.

In: Alcohol-Related Cognitive Disorders   ISBN: 978-1-60741-730-9
Editors: L. Sher, I. Kandel, J. Merrick pp. 199-209   © 2009 Nova Science Publishers, Inc.

Chapter 12

CAFFEINE AND ALCOHOL: CONTROL OF BEHAVIOR

Karen E. Grattan-Miscio

ABSTRACT

This chapter describes an experiment designed to examine the effects of caffeine expectancy on intentional control of behavior under alcohol. A process dissociation paradigm was used to measure the separate influence of automatic and intentional controlled processes on performance of a word-stem completion task. Forty social drinkers studied a list of words, received either alcohol or a placebo, and then performed a word-stem completion task designed to measure intentional control of behavior. Before performing the task, two groups (i.e., one alcohol and one placebo group) also received decaffeinated coffee, which has been shown effectively to establish caffeine expectancy. The results indicated that the expectation of receiving caffeine was sufficient to counteract the impairment of intentional control seen under alcohol. Those individuals who received both alcohol and decaffeinated coffee demonstrated better intentional control than those who received alcohol alone. Moreover, the performance of the alcohol-decaffeinated coffee group did not differ from placebo. No treatment significantly affected automatic processes. The expectation of receiving caffeine under alcohol was sufficient to counteract the impairing effects of the drug.

INTRODUCTION

When individuals are under the influence of alcohol, do they lose intentional control or do they retain the ability to control their behavior? Recent research has shown that alcohol can impair many types of psychomotor and mental tasks [1]. The possibility that these effects are due to impaired self-control is raised by observations that drinkers may display extreme behavior, including hazardous and antisocial acts that would not normally be displayed when sober [2,3]. A good deal of folklore is also consistent with this opinion. For instance, it is often claimed that a good way to get people to reveal a secret, or to say what they really think, is to get them drunk. In addition, individuals commonly report that they did not know what they were doing because they were drinking. Although these sorts of observations convince some that alcohol impairs intentional control of behavior, this belief is far from unanimous.

Others have argued that intentional control of behavior can be retained under alcohol. This idea was advanced over a century ago. "The mind exercises a considerable effect upon drunkenness and may control it powerfully" [4]. McNish's claimed that drinkers can control behavioral symptoms of intoxication is consistent with stories of drinkers who report suddenly "sobering up", when advantageous to do so. Intentional control of behavior under alcohol has also been implicated in studies showing that trained observers are unlikely to detect symptoms of intoxication in suspected impaired drivers, even though the blood alcohol concentrations of the suspects are over 100 mg/100 ml [5,6]. Langen-Bucher and Nathan [7] observed that the behavioral effects of alcohol were extremely difficult to detect in social drinkers and alcoholics, particularly when the symptoms of intoxication were socially unacceptable and sobriety was advantageous. Apparent goal-directed behavior might commonly be thought to be intentional and to support the claim that attributing behavior to the effect of alcohol simply excuses deliberate behavior that achieves some desired outcome [8].

Some recent research has attempted to provide a resolution to the debate over intentional control of behavior under alcohol. Experiments using different tasks and experimental paradigms indicate that the administration of doses of alcohol ranging from 0.57 to 0.62 g/kg impair social drinkers' intentional responses but do not alter their automatic responses. For example, alcohol has been found to impair controlled (effortful) memory processes and to leave automatic memory processes unaffected [9]. The process-dissociation paradigm has been widely used in basic and applied research on intentional control [10]. The process dissociation paradigm is based on the rationale that no intentional control of behavior is displayed if a response is as likely to occur whether a person is trying or is not trying to make the response. In this paradigm, an individual performs a task under two conditions: when automatic and controlled processes act collaboratively and when they act in opposition. Performance is facilitated when the two processes act in concert to generate the same response. However, when the two processes act in opposition, the responses generated by automatic processes oppose those of the controlled processes, so that errors, or inappropriate 'action slips' are exhibited and intentional behavior is compromised. The proportion of correct responses when automatic and controlled processes operate in concert and the proportion of action slips when the two processes are opposed are used to estimate the separate influence of automatic and controlled processes on a person's performance of a task. The process-dissociation paradigm has been frequently used in research to demonstrate the selective impairment of intentional behavior by alcohol [11-13].

However, the debate regarding intentional control is deepened by other 'myths' concerning alcohol consumption. One of the myths, which may actually contain some truth, contends that caffeine reduces the impairing effects of alcohol. It is not uncommon for social drinkers to report consuming several cups of coffee in an attempt to 'sober up'. In laboratory settings, caffeine alone has been shown to counteract the impairing effects of alcohol on both cognitive [13] and motor skills [14]. However, when drinkers self-medicate with coffee, it is done with the added expectation that the caffeine will restore sobriety.

ASSOCIATE LEARNING

Research on alcohol has shown that the drug might affect multiple neurotransmitters and systems that control complex brain functions, such as those involved in memory, consciousness, alertness, and learning. Alcohol-induced changes in these biological processes might account for some of the behavioral effects of the drug. However, research has demonstrated that associative learning (i.e., expectancies) concerning the relation between drug and stimuli in the setting can interact to determine the behavioral effects of alcohol. For example, research at the cellular level has shown that the intensity of the drug effects is dose-related, and that prolonged exposure to alcohol often results in a reduction in these effects (i.e., tolerance) [15]. However, measures on behavioral tolerance to alcohol, as well as other psychoactive drugs, have indicated that tolerance does not depend solely on drug exposure, but that the context in which the dose exposure occurs must also be considered. For instance, research by Seigel [16] demonstrated that when the drug exposure is held constant, animals display greater tolerance to a dose when it is administered in the presence of the usual pre-drug cues as compared to a novel environment. The results of that study were predicted based on learned associations between pre-drug and drug stimuli, such that pre-drug cues signal the occurrence of the drug and, thereby, lead to the expectation of receiving the drug.

The learning interpretation of expectancies regarding the effects of alcohol is congruent with the associative learning theory. This theory defines expectancy as the acquisition of information regarding the relation between two events [17], such that whenever one event is repeatedly followed by a second event, an opportunity exists to learn to expect this second event whenever the first one occurs. For instance, "if I drink this, then that will happen." These learned expectations can be acquired by first-hand experience, as well as through the media and the observations of other drinkers. Some researchers report that children who have not yet consumed alcohol readily report expectancies about the drug's effects [18]. Others have found that more pleasant expectations predict the onset of social and problem drinking once adolescents begin consuming the drug [19].

Applications of associative learning theory to drug-taking situations have identified three types of expectancies that can affect the behavioral response to a drug [20]. One such expectancy is based on the association between the drug stimuli and its behavioral effects. Individuals engage in a variety of activities after drinking that might provide an opportunity to learn the type of effect alcohol exerts on a given activity. Experiments using simple and complex motor-skill tasks have demonstrated that drinkers' expectancies concerning the degree of impairment alcohol exerts on a task predict individual differences in the amount of impairment displayed under both alcohol and a placebo [21]. Moreover, this research has indicated that the expectancy effect can be expanded to explain the relation between receiving other performance-altering drugs, such as caffeine, and performance under alcohol.

This research has demonstrated that the expectation of receiving caffeine can counteract the impairing effects of alcohol on cognitive (e.g., inhibitory control) tasks. Additionally, these expectations appear to counteract impairment under alcohol to levels equivalent to that of the stimulant drug alone, and the combination of these two factors has been shown to restore performance to levels greater than that of sober performance [14].

OUR STUDY

Forty healthy undergraduate university students (24 males and 16 females; ages 19-25 years) were randomly assigned to one of four groups (n=10; 6 males and 4 females per group): Alcohol Only (A); Placebo Only (P); Alcohol with caffeine expectancy (AE); and Placebo with caffeine expectancy (PE). All participants had normal color vision, and no one was taking any medication. They fasted for four hours, and abstained from alcohol and all other drugs for at least 24 hours before the alcohol session.

A set of 90, five-letter, English common nouns (e.g., bunny) was used to create two lists identical to those used in other research [12]. The words were drawn from a list developed by Merikle and Stolz [22] who presented normative data on male and female college students showing that each three-letter stem for a word could be completed with at least four five-letter words. The words were divided into two lists of 40, plus five buffer words at the beginning and at the end of the list to prevent primacy and recency effects. Buffer words were identical for both lists. No words from either list had the same word-stem, and the chance of completing a word-stem with words from each list was equated. A participant was presented with only one list of words. A PC computer using MEL software (Micro Experimental Laboratory, 1998) presented words in lowercase lettering, using 12 point Times New Roman font, in the center of the computer screen. Words were displayed individually for 1.5 s, followed by a 2 s blank screen before the next word was presented.

The task presented the three-letter stems corresponding to the 80 words from the two lists. The fourth and fifth letters appeared as dashes (e.g., bun- -), which could be completed with at least four five-letter nouns (e.g., bunny, bunch, bunks, bunts). Forty of these word-stems (i.e., 20 colored red and 20 colored green) corresponded to the 40 familiar words from the list that the person had previously seen. The remaining 40 stems (i.e., 20 red and 20 green) corresponded to new words from the other list that had not been presented. The 80 word-stems appeared on the computer screen one at a time. Word-stems were presented randomly with the constraint that no more than four words from the same list or the same color appeared consecutively. Participants were asked to complete a green stem with a word from the familiar list. Red stems were to be completed with any other noun that fit the stem. All responses were given verbally and participants had 15 s to complete each stem. If a word-stem was completed before 15 s, the next stem was presented immediately.

A Drinking Habit Questionnaire (15) was completed by each participant to provide three measures of current typical drinking habits: frequency (i.e., the number of drinking occasions per week), dose (i.e., milliliters of absolute alcohol per kilogram of body weight typically consumed during a single drinking occasion), and duration (i.e., time span in hours of a typical drinking occasion). Two additional items were included to identify and exclude participants who may have alcohol-related problems. However, no participants in this study reported any problems related to alcohol.

Participants also completed a questionnaire that provided a measure of their caffeine consumption based on their reports of the amount of various beverages and foods containing caffeine consumed during a week. Estimates of the caffeine content in the foods and beverages were obtained from Barone and Roberts [23].

A Beverage Rating Scale was used to determine whether participants who received a placebo perceived that their drinks had contained no alcohol. Participants were asked to rate the content of their beverages in terms of bottles of 5% alcohol beer on a scale ranging from zero to 10, divided into 0.5 increments. Ratings of the amount of alcohol consumed during the experiment ranged from 0.5 to 6.0 bottles of 5% beer. Blood alcohol concentrations (BACs) were determined from breath samples measured by a Breathalyser, Model 900A (Smith and Wesson, Eatontown, NJ).

Participants were told that the study concerned the effects of alcohol and caffeine on responses to information presented on a computer screen. At the start of the session, participants provided informed consent, and completed the questionnaires on drinking habits and caffeine use. Participants then provided a breath sample to verify that their BACs were zero. Participants then received information presented in the form of a word list. They were told that words would be presented on the screen, one at a time. They were to read each word aloud and try to remember it for a later task. Presentation of the lists was counterbalanced within groups, with half of each group learning words from one list and the other half learning words from the other list.

After the word list had been presented, the word-stem completion task was explained and participants had a brief practice on the task to ensure that they fully understood the task requirements before receiving any treatment. The 10 word-stems that corresponded to the 10 buffer words in the study lists were presented on the screen one at a time. Half of the word-stems were colored green and participants were told to complete these stems with the familiar word from the list they had seen. If they could not think of the list word, they were to complete the stem with the first word that came to mind that fit the stem. The remaining five word-stems were presented in red. Participants were told to complete the red word-stems with any five-letter noun that had not been on the list, and if they could not think of a word that was not in the list, they should complete the stem with the first word that came to mind. They were also instructed not to use proper nouns, such as names of people, places, or companies, to complete any of the stems. Participants in each group then received their respective treatments.

Treatment in Our Experiment

After the familiarization, the groups received their respective treatments. Those in the two alcohol groups (A and AE) received 0.62 g/kg absolute alcohol in a beverage containing two parts carbonated beverage to one part alcohol. For a 75 kg person, this dose is equivalent to 3.5 12-oz. bottles of 5% beer. To keep BACs equivalent to males in this study, the females received 87% of the dose for males (i.e., 0.54 g/kg). The beverage was administered in two equal volume drinks, served five minutes apart. Participants were asked to finish each drink within one minute.

Participants in the P and PE groups were told that they would receive alcohol, but instead received two placebo drinks containing the carbonated beverage, with a per body weight volume equal to that of the alcohol drinks. A few drops of alcohol were floated on the surface of each drink, and the serving glasses were sprayed with an alcohol mist of 50% water - 50% alcohol. The mist appeared as condensation and provided a strong alcohol scent to add to the credibility of the placebo drink. Previous studies have demonstrated that this is an effective placebo [21].

The caffeine expectancy groups (AE and PE) received a 150 ml cup of decaffeinated coffee. This amount of decaffeinated coffee has been shown to be effective in eliciting caffeine expectations [24]. The groups receiving no caffeine expectancy received an additional 150 ml of carbonated beverage added to their alcohol drinks.

After consuming their drinks, participants rested for 21 minutes to soft music. After this rest, all participants' BACs were measured, and participants rested again for another 6 minutes. Thirty minutes after drinking commenced, BACs were measured again and the word-stem task was performed. BACs were measured again when the task concluded (i.e., 45 min after drinking started). Thereafter, BACs were monitored, as needed, to determine when participants' BACs had declined to a safe level. During this time they completed the Beverage Rating Scale, were fully debriefed, and paid for their participation.

The dependent measures of primary importance were based on the responses to the 40 word-stems that corresponded to the 40 familiar words from the list that participants had studied. The proportion of responses to the 20 green stems that were completed with familiar words measures correct responses (CR), when controlled and automatic processes act collaboratively. The proportion of responses to the 20 red word-stems that were incorrectly completed with familiar words measures action slips (AS) when the two processes are opposed.

The influence of controlled and automatic processes is calculated algebraically. Controlled processes (CP) are estimated by subtracting the proportion of action slips (AS) from the proportion of correct responses (CR). This equation is $CP = CR - AS$. The influence of automatic processes (AP) is estimated by the proportion of action slips when controlled processes fail to influence the response (i.e., $1 - CP$). This is calculated by the equation $AP = AS/(1 - CP)$.

Evidence of an automatic influence on responding requires that the estimate of the automatic process is higher than the baseline (chance) probability of completing the word-stems with words from a list that was not studied [10]. The proportion of the 40 word-stems completed with words from the list a participant had not seen was used to estimate the baseline probability of completing stems with list words by chance.

Treatment effects on each dependent measure were tested by an analysis of variance (ANOVA). Specific comparisons between treatments were made by planned comparisons using the mean square error term from the appropriate ANOVA.

OUR FINDINGS

Separate one-way ANOVAs of each of the drinking habit measures reported by participants obtained no significant group differences (ps > 0.487). The entire sample reported a mean frequency of 1.70 (SD = 1.54) weekly drinking occasions, with a mean duration of 4.38 hrs (SD = 1.59) per occasion. Their mean typical dose per occasion was 1.26 ml alcohol/ kg (SD = 0.54). This dose would be the equivalent of approximately bottles 5 of 5% alcohol beer for an individual weighing 70 kg. A one-way ANOVA of the typical weekly use of foods and beverages containing caffeine revealed no group differences (F(3, 36) = 0.31, p = 0.991). The mean caffeine consumed per occasion was 94.5 mg (SD = 44.16). This amount would approximate one cup of ground roasted coffee.

The BACs were measured at 21, 30, and 45 min after drinking commenced. The placebo group (P) had no detectable BACs. None of the members of this group rated the alcohol content of their drink as zero, so it appears that the placebo was credible. A 2 x 3 (Alcohol group × Time) ANOVA of BACs revealed no significant main effects or interactions, ps > 0.150. During the 21 to 30 min resting period, the mean BAC rose from 58 (SD = 23) to 64 (SD = 15) mg/100. While the word-stem task was performed from 30 to 45 min, the mean BAC rose from 64 (SD = 15) to 67 (SD = 12) mg/100 ml.

The ANOVA of the CP measures indicated a significant interaction of Drug x Expectancy (F(3, 36) = 9.57, p = 0.004). The interaction presented in figure 1 suggests that a moderate dose of alcohol-impaired intentional control of behavior, but the expectation of receiving caffeine was able to counteract this impairment. Comparison of the A and P groups showed the influence of CP was weaker in the A group (p < 0.001). Likewise, comparisons of the AE, A and P groups indicated that expectations of receiving caffeine were able to improve performance under alcohol (p < 0.001); this improvement was comparable to sober performance (p = 0.344).

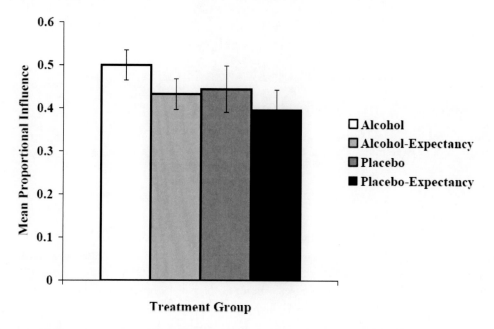

Figure 1. Mean estimated influence of controlled processes in alcohol and placebo groups with or without caffeine expectancy. Vertical bars represent standard errors of the means.

The ANOVA of measures of automatic processes obtained no significant group differences (ps > 0.14). Multiple comparisons of the scores of automatic processing, using the Tukey's HSD (p < 0.05), showed that none of the groups receiving alcohol differed from the placebo group (ps > 0.28). The mean proportional influence of AP in each group is presented in figure 2.

The mean baseline proportions of red and green word-stems completed with words from the list that had not been seen were similar (0.320 and 0.306 respectively). A one-way ANOVA of the baseline scores obtained no significant group effects (F(3, 36) = 1.40, p = 0.258), and indicated that solutions to stems of new words were unaffected by the treatments.

The mean automatic and baseline scores for the entire sample (N = 40) were 0.446 (SD = 0.13) and 0.313 (SD = 0.11) respectively, and a paired sample t test confirms that the influence of AP was higher than baseline chance responding (t(39) = 5.20, p = 0.001).

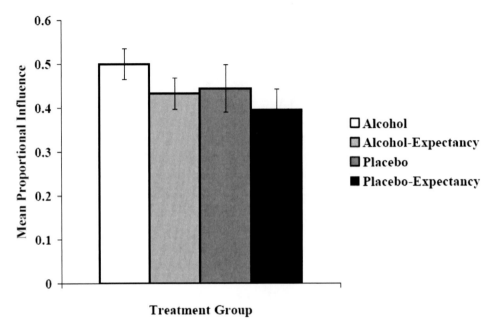

Figure 2. Mean estimated influence of automatic processes in alcohol and placebo groups with or without caffeine expectancy. Vertical bars represent standard errors of the means.

DISCUSSION

This experiment tested the effect of caffeine expectancy on controlled and automatic processes under alcohol. This treatment was predicted to increase controlled processes to drug-free levels. A process-dissociation paradigm was used to estimate the separate influence of controlled and automatic processes, thought to govern intentional and unintentional responding, respectively. In accord with the hypotheses, weakened controlled processes under alcohol were strengthened to drug-free levels by caffeine expectancy. Those individuals who received both alcohol and decaffeinated coffee demonstrated better intentional control than those who received alcohol alone. Moreover, the performance of the alcohol-decaffeinated coffee group did not differ from placebo. No treatment significantly affected automatic processes. This finding supports previous research that has shown that treatments, such as an acute dose of alcohol, caffeine, or reward, selectively attack controlled processes and leave automatic processes unaffected [11-13].

The finding that caffeine expectation counteracts the impairing effects of alcohol on intentional control supports previous research that indicates a motivating treatment (e.g., reward) with expectancy counteracts intentional control of behavior [12,13], as well as research examining the influence of caffeine expectation on other cognitive tasks (e.g., inhibitory control) [14]. Some recent research has demonstrated that drinkers who expect an antagonistic effect of caffeine will display greater impairment from alcohol on a psychomotor task compared with those who were led to expect no antagonist effect of caffeine [25]. Research by Fillmore et al [24] demonstrated an antagonist effect of caffeine expectancy on psychomotor performance, but only when the expectancy was not combined with an alcohol treatment. In the current research study, the expectation related to the caffeine expectancy treatment was not directly manipulated. However, some research indicates that performance on psychomotor tasks and cognitive tasks differ in sensitivity to alcohol impair-ment [26]. Thus, possibly intentional control is not susceptible to similar expectation effects as found by Fillmore et al [25]. Further research should be done to manipulate the various expectancies related to caffeine to obtain a better understanding of drug effects on intentional control of behavior.

Although caffeine expectancy strengthened con-trolled processes under alcohol, the anticipation did not affect controlled processes under the placebo. The performance under a placebo is analogous to the performance in a drug-free state. Some research in cognition has tested the effect of other treatments on controlled and automatic processes when a stem-com-pletion task is performed drug-free and obtained similar results to those of the current research study [12].

Although the present research included male and female social drinkers, the study was not designed to assess possible sex differences. Basic research using the process paradigm task has not reported any gender differences, but it is necessary determine whether alcohol and caffeine expectations differently affect the intentional control of behavior by men and women. The results of the research are also limited to relatively young social drinkers, and to investigate the effects of an acute dose of alcohol on the intentional control of older more experienced social drinkers, especially those who drink more heavily, would be important.

The finding that an individual can resist the impairing effects of alcohol on intentional control is of incredible importance to society, particularly the justice system. Typically, the justice system will administer a more severe penalty for an offense if an act can be demonstrated to have been intentional. If a defendant had been drinking at the time of the offense, the possibility that alcohol impairs intentional control may be used as a defense. The current research supports past findings that indicate that an individual can resist the impairing effects of alcohol on intentional controlled performance, if that individual has some expectation to motivate himself/herself toward successful achievement of a goal. Hence, the argument that alcohol removed intent to commit an offense may not be valid if the crime achieved some beneficial goal for the accused.

More generally, our findings showed that the depressing effect of alcohol on controlled processes can be counteracted by the expectation of receiving a stimulant drug, caffeine. The findings are consistent with folklore concerning the effects of such treatments in restoring self-control during intoxication, and provide a basis for further research on these treatments and the processes underlying their effects.

REFERENCES

[1]   Holloway FA. Low-dose alcohol effects on human behavior and performance. *Alcohol Drugs Driving* 1995;11(1):39-55.

[2] Bushman BJ, Cooper HM. Effects of alcohol on human aggression: An integrative research review. *Psychol. Bull* 1990;107(3):341-54.

[3] Steele CM, Southwick L. Alcohol and social behavior I: The psychology of drunken excess. *J. Pers Soc. Psychol.* 1985;48(1):18-34.

[4] McNish R. *The anatomy of drunkeness*, Fourth ed. Glasgow, UK: McPhun Press, 1832.

[5] Jones IS, Lund AK. Detection of alcohol-impaired drivers using a passive alcohol sensor. *J. Police Science Admin.* 1979;14:153-60.

[6] Zusman ME, Huber, JD. Multiple measures and the validity of response on drinking drivers. *J. Safety Res.* 1979;11:132-7.

[7] Langenbucher JW, Nathan, PE. Psychology, public policy, and the evidence for alcohol intoxication. *Am. J. Psychol.* 1983;38:1070-7.

[8] Critchlow B. Blaming the booze: The attribution of responsibility for drunken behavior. *Pers. Soc. Psychol. Bull* 1983;9(3):451-73.

[9] Tracy JI, Bates ME. The selective effects of alcohol on automatic and effortful memory pro-cesses. *Neuropsychology* 1999;13:282-90.

[10] Jacoby LL, Jennings JM, Hay JF. Dissociating automatic and consciously controlled processes: Implications for diagnosis and rehabilitation of memory deficits. In: Herrman D, McEvoy C, Hertzog C, Hertal P, Johnson MK, eds. *Basic and applied memory research: Theory in context.* Vol. 1. Hillsdale, NJ: Lawrence Erlbaum, 1996:161-93.

[11] Fillmore MT, Vogel-Sprott M, Gavrilescu D. Alcohol effects on intentional behavior: Dissociating controlled and automatic influences. *Exp. Clin. Psychopharmacol* 1999;7:372-8.

[12] Grattan KE, Vogel-Sprott M. Maintaining intentional control of behavior under alcohol. *Alcohol Clin. Exp. Res.* 2001;25:192-7.

[13] Grattan-Miscio KE, Vogel-Sprott M. Alcohol, intentional control and inappropriate behavior: Regulation by motivation or caffeine. *Exp. Clin. Psychopharmacol* 2005;13(1):48-55.

[14] Fillmore MT, Vogel-Sprott M. Psychomotor per-formance under alcohol and under caffeine: Expectancy and pharmacological effects. *Exp. Clin. Psychopharmacol.* 1994;2: 319-28.

[15] Vogel-Sprott M. *Alcohol tolerance and social drinking: Learning the consequences.* New York, NY: Guillford, 1992.

[16] Seigel S. Pharmacological conditioning and drug effects. In: Goudie AJ, Emmet-Oglesby MW, eds. *Psychoactive drugs: Tolerance and sensitization.* Clifton, NJ: Humana Press, 1989.

[17] Bolles RC. *Learning theory*, Second ed. New York, NY: Holt Rhinehart Winston, 1979.

[18] Christiansen BA, Goldman MS. Alcohol-related expectancies versus demographic/background var-iables in the prediction of adolescent drinking. *J. Consult Clin. Psychol.* 1983;51:249-57.

[19] Smith GT, Roehling PV, Christiansen BA, Gold-man MS. Alcohol expectancies predict early adolescent drinking: A longitudinal study. *Paper presented at the 94th Ann. Conv Am. Psychol. Assoc,* Washington, DC, USA, 1986.

[20] Vogel-Sprott M. Drugs, behavior and environ-mental sources of motivation: Bridging a gap. In: Bevans R, Bardo M, eds. *Motivational factors in the etiology of drug abuse.* 50th Ann Nebraska Symp Motivation. Lincoln, NE: Univ Nebraska Press, 2004:235-60.

[21] Fillmore MT, Vogel-Sprott M. Expectancies about alcohol-induced motor impairment predict indi-vidual differences in responses to alcohol and placebo. *J. Stud. Alcohol.* 1995;56:90-8.

[22] Merikle PM, Stolz J. [Norms for 3-letter stem-completions of 5-letter words based on male and female college students]. Unpublished raw data, 1998.

[23] Barone JJ, Roberts HR. Caffeine consumption. *Food Chem. Toxicol* 1996;34:119-29.

[24] Fillmore MT, Mulvihill LE, Vogel-Sprott M. The expected drug and its expected effect interact to determine placebo responses to alcohol and caffeine. *Psychopharmacol* 1994;115:383-8.

[25] Fillmore MT, Rice JT, Roach EL. Does caffeine counteract alcohol-induced impairment? The ironic effects of expectancy. *J. Stud. Alcohol.* 2002;63:745-54.

[26] Fogarty J, Vogel-Sprott M. Cognitive processes and motor skills differ in sensitivity to alcohol impairment. *J. Stud. Alcohol.* 2002;63:404-11.

In: Alcohol-Related Cognitive Disorders   ISBN: 978-1-60741-730-9
Editors: L. Sher, I. Kandel, J. Merrick pp. 211-220   © 2009 Nova Science Publishers, Inc.

Chapter 13

ALCOHOL AND MEMORY

Miriam Z. Mintzer

ABSTRACT

With the widespread use of alcohol in our society, research on the effects of alcohol on memory has clinical importance. In addition, an investigation of the amnesia produced by alcohol can be a powerful tool for elucidating normal and abnormal memory mechanisms. The purpose of this chapter was to provide a review of placebo-controlled laboratory studies of the acute effects of alcohol administration on memory in healthy adult social drinkers. Acute alcohol administration impairs working memory, episodic memory, and semantic memory, but does not appear to impair implicit memory or automatic, non-conscious memory processes. Alcohol produces relatively greater impairment of episodic memory encoding than retrieval processes. Whereas episodic memory is impaired following acute alcohol administration (anterograde amnesia), episodic memory for information presented prior to alcohol administration is enhanced under certain conditions (retrograde facilitation). Although extensive research has been conducted on the acute effects of alcohol on memory, many interesting questions surrounding the effects of alcohol on memory (e.g., the selectivity of alcohol's effects on different working memory processes; the conditions under which episodic memory retrieval is impaired; the mechanisms underlying retrograde facilitation; the effects of ascending versus descending blood levels on different memory processes), as well as the relationship between memory effects and emotion/mood, remain to be explored. Further hypothesis-driven memory research with alcohol using behavioral and neuroimaging techniques has the potential both to enhance the understanding of the clinical implications of alcohol use and to elucidate basic cognitive and brain mechanisms.

INTRODUCTION

The acute effects of alcohol on human memory have been studied extensively. Given the widespread use of alcohol in society, this research has important clinical utility. In addition, like neuropsychological studies of brain-damaged patients, which have played a critical role in advancing the understanding of normal and abnormal memory mechanisms, investigation of the amnesia produced by alcohol and other drugs (e.g., benzodiazepines, scopolamine) can also be a powerful tool for elucidating memory mechanisms. In fact, investigation of drug-induced amnesia has several distinct advantages over traditional studies of amnesic patients. Most important, unlike the memory deficits found in amnesic patients, the effects of drugs on memory processes are reversible and can be empirically manipulated in controlled laboratory experiments with large numbers of healthy volunteers. Findings of selective effects of drugs on particular aspects of memory performance but not others can provide converging evidence with data from non-pharmacological studies for the dissociability of specific processes or subcomponents.

The purpose of this chapter was to provide a review of human laboratory studies of the acute effects of alcohol administration on memory. The effects of alcohol relative to placebo are summarized based on published placebo-controlled laboratory studies in healthy adult social drinkers. Studies in heavy alcohol users or other drug abusers are excluded. To examine the selectivity of alcohol's effects, we have summarized the effects on different types of memory using a memory systems framework [1,2]. Five memory systems have been identified (working memory, episodic memory, semantic memory, procedural learning, the perceptual representation system) that are purportedly subserved by distinct brain mechanisms.

EFFECTS ON MEMORY SYSTEMS

Working Memory

This type of memory enables one to hold onto and manipulate small amounts of information for short periods of time and is critical to the performance of many basic daily tasks, such as holding in mind the beginning of a sentence until the end of the sentence in conversation or reading, retaining a phone number until it is dialed, or performing mental arithmetic. Working memory is commonly measured in the laboratory by presenting a small number of items (usually digits or letters) to the participant followed by immediate memory testing.

Following acute administration, alcohol has been shown to produce dose-related impairment of working memory performance on a variety of different tasks. In the digit span task [3], digits are presented in successive trials and participants are asked to recall the digits in the order of presentation (forward digit span) or in the reverse order (backward digit span). On each successive trial, the number of digits presented is increased by one and the outcome measure is the number of trials completed before an error occurred. Alcohol has been shown to impair digit span performance [4-5] suggesting that working memory capacity is reduced. Interestingly, Finn et al [5] reported that alcohol impaired digit span performance (backward) only in participants with a high working memory capacity.

Other studies have examined effects of alcohol on the Sternberg task [6]. Small sets of letters (typically 4-7 letters) are presented briefly, after which participants are presented with a probe letter and asked to indicate whether the probe letter was included in the presentation set. Alcohol has been shown to increase the number of errors and reaction time (RT) on the

Sternberg task, although the effect on RT is not consistently observed [7-9]. In one study testing participants during both the ascending and descending limbs of the blood alcohol concentration curve, the number of errors was impaired on both limbs, whereas RT was impaired only on the ascending limb [7]. Incentives for good performance were shown to counteract the impairment in RT but not the number of errors [7]. The impairment appears to increase as a function of presentation set size, which again suggests that alcohol reduces working memory capacity [7]. Echeverria et al [4] reported no effect of alcohol on the Sternberg task; however, there is not sufficient detail regarding task procedures to enable speculation regarding the lack of effect in that study.

Alcohol also has been shown to impair the immediate ordered recall of eight digit numbers presented visually or auditorally in a practical number-dialing task [10] and to impair performance on visuospatial working memory tasks [9,11]. However, Weissenborn et al [12] found no effect of alcohol on a different visuospatial working memory task. Interestingly, in that study, participants who reported 'binge drinking' performed worse in the visuospatial working memory task than 'non-bingers', although no differences were seen between the groups in the acute effects of alcohol on the task.

Dougherty et al [13] tested the effects of alcohol on a working memory task in which participants were presented with single digits successively and asked to respond when the current digit was identical to the one that preceded it. The authors reported that alcohol decreased the number of responses to target stimuli, decreased the number of commission errors (i.e., responses to non-target digits), decreased the ability to discriminate between targets and non targets, and induced a more conservative response bias. In a recent fMRI study, alcohol attenuated the activation in the dorsolateral prefrontal cortex that is associated with working-memory load during a visual working memory task, although task performance was not impaired by alcohol [14]. The results of this study suggests that acute alcohol administration affects the brain processes underlying working memory performance.

Episodic Memory

Episodic memory (sometimes labeled explicit memory) refers to conscious long-term memory for a personally experienced event that occurred at a specific time and place (e.g. what you had for dinner last night) and is measured in the laboratory by presenting information (most commonly, a list of words) to the participant (study phase) and testing memory for that information following a delay (most commonly, at least 10 minutes) (test phase). Information is most commonly tested by asking the participant to recall the words from the study phase (recall) or by presenting the participant with words from the study phase (old) along with words that were not presented during the study phase (new) and asking the participant to distinguish between old and new words.

A large body of research has been conducted on the acute effects of alcohol on episodic memory. A comprehensive review of this literature is beyond the scope of this chapter. Below, a summary of the effects and hypothesized underlying cognitive mechanisms is provided, and sample publications are cited.

Following acute administration, alcohol has been shown to dose-dependently decrease the number of old words produced on recall tasks [15-16]. On recognition memory tasks, alcohol has generally been shown to decrease hit rates (proportion of old words identified as old) and d' (signal detection measure of sensitivity in distinguishing between old and new words) and to induce a more conservative response bias (i.e., decreased likelihood of responding old) in some cases, but to have no effect on false alarm rates (proportion of new words identified as old) [16-20]. However, in contrast to effects on recall, the effects of alcohol on recognition memory are not consistently observed across studies [21-22]. One factor that appears to increase the likelihood of alcohol-induced impairment of recognition memory is the degree to which the recognition memory judgment is based on context-specific retrieval of the study phase episode [20]. For example, when participants are asked during recognition memory tasks to make remember/know judgments indicating whether they have a specific recollection of the word's presentation during the study phase ("remember"; recollection-based recognition) or responded "old" because the word seemed familiar ("know"; familiarity-based recognition) (2), alcohol has been shown to reduce the remember responses but not the know responses [23].

Alcohol has been generally shown to produce relatively greater impairment of episodic memory encoding (cognitive processes engaged during an initial event that lead to the creation of a representation or trace of the event in memory) than retrieval (cognitive processes engaged to access or bring back into consciousness the memory representation associated with a previously encoded event) [21,24]. Nevertheless, impairment of retrieval has been observed under certain conditions [16,25]. Soderlund et al [16] reported that alcohol impaired retrieval on the ascending limb of the blood alcohol concentration curve but not on the descending limb, whereas encoding was impaired on both limbs. The authors speculated that acute tolerance might have developed to the effects of alcohol on retrieval. Asymmetric state-dependent effects have been observed such that performance is better when participants are under the influence of alcohol during both encoding and retrieval (alcohol-alcohol) than when participants are under the influence of alcohol during encoding, but not retrieval (alcohol-placebo), whereas no performance difference is observed between placebo-placebo and placebo-alcohol conditions; however, state dependent effects are not consistently observed (for reviews of the early literature in this area, see 26, 27). In fact, under conditions in which alcohol impairs retrieval, performance can actually be worse in the alcohol-alcohol condition relative to all other conditions [16,25].

Different hypotheses have been proposed regarding the cognitive mechanisms underlying alcohol-induced episodic memory impairment. For example, it has been proposed that alcohol impairs context-specific memory [20], the ability to process information at a deep level during encoding [28], and effortful, controlled, or conscious memory processes (versus automatic or non-conscious processes that generally are not impaired)[29-31]. That alcohol impairs inhibitory processes that are used during retrieval to suppress information that is not wanted has also been suggested [32].

As reviewed above, episodic memory is impaired under various conditions following acute alcohol administration (anterograde amnesia). However, episodic memory for information presented before the admin-istration of alcohol is dose-dependently enhanced under certain conditions (retrograde facilitation) [33-36]. Two leading hypotheses regarding the mechanisms underlying this effect are (1) that alcohol directly enhances consolidation processes, and (2) that alcohol improves memory for information presented before administration indirectly by impairing memory for information that is presented after administration (anterograde amnesia), thereby reducing retroactive interference effects. Contrary to the consolidation hypothesis, evidence has been provided that the retrograde facilitation effect is not affected by the consolidation interval (i.e., the interval between the study phase and alcohol administration), and consolidation is thought to be time limited [36]. However, the tested intervals (immediate versus 40 min) are not sufficient to rule out conclusively the consolidation hypothesis, and further research in which additional intervals are tested is necessary.

Contrary to the interference hypothesis, retrograde facilitation occurs even when no specific interfering information is presented after alcohol administration [35]. However, it is possible that alcohol enhances memory by reducing nonspecific interference. In fact, in the context of a general theory of forgetting, Wixted [37] proposed that alcohol, benzodiazepine drugs, and sleep might enhance memory by temporarily closing the hippocampus to new information, thereby protecting recently formed memories from nonspecific retroactive interference that is associated with the process of memory formation itself.

Semantic Memory

Semantic memory refers to conscious, long-term memory for conceptual and factual knowledge that is not associated in memory with a specific time and place (e.g., Washington DC is the capitol of the United States; a dog is an animal).

Few studies have examined the effects of alcohol on semantic memory. On the fluency task, in which participants are asked to produce as many items as possible from a specified category (e.g., fruits, words beginning with the letter "A") within a given period of time, alcohol was shown to reduce the number of correct responses produced and to reduce activation in the left dorsolateral prefrontal cortex during the task [38]. Likewise, on a general information task, alcohol reduced the number of questions correctly answered [39]. On a mediated semantic priming task in which target words were preceded by prime words that were either unrelated or indirectly related to the target, alcohol was shown to reduce the priming effect (i.e., the difference in response time to targets preceded by related vs. unrelated primes), suggesting that alcohol limited the spread of activation of associated information [40]. Interestingly, the reduced priming effect was observed in participants without a family history of alcoholism but not in participants with a family history of alcoholism.

Implicit Memory (Perceptual Representation System/ Procedural Learning)

Implicit memory refers to long-term memory for a previous experience that is expressed unintentionally or without conscious recollection of the experience. Within the memory systems framework, procedural learning and the perceptual representation system are both implicit or non-declarative memory systems. In the acute alcohol administration literature, research has focused primarily on perceptual priming tasks, which are thought to tap the perceptual representation system. For example, in the word-stem completion task, participants are presented with a list of words. Following a delay, the participants are presented with word stems (e.g., STR _ _ _) and instructed to complete each stem with the first word that comes to mind (e.g., STREAM). Implicit memory is manifested by the degree of priming, which refers to increased rates of completing stems with words from the presentation list, relative to words that had not been presented.

Alcohol has been shown not to impair priming on implicit memory tasks [15,22,41-43]. The observation of intact implicit memory in conjunction with impaired explicit memory (see Episodic memory above) following alcohol administration provides further evidence for the distinction between implicit and explicit memory that is supported by dissociations in performance on implicit versus explicit memory tasks as a function of a variety of subject and independent variables (e.g., brain damage; aging; encoding conditions; benzodiazepine drugs; for reviews, see [44-45]). The dissociation between the effects of alcohol on conscious (or controlled) versus non-conscious (or automatic) memory processes is also supported by the results of studies in which these two processes were separated within a single task using the process dissociation procedure [29-30,46].

DISCUSSION

In summary, acute alcohol administration impairs working memory, episodic memory, and semantic memory but does not appear to impair implicit memory or automatic, non-conscious memory processes. Alcohol produces a relatively greater impairment of episodic memory encoding than of retrieval processes. Whereas episodic memory is impaired following acute alcohol administration (anterograde amnesia), episodic memory for information presented prior to alcohol administration is enhanced under certain conditions (retrograde facilitation). It is important to note is that although the memory systems approach provides a useful framework for reviewing the effects of alcohol and is widely accepted, different theories exist regarding the sub-components into which memory should be fractionated. In addition, most laboratory tasks tap multiple systems, and there is overlap between memory systems in terms of the cognitive processes involved. Indeed, some hypotheses mentioned above regarding the mechanisms underlying alcohol-induced episodic memory impairment involve cognitive processes that cut across memory systems (e.g., controlled processes, inhibitory processes).

It appears that alcohol reduces working memory capacity and affects the brain processes underlying working memory performance. However, the selectivity of alcohol's effects on different working memory processes is difficult to infer from between-study comparisons. Further hypothesis-driven research in which specific variables (e.g., spatial versus verbal materials; storage vs. rehearsal processes; maintenance vs. manipulation processes) are manipulated within single working-memory studies is needed. Within episodic memory, many issues remain to be explored, including the conditions under which episodic memory retrieval is impaired and the mechanisms underlying retrograde facilitation. The observation that alcohol is associated with the adoption of a more conservative response bias is of potential theoretical interest because response bias is considered a measure of participant control, which is a component of metamemory (an individual's knowledge and awareness of his or her own memory) [47-49]. Benzodiazepines, which also produce anterograde amnesia, have been associated with the adoption of a less conservative response bias [50-51]. Thus, comparative studies of the effects of alcohol and other drugs on metamemory could enhance the understanding of cognitive as well as pharmacological mechanisms.

With respect to the time-course of the effects of alcohol, further research is needed to understand the effects of ascending versus descending blood levels on different memory processes. The few studies that have compared memory performance between limbs have generally shown relatively greater impairment on the ascending versus descending limb at comparable blood levels [7,52]. Schweizer et al [11] reported differences among memory tasks such that impairment on some tasks occurred only on the ascending limb whereas impairment on others occurred only on the descending limb. One pattern that is supported by two different studies is that effects on accuracy (number of errors) are observed on both limbs whereas effects on RT are limited to the ascending limb [7,11]. As mentioned earlier, one possible mechanism for the finding of relatively less impairment on the descending limb is the development of acute tolerance to the effects. Consistent with this hypothesis, in a study in which testing limb was manipulated between subjects such that participants were not tested on both limbs, greater impairment (in executive functions) was actually observed on the descending than on the ascending limb [53].

The ascending versus descending limbs are also generally associated with different subjective effects, such that the ascending limb is associated with feelings of euphoria and arousal whereas the descending limb is associated with feelings of depression and sedation [54]. Thus, another interesting area to be explored is the relationship between the subjective and memory effects of alcohol. A related issue is the relationship between the emotional content of to be remembered information and the effects of alcohol on memory. Interestingly, both alcohol-induced memory impairment for infor-mation presented after administration (anterograde amnesia) and alcohol-induced memory enhancement for information presented before administration (retrograde facilitation) have been shown to be relatively greater for emotional than for neutral material [55-56].

CONCLUSIONS

In conclusion, although extensive research on the acute effects of alcohol on memory has been conducted, many interesting questions surrounding the effects of alcohol on memory, as well as the relationship between memory effects and emotion/mood, remain to be explored. Further hypothesis-driven research in which the effects of alcohol on memory are studied using behavioral and neuroimaging techniques has the potential both to enhance the understanding of the clinical implications of alcohol use in society and to elucidate basic cognitive and brain mechanisms.

ACKNOWLEDGMENT

The author was supported by National Institute on Drug Abuse Research Grant DA-11936 during the preparation of this manuscript.

REFERENCES

[1]   Schacter DL, Tulving E. *Memory systems*. Cambridge, MA: MIT Press, 1994.
[2]   Tulving E. How many memory systems are there? *Am. Psychol*. 1985;40:398.

[3]   Wechsler D. Manual for the wechsler adult intelligence scale. New York: *Psychol. Corp,* 1981.

[4]   Echeverria D, Fine L, Langolf G, Schork T, Sampaio C. Acute behavioural comparisons of toluene and ethanol in human subjects. *Br. J. Ind. Med.* 1991;48(11):750-61.

[5]   Finn PR, Justus A, Mazas C, Steinmetz JE. Working memory, executive processes and the effects of alcohol on Go/No-Go learning: testing a model of behavioral regulation and impulsivity. *Psychopharmacol* (Berl) 1999;146(4):465-72.

[6]   Sternberg S. The discovery of processing stages: Extensions of Donder's method. *ACTA Psychologica* 1969;30:276-315.

[7]   Grattan-Miscio KE, Vogel-Sprott M. Effects of alcohol and performance incentives on immediate working memory. *Psychopharmacol* (Berl) 2005; 181(1):188-96.

[8]   Kennedy RS, Turnage JJ, Wilkes RL, Dunlap WP. Effects of graded dosages of alcohol on nine computerized repeated-measures tests. *Ergonomics* 1993;36(10):1195-1222.

[9]   Tiplady B, Franklin N, Scholey A. Effect of ethanol on judgments of performance. *Br. J. Psychol.* 2004; 95(Pt 1):105-18.

[10]   Nordby K, Watten RG, Raanaas RK, Magnussen S. Effects of moderate doses of alcohol on immediate recall of numbers: some implications for information technology. *J. Stud. Alcohol.* 1999;60(6):873-8.

[11]   Schweizer TA, Vogel-Sprott M, Danckert J, Roy EA, Skakum A, Broderick CE. Neuropsychological profile of acute alcohol intoxication during ascen-ding and descending blood alcohol concentrations. *Neuropsychopharmacol* 2006;31(6):1301-9.

[12]   Weissenborn R, Duka T. Acute alcohol effects on cognitive function in social drinkers: their relation-ship to drinking habits. *Psychopharmacol* (Berl) 2003;165(3):306-12.

[13]   Dougherty DM, Marsh DM, Moeller FG, Chokshi RV, Rosen VC. Effects of moderate and high doses of alcohol on attention, impulsivity, discriminability, and response bias in immediate and delayed memory task performance. *Alcohol. Clin. Exp. Res.* 2000; 24(11):1702-11.

[14]   Paulus MP, Tapert SF, Pulido C, Schuckit MA. Alcohol attenuates load-related activation during a working memory task: relation to level of response to alcohol. *Alcohol Clin. Exp. Res.* 2006;30(8):1363-71.

[15]   Lister RG, Gorenstein C, Fisher-Flowers D, Wein-gartner HJ, Eckardt MJ. Dissociation of the acute effects of alcohol on implicit and explicit memory processes. *Neuropsychologia* 1991;29(12):1205-12.

[16]   Soderlund H, Parker ES, Schwartz BL, Tulving E. Memory encoding and retrieval on the ascending and descending limbs of the blood alcohol concen-tration curve. *Psychopharmacol* (Berl) 2005;182(2): 305-17.

[17]   Maylor EA, Rabbitt PM. Effect of alcohol on rate of forgetting. *Psychopharmacol* (Berl) 1987;91(2): 230-5.

[18]   Mintzer MZ, Griffiths RR. Alcohol and false recognition: a dose-effect study. *Psychopharmacol* (Berl) 2001;159(1):51-7.

[19]   Mintzer MZ, Griffiths RR. Alcohol and triazolam: differential effects on memory, psychomotor per-formance and subjective ratings of effects. *Behav. Pharmacol* 2002;13(8):653-8.

[20]   Ray S, Bates ME. Acute alcohol effects on repetition priming and word recognition memory with equivalent memory cues. *Brain Cogn.* 2006; 60(2):118-27.

[21] Goodwin DW, Powell B, Bremer D, Hoine H, Stern J. Alcohol and recall: state-dependent effects in man. *Science* 1969;163(873):1358-60.

[22] Hashtroudi S, Parker ES, DeLisi LE, Wyatt RJ, Mutter SA. Intact retention in acute alcohol amnesia. *J. Exp. Psychol. Learn Mem. Cogn.* 1984; 10(1):156-63.

[23] Curran HV, Hildebrandt M. Dissociative effects of alcohol on recollective experience. *Conscious Cogn* 1999;8(4):497-509.

[24] Birnbaum, Isabel M., Parker, Elizabeth S., Hartley, Joellen, T., Noble, Ernest P. Alcohol and memory: Retrieval processes. *J. Verbal Learning Verbal Behav.* 1978;17:325-35.

[25] Weissenborn R, Duka T. State-dependent effects of alcohol on explicit memory: the role of semantic associations. *Psychopharmacol* (Berl) 2000;149(1): 98-106.

[26] Eich JE. State-dependent retrieval of information in human episodic memory In: Birnbaum IM, Parker ES, eds. *Alcohol and human memory.* Hillsdale, NJ: Erlbaum, 1977:141-58.

[27] Weingartner H, Murphy DL. State-dependent storage and retrieval of experience while intoxi-cated. In: Birnbaum IM, Parker ES, eds. *Alcohol and human memory.* Hillsdale, NJ: Erlbaum, 1977: 159-73.

[28] Craik FMI. Similarities between the effects of ageing and alcoholic intoxication on memory per-formance, construed with a "levels of processing" framework. In: Birnbaum IM, Parker ES, eds. *Alcohol and human memory.* Hillsdale NJ: Erlbaum, 1977:9-21.

[29] Fillmore MT, Vogel-Sprott M, Gavrilescu D. Alcohol effects on intentional behavior: dissoc-iating controlled and automatic influences. *Exp. Clin. Psychopharmacol.* 1999;7(4):372-8.

[30] Kirchner TR, Sayette MA. Effects of alcohol on controlled and automatic memory processes. *Exp. Clin. Psychopharmacol.* 2003;11(2):167-75.

[31] Tracy JI, Bates ME. The selective effects of alcohol on automatic and effortful memory processes. *Neuropsychology* 1999;13(2):282-90.

[32] Lombardi WJ, Sirocco KY, Andreason PJ, George DT. Effects of triazolam and ethanol on proactive interference: evidence for an impairment in retrieval inhibition. J Clin Exp *Neuropsychol.* 1997;19(5):698-712.

[33] Mueller CW, Lisman SA, Spear NE. Alcohol enhancement of human memory: tests of consoli-dation and interference hypotheses. *Psychopharma-col* (Berl) 1983;80(3):226-30.

[34] Parker ES, Birnbaum IM, Weingartner H, Hartley JT, Stillman RC, Wyatt RJ. Retrograde enhance-ment of human memory with alcohol. *Psychophar-macol* (Berl) 1980;69(2):219-22.

[35] Parker ES, Morihisa JM, Wyatt RJ, Schwartz BL, Weingartner H, Stillman RC. The alcohol facili-tation effect on memory: a dose-response study. *Psychopharmacol* (Berl) 1981;74(1):88-92.

[36] Tyson PD, Schirmuly M. Memory enhancement after drinking ethanol: consolidation, interference, or response bias? *Physiol. Behav.* 1994;56(5):933-7.

[37] Wixted JT. A theory about why we forget what we once knew. *Curr. Direct Psychol. Sci.* 2005;14(1):6-9.

[38] Wendt PE, Risberg J. Ethanol reduces rCFB activation of left dorsolateral prefrontal cortex during a verbal fluency task. *Brain Lang* 2001; 77(2):197-215.

[39] Nelson TO, McSpadden M, Fromme K, Marlatt GA. Effects of alcohol intoxication on meta-memory and on retrieval from long-term memory. *J. Exp. Psychol. Gen.* 1986;115(3):247-54.

[40] Sayette MA, Martin CS, Perrott MA, Wertz JM. Parental alcoholism and the effects of alcohol on mediated semantic priming. Exp Clin Psychopharmacol 2001;9(4):409-17.

[41] Duka T, Weissenborn R, Dienes Z. State-dependent effects of alcohol on recollective experience, familiarity and awareness of memories. *Psychopharmacol* (Berl) 2001;153(3):295-306.

[42] Nilsson LG, Backman L, Karlsson T. Priming and cued recall in elderly, alcohol intoxicated and sleep deprived subjects: a case of functionally similar memory deficits. *Psychol. Med.* 1989;19(2):423-33.

[43] Ray S, Bates ME, Ely BM. Alcohol's dissociation of implicit and explicit memory processes: implications of a parallel distributed processing model of semantic priming. *Exp. Clin. Psychopharmacol.* 2004;12(2):118-25.

[44] Roediger HL, McDermott KB. Implicit memory in normal human subjects. In: Spinnler H, Boller F, eds. *Handbook of neuropsychology.* Amsterdam: Elsevier, 1993:61-131.

[45] Schacter DL, Chiu CY, Ochsner KN. Implicit memory: a selective review. *Ann. Rev. Neurosci.* 1993;16:159-82.

[46] Jacoby LL, Toth JJP, Yonelinas AP. Separating conscious and unconscious influences of memory: Measuring recollection. *J. Exp. Psychol. Gen.* 1993;122:139-54.

[47] Flavell JH. What is memory development the development of? *Human Dev* 1971;14:272-8.

[48] Metcalfe J, Shimamura AP. *Metacognition: Knowing about knowing.* Cambridge: MIT Press, 1994.

[49] Koriat A, Goldsmith M. Monitoring and control processes in the strategic regulation of memory accuracy. *Psychol. Rev.* 1996;103(3):490-517.

[50] Mintzer MZ, Griffiths RR. Triazolam and zolpidem: effects on human memory and attentional processes. *Psychopharmacol* (Berl) 1999;144(1):8-19.

[51] Mintzer MZ, Griffiths RR. Acute effects of triazolam on false recognition. *Mem. Cognit* 2000; 28(8):1357-65.

[52] Jones BM. Memory impairment on the ascending and descending limbs of the blood alcohol curve. *J. Abnorm. Psychol.* 1973;82(1):24-32.

[53] Pihl RO, Paylan SS, Gentes-Hawn A, Hoaken PN. Alcohol affects executive cognitive functioning differentially on the ascending versus descending limb of the blood alcohol concentration curve. *Alcohol Clin. Exp. Res.* 2003;27(5):773-9.

[54] Martin CS, Earleywine M, Musty RE, Perrine MW, Swift RM. Development and validation of the biphasic alcohol effects scale. *Alcohol Clin. Exp. Res.* 1993;17(1):140-6.

[55] Bruce KR, Pihl RO. Forget "drinking to forget": enhanced consolidation of emotionally charged memory by alcohol. *Exp. Clin. Psychopharmacol.* 1997;5(3):242-50.

[56] Knowles SK, Duka T. Does alcohol affect memory for emotional and non-emotional experiences in different ways? *Behav. Pharmacol.* 2004;15(2):111-21.

In: Alcohol-Related Cognitive Disorders   ISBN: 978-1-60741-730-9

Editors: L. Sher, I. Kandel, J. Merrick pp. 221-231   © 2009 Nova Science Publishers, Inc.

Chapter 14

DRIVING AND FLYING WITH A HANGOVER

Joris C. Verster

ABSTRACT

Driving and flying are common ways of transportation. The impairing effects of alcohol intoxication on driving and flying skills have been extensively studied. It has been shown that driving and flying skills are impaired in a dose-dependent manner. Public health campaigns have drawn attention to the dangers of drunk driving and strict flying rules regarding alcohol use have been established. In contrast, driving and flying during alcohol hangover (ie, when blood alcohol concentrations are zero) received relatively little scientific attention. A literature review was performed to identify all clinical trials that examined the impact of alcohol hangover on driving and flying. The few studies that have been published (N=11) showed that driving performance and flying during alcohol hangover were significantly impaired. Public health campaigns should therefore point at the risks of driving the day after a heavy drinking session and flying regulations should adopt a strict zero alcohol policy.

INTRODUCTION

Driving and flying are popular ways of transportation. The effects of alcohol intoxication on driving and flying have been thoroughly investigated. With increasing blood alcohol concentrations performance becomes worse and the risk of accidents increases.

Driving

Drinking and driving is a dangerous combination. Public awareness campaigns repeatedly point at the dangers of driving when intoxicated. Apart from a small number of persistent drunk drivers, most drivers abstain from alcoholic beverages before driving or limit their consumption to stay below the legal limits for driving. Such limits vary across countries from zero up to 0.10%, most commonly set at 0.02%, 0.05%, 0.08%, or 0.10%. There is a trend to lower current limits because epidemiologic evidence proves that the reduction saves lives. The number of traffic deaths is increasing yearly, and the World Health Organization has estimated that in 2020, traffic deaths will outnumber those who are killed in war [1]. The number of alcohol-related accidents decreased until the mid-1990s, suggesting that public awareness on alcohol and driving was growing. Thereafter, however, from 1995 to date, self-reported episodes of driving after having used alcohol are increasing again. Data from the United States (US) National Highway Traffic Safety Administration revealed that 9% of all crashes are alcohol-related, and that 35% percent of intoxicated drivers involved in a crash had a blood alcohol level above 0.08 percent. The predictors of drunk driving include having alcohol related problems, being male, being young, an early age of drinking onset, and previous convictions of driving while intoxicated [2]. Alcohol is the number one cause of death of young adults. In 2002, 41% of traffic deaths among people younger than 34 years old were alcohol related [3].

Because most people are aware that driving while intoxicated is risky, they seek alternatives. For example, the majority of Dutch students report that they do not travel home by car, but use a bicycle to get home from the pub. That this is far from safe was shown by a survey among 800 Dutch college students [4]. This survey revealed that on average students who returned home by bicycle had a blood alcohol concentration of 0.095%, i.e. approximately five times the legal limit for participating in traffic for novice drivers in the Netherlands. An exponential relationship between blood alcohol concentration and the risk of having a bicycle accident was found, illustrated in figure 1. The outcome of this survey points at the fact that prevention campaigns should broaden their view to other modes of transportation besides driving a car when intoxicated.

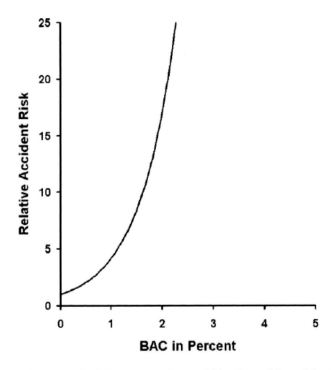

Figure 1. The relation between alcohol consumption and bicycle accident risk after an evening of alcohol consumption [4].

Because of safety concerns, ethical committees and lawmakers often prohibit investigators from conducting experiments in which intoxicated drivers are tested on the road during normal traffic. The legislative restrictions of most countries prohibit experiments with alcohol and medicinal drugs in real traffic. Currently such studies are performed only in the Netherlands.

As an alternative, studies examining the effects of alcohol on driving performance are conducted on closed roads or use driving simulators in a laboratory setting. Although these settings seem favorable in terms of safety, predicting actual driving performance from laboratory test battery results or driving simulators has been shown to be not always reliable [5]. Nevertheless, most researchers test driving-related skills instead of real driving. For example, tracking tests have been used to predict lane-keeping, whereas other tests examine the skills needed during driving, such as fast decision making or the ability to react to events that happen on the road (e.g., reaction time tests, psychomotor tests, and divided attention tests), sustained attention needed during prolonged driving (e.g. vigilance tests), working memory, or visual functioning.

Figure 2 gives an overview of a various driving-related skills and abilities that have been tested under controlled circumstances in laboratory settings, as reviewed by Moskowitz and Fiorentino [6]. The authors reviewed 112 trials performed from 1981 to 1998 that examined driving-related skills. Figure 2 shows blood alcohol concentrations at which at least 50% of tests showed significant performance impairment on the behavioral tests. Not all skills and abilities are equally impaired at a particular blood alcohol concentration: significant performance impairment on the laboratory tests is evident at blood alcohol concentrations ranging from almost zero for divided attention up to 0.10% for simple reaction time tasks.

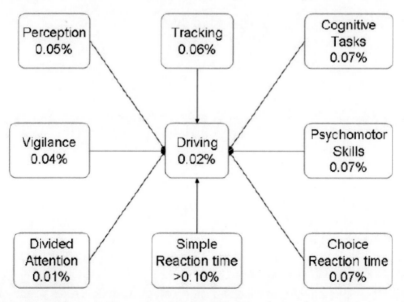

Figure 2. Skills and abilities related to driving and blood alcohol concentrations at which 50% of more of behavioral tests indicated consistent impairment [6].

On-the-road tests show that actual driving is significantly worse than placebo with blood alcohol concentrations of 0.02-0.04% [7]. Thus, one can conclude that not all skills and abilities are equally important during actual driving. The data summarized in figure 2 also make clear that extrapolating laboratory test results to actual (complex) behavior like driving may not be an adequate reflection of reality.

Flying

Our 24-hour economy puts high demands on flight personnel. The pilots are put under increased stress, which may provoke alcohol use when off duty. Many flights return from their destination within several hours after landing, or the next day after a night of sleep. During these boring waiting hours, flight personnel are often constricted to the airport launch or hotel bar. In this environment, killing time by drinking is a risky temptation. Like car driving, flying is an example of a complex task in which subtasks compete for limited processing capacity [8]. Continuous demands are made on working memory, and attention must be divided among various mental tasks, especially during take off and landing. In addition, pilots rely heavily on radio communication to be updated on changing weather conditions, other traffic and flight instructions.

A generally acknowledged point of view is that blood alcohol levels should be zero in persons who have responsibility over the lives of such a great number of passengers. In this context, not surprisingly, considerable concerns have been expressed regarding the use of alcohol by flight personnel. As a result, the regulations and testing for alcohol use of flight personnel have been strengthened over the last decades. Currently, the US Federal Aviation Administration (FAA) regulations concerning alcohol use state that flying is prohibited in one or more of the following instances:

- Blood alcohol concentration (BAC) > 0.04%
- A pilot has been drinking within 8 hours before flying
- A pilot feels 'impaired'.

The European guidelines for aircraft personnel are even stricter and prohibit being on duty when the BAC is > 0.02 percent. Being on duty also includes pre-flight preparations.

Views of Flight Personnel Regarding Alcohol Use

Flight personnel often underestimate the risks of flying and drinking. For example, a 1978 survey showed that over 50% of pilots' view that flying within four hours after drinking some alcohol was safe [9]. From other reports it is evident that after drinking, pilots were unable to determine when their blood alcohol level has fallen below 0.02%. Additionally, a large number of them felt it was safe to fly with blood alcohol concentrations higher than 0.02% [10]. Most pilots overestimated the number of alcoholic drinks needed to reach a certain peak blood alcohol level. At the same time, they underestimated the rate at which blood alcohol levels decrease over time [11]. Unfortunately, these errors were most pronounced in moderate and heavy drinkers. Moderate and heavy drinkers are also more tolerant when it comes to alcohol use and flying [12]. This situation is of great concern because it suggests that those who consume the most alcohol are more likely to disobey flight rules regarding alcohol use. Little scientific evidence has emerged that the results from these surveys have changed. On the contrary, the results from a recent survey among United Kingdom civil aviation pilots show that flight personnel do not take the European alcohol policy too seriously. That over than 50% of these pilots reported that they have been on duty with higher blood alcohol concen-trations than allowed is indeed of great concern [13].

In contrast to the acute effects of alcohol, the after effect of alcohol consumption, i.e. the hangover phase, has received relatively little scientific attention. Often it is assumed that when alcohol is no longer present in the blood, negative effects on performance are unlikely. As will become evident from the following literature review, this is a misjudgment that can have serious safety consequences.

A LITERATURE REVIEW

A literature search was performed using Medline (from 1966), Embase (from 1974), and the Cochran clinical trials database (searched April, 2007), to collect clinical trials that examined alcohol hangover effects on driving and flying. Keywords were "alcohol" and "hangover" combined with "driving" or "flying". Cross-references were checked as well. Studies using laboratory tests other than driving or flight-simulators were excluded. Together this search yielded two studies that examined driving ability during hangover and nine studies that examined flying ability.

Driving during Alcohol Hangover

In most public awareness campaigns that address drinking and driving, alcohol hangover is not an issue. Hence, most people presume that it is safe to drive a car as soon as blood alcohol levels reach zero or are below the legal limits. Yet, scientific evidence for this assumption is lacking.

Laurell and Törnros [14] conducted two studies to examine driving ability during alcohol hangover on a closed road and in a driving simulator. In their first study on a closed road, 22 healthy volunteers had to perform a driving task. They were instructed to make 10 difficult avoidance maneuvers without knocking down pylon cones that were positioned along the circuit. On each side of the car, a 15 cm space was left to perform the maneuver without hitting the cones. The night before performing this test, the participants consumed alcohol in a party-like atmosphere to reach a peak BAC of around 0.15%. The tests started the following morning, after 8-9 hours of sleep, as soon as blood alcohol concentrations reached zero. Three hours thereafter, a second test session was scheduled. The results from both sessions showed that all subjects performed worse relative to the control session. Overall, the hangover state caused a significant performance reduction of approximately 20%. Interestingly, hangover severity did not correlate significantly with performance reduction on the driving test. Participants were unable to estimate their BAC levels or the time when BAC reached zero [15]. A limitation of this study may be the nature of the test: maneuvering along cones does not resemble normal driving, and no other traffic was present at the closed circuit. Additionally, the participants were aware that they had consumed alcohol: on the alcohol session they slept at the Institute, whereas at the control session (no alcohol) they slept at home the night before testing.

A second study by the same investigators was performed in a driving simulator [16]. The task comprised operating the vehicle over a 20 km hilly and curved circuit. The subjects were instructed to drive as fast as possible and take the risk of crashing. Leaving 'the road' was counted as a crash and resulted in a time-penalty of 20 seconds.

Twenty-four healthy volunteers participated in this study. All participants knew each other well, and alcohol was consumed freely in a party-like atmosphere until midnight. The peak BAC was 0.18 percent. Eleven participants (out of 12) completed the driving simulator test when intoxicated and performed significantly worse than in the sober condition. The following day, tests were performed every 2.5 hours. Despite the various practice sessions, on every subsequent test, the subjects in both conditions performed better, suggesting a learning/practice effect. A significant difference between the hangover and control session was found only on the first test after awakening: the subjects who consumed alcohol performed significantly worse relative to the sober condition. At the time of testing, the BAC was not zero, but approximately 0.04%. The BAC levels gradually decreased during the day and reached zero just before the fourth session (4.30 AM). At that time, no significant effects were found. After this day, the participants remained at the Institute for a second night of sleep. No alcohol was consumed on the second evening, and the following morning all previously reported hangover symptoms were absent and their performance on the simulator test was unimpaired. A possible limitation of this study is that the subjects had to drive as fast as possible. In real traffic, this behavior is not advisable. The authors admitted that this test of extreme driving puts very high demands on subjects [17], and the test results therefore may apply more to rally racing than to normal driving.

Flying during Alcohol Hangover

Several studies examined the effects of alcohol hangover in flight simulators, both at ground level and at simulated high altitudes. In the 1970s, Dowd and colleagues [18] examined alcohol hangover in a 'spatial orientation trainer', a simulator used to teach pilots how to fly. Seven pilots completed this not-blinded study. The pilots consumed 0.85 or 1.71 g/kg alcohol mixed with soft drinks. In the simulator, a pitch illusion task representing flight take-off was performed in which the pilots had to return the plane to a straight level as quickly as possible. Although their blood alcohol levels were not zero after a 7-hours night sleep, their performances on this relatively simple orientation test were not significantly affected. Unfortunately, practice effects made the test results difficult to interpret (pilots performed better on each subsequent session), and no control group was used to correct for these effects.

Yesavage and Leirer [19] examined the alcohol hangover effects 14 hours after alcohol consumption (1.0 g/kg). Ten aircraft pilots participated in this placebo controlled crossover study. The participants performed two simulator flights in which take-off maneuvers and landing skills were assessed. To make circumstances difficult for the pilots, the flight simulation was complicated by losing two of four engines on one side of the aircraft. During alcohol hangover, both take-off and landing maneuvers were significantly affected. Of concern, some pilots were not aware of their perfor-mance impairment during hangover.

Level of Intoxication

Petros and colleagues [20] of the University of North Dakota examined the impact of alcohol dosage on the severity of impairment during alcohol hangover. The investigators recruited 36 pilots who performed simulated flights after drinking different dosages of alcohol. In their study, 2 or 3 ml/kg vodka was administered to reach peak blood alcohol levels of 0.07% or 0.10%, respectively. Eleven hours after alcohol intake or placebo, when blood alcohol concentrations were zero, the pilots performed two 75-minute flights in the simulator. Pilots that received the higher alcohol dose performed significantly worse in turning and landing maneuvers than those who consumed no alcohol. Deviations from optimal heading, speed, and altitude were not affected during hangover. Working memory for the given instructions by ground personnel were not affected either, however, executing these instructions was significantly impaired (they were able to recall the instructions, but during the flight they carried out significantly fewer directives when compared with the placebo group). In contrast, impairment was not significant in pilots that received the lower dose of vodka. The findings suggest that in determining whether hangover effects significantly impair cognitive performance, the level of intoxication plays a role as well.

Men Versus Women

Sometimes it is speculated that men and women differ in flying skills. On first sight, this popular belief seemed to be supported by McFadden [21]. Examining the number of accidents made from 1986 to 1992 by US airline pilots revealed that women employed by major airlines had significantly higher accident rates than male pilots. However, after adjusting for flying experience (total number of flying hours were much higher in men) the difference between male and female pilots was no longer significant.

Taylor and colleagues [22] compared flight simulator performance of male and female pilots. In a daytime study, alcohol was administered in the morning to reach a peak BAC of 0.08 percent. In the afternoon, 8 hours after alcohol administration, flight simulator tests were performed. The simulator test was made difficult by severe turbulence during the flying period and crosswind while landing. Test performance was significantly impaired during acute intoxication. In contrast, when blood alcohol levels were zero no significant effects were found on take off ability, air traffic control, line-up with the runway, and landing maneuvers. Men and women did not significantly differ on any test parameter during hangover. Taken together, no scientific proof of gender differences was found, neither when sober, during intoxication, nor during alcohol hangover.

Aging

Aging is often associated with cognitive decline. Therefore, the Age 60 Rule that prohibits civil aircraft pilots over 60 years of age from flying is effective. Although the Age 60 Rule was enforced to increase safety, from its introduction its existence has been under debate. For example, it has been claimed that young pilots have much less flying experience than do older pilots. Additionally, it has been argued that cognitive decline may differ greatly between aging individuals, and the chosen age of 60 thus seems arbitrary.

A recent study in 100 aircraft pilots examined the relation between age and simulated flight performance (without alcohol administration or other experimental manipulation). Increased age was significantly associated with decreased test performance [23]. Age, however, explained only 22% of the variance in flying performance, suggesting that other factors than age may have a bigger impact on performance levels. Alcohol may be a likely candidate, and its interaction with age on flight simulator performance during intoxication and hangover has been scientifically examined.

For example, Morrow and colleagues [8] examined the effects of alcohol on flight simulator performance in a placebo-controlled crossover study in seven young and seven older pilots. All pilots had similar flying experience. The tests were performed during daytime at peak BAC levels of 0.04% and 0.10%, and 2, 4, 8, 24 and 48 hours thereafter. Various flying-related skills were examined in the simulator task, including near target avoidance, far target detection, engine emergency detection, take-off, approach, and landing. During the performance of the simulator test, radio communication with ground control and course errors were assessed as well. Cognitive demands during flying were increased by simulated turbulence and heavy crosswind. During alcohol intoxication (after administration of the high alcohol dosage), radio communication errors and course errors (heading and altitude) were significantly increased in old pilots but not in young pilots. After 8 hours (BAC was zero), all pilots made significantly more radio communication errors, but no effect on course errors was found.

Yesavage and colleagues [24] examined flight simulator performance in 14 young (mean age 27) and older pilots (mean age 60). All pilots were trained extensively on a complex flight simulator test, including take-off ability, communication, traffic avoidance, cockpit monitoring, visual approach and landing maneuvers. Performance was scored and summarized into an overall flying ability score. Simulator performance was tested at baseline, during intoxication (peak BAC of 0.08%) and alcohol hangover. No sleeping was allowed on this test day. Flying ability was significantly impaired during intoxication and hangover for all pilots, but the age groups did not differ from each other. Ten months later, whether the older pilots had forgotten more about this task and had increased skills decrements relative to younger pilots was examined. The same test was performed during baseline, alcohol intoxication (peak BAC of 0.10%) and hangover. Again, flying ability was significantly impaired during intoxication and hangover for all pilots. Again, no significant differences were found between young and older pilots. According to the authors, the relatively small number of subjects and because the performance decrement in older pilots may have been compensated by having much more flying experience than younger pilots may account for the absence of differences in overall flying skills between the age groups. Re-analysis of the data in more detail by Taylor and co-workers [25] revealed that the young pilots were specifically impaired in cockpit monitoring and made significantly more communication errors during intoxication. The communication errors were also evident during alcohol hangover. Older pilots produced more communication errors than did young pilots, but this effect did not reach statistical significance.

Taken together, some evidence has been found that older pilots may perform worse when compared with young pilots. However, a great variability was observed in the performance of older pilots. Therefore, the Age 60 Rule seems unfortunate for a number of highly experienced and qualified over-60 pilots. Individual testing of older pilots therefore seems wiser than using an arbitrary age rule.

Performance at High Altitude

Studies have shown that just being at a high altitude can already affect cognition and psychomotor performance. Results from flight simulator tests performed at ground level may thus be of limited value. Carroll and colleagues [26] conducted an experiment in a decompression chamber, examining tracking ability and monitoring performance (responding to peripheral light signals) during alcohol hangover at ground level and at a simu-lated altitude of 8,000 and 13,000 feet. Surprisingly, relative to ground level, high altitudes did not affect performance on the tests during hangover. Collins [27] also examined the effects of alcohol intoxication and hangover on psychomotor performance and cognitive functioning at ground level and 12,000 feet. In a placebo-controlled crossover design, eight pilots were tested until 02:30 AM after consuming alcohol (mixed with 7-Up) to reach a peak BAC of 0.09%. During intoxication, both reaction speed and tracking perfor-mance were significantly affected by alcohol. Relative to ground level, at high altitude reaction speed and tracking performance were worse after both placebo and alcohol. The pilots were awakened at 6:45 AM and after a standardized breakfast, the test procedures were repeated at 07:30 AM. During this hangover state, 8 hours after drinking, their mean BAC was 0.012%. Their performance on the tests was not significantly affected during hangover, and performance at high altitude did not differ from ground level. In addition to the limited number of participants in these studies, whether the observed effects are due to alcohol hang-over, sleeping for only few hours, or a combination of both remains unsure.

In sum, the evidence that performance under the influence of alcohol may differ at high altitudes is limited and deserves further examination.

CONCLUSIONS

Limited research has been done examining the effects of alcohol hangover on driving and flying. From these studies and can be concluded that:

- The results from the studies conducted by Laurell and Törnros [14] support the idea that driving ability is impaired during alcohol hangover. Additional research is necessary, however, preferably performed on-the-road during normal traffic.
- The FAA guidelines regarding alcohol use for aircraft personnel are insufficient because flight simulator performance has been show to be:
    - impaired at BAC < 0.04%,
    - still significant 8 hours after consumption,
    - significantly impaired when pilots report being unimpaired
- Aging has a negative impact on performance, which may aggravate the performance decrement during intoxication and alcohol hangover. The Age 60 Rule is arbitrary, and each pilots' ability to fly should be judged on an individual basis.

- Limited evidence suggests no differences in flight performance between men and women, both during alcohol intoxication and hangover. As an increasing number of pilots are women, future studies should further examine possible sex differences on flying ability.
- No convincing evidence has been found that alcohol hangover effects differ significantly at high altitude relative to ground level.

Taken together, the present data suggest that a zero alcohol policy for flight personnel seems the only safe recommendation to be adopted by the FAA and other flight associations.

REFERENCES

[1]   Peden M, Scurfield R, Sleed D, et al. *World Report on Road Traffic Injury Prevention*. Geneva: World Health Organization, 2004.
[2]   Hingson R, Winter M. Epidemiology and cones-quences of drinking and driving. *Alcohol. Res. Health 2003*;27:63-78.
[3]   Quinlan KP, Brewer RD, Siegel P, Sleet DA, Mokdat AH, Shults RA, Flowers N. Alcohol-impaired driving among U.S. adults 1993-2002. *Am. J. Prev. Med.* 2005;28:346-50.
[4]   Verster JC, Van Herwijnen J, Olivier B, Volkerts ER. Bicycle accident risk after an evening of alcohol consumption. *J. Psychopharmacol.* 2006;20(Suppl5): A49.
[5]   Verster JC. *Measurement of the effects of psycho-active drugs on driving ability and related psycho-logical processes*. Thesis. Utrecht, the Netherlands, 2002.
[6]   Moskowitz H, Fiorentino D. A review of the literature on the effects of low doses of alcohol on driving-related skills. US Department of Transpor-tation. National Highway Traffic Safety Administra-tion. *Report DOT HS* 809 028, 2000.
[7]   Verster JC, Volkerts ER, Schreuder AHCML, Eijken EJE, Van Heuckelum JHG, Veldhuijzen DS, Verbaten MN, Patat A, Paty I. Residual effects of middle-of-the-night administration of zaleplon and zolpidem on driving ability, memory functions and psychomotor performance. *J. Clin. Psychopharmacol.* 2002;22:576-83.
[8]   Morrow DG, Leirer VO, Yesavage JA. The influence of alcohol and aging on radio communi-cation during flight. *Aviat Space Environ. Med.* 1990;61:12-20.
[9]   Damkot DK, Osga GA. Survey of pilot's attitudes and opinions about drinking and flying. *Aviat Space Environ. Med.* 1978;49:390-4.
[10] Widders R, Harris D. Pilots' knowledge of the relationship between alcohol consumption and levels of blood alcohol concentration. *Aviat Space Environ. Med.* 1997;68:531-7.
[11] Ross SM, Ross LE. Pilots' knowledge of blood alcohol levels and the 0.04% blood alcohol con-centration rule. *Aviat Space Environ. Med.* 1990; 61:412-7.
[12] Ross LE, Ross SM. Pilot's attitudes toward alcohol use and flying. *Aviat Space Environ. Med.* 1988; 59:913-9.
[13] Maxwell E, Harris D. Drinking and flying: a structural model. *Aviat Space Environ Med.* 1999; 70:117-23.

[14] Laurell H, Törnros J. Investigation of alcoholic hang-over effects on driving performance. *Blutalcohol.* 1983;20:489-99.

[15] Frank DH. 'If you drink, don't drive' motto now applies to hangovers as well. *JAMA* 1983;250: 1657-8.

[16] Törnros J, Laurell H. Acute and hang-over effects of alcohol on simulated driving performance. *Blutalcohol* 1991;28:24-30.

[17] Törnros J. Hangover effects of alcohol and carry-over effects of certain benzodiazepine hypnotics on driving performance. Uppsala, Sweden: *Acta Universitatis Upsaliensis* 102, 2001.

[18] Dowd PJ, Wolfe JW, Cramer RL. Aftereffects of alcohol on the perception and control of pitch attitude during centripetal acceleration. *Aerospace Med.* 1973;44:928-30.

[19] Yesavage JA, Leirer VO. Hangover effects on aircraft pilots 14 hours after alcohol ingestion: a preliminary report. *Am. J. Psychiatry* 1986;143: 1546-50.

[20] Petros T, Bridewell J, Warren J, Ferraro FR, Bates J, Moulton P, et al. Post-intoxication effects of alcohol on flight performance after moderate and high blood alcohol levels. *Int .J. Aviat Psychology* 2003;13:287-300.

[21] McFadden KL. Comparing pilot-error accident rates of male and female airline pilots. *Omega Int. J. Mgmt. Sci.* 1996;24:443-50.

[22] Taylor JL, Dolhert N, Friedman L, Mumenthaler M, Yesavage JA. Alcohol elimination and simulator performance of male and female aviators: a pre-liminary report. Aviat Space Environ Med 1996; 67:407-13.

[23] Yesavage JA, Taylor JL, Mumenthaler MS, Noda A, O'Hara R. Relationship of age and simulated flight performance. *J. Am. Geriatr. Soc.* 1999;47:819-23.

[24] Yesavage JA, Dolhert N, Taylor JL. Flight simulator performance of younger and older aircraft pilots: effects of age and alcohol. *J. Am. Geriatr. Soc.* 1994; 42:577-82.

[25] Taylor JL, Dolhert N, Friedman L, Yesavage JA. Acute and 8-hour effects of alcohol (0.08% BAC) on younger and older pilots' simulator performance. *Aviat Space Environ. Med.* 1994;65:718-25.

[26] Carroll JR, Ashe WF, Roberts LB. Influence of the aftereffects of alcohol combined with hypoxia on psychomotor performance. *Aerospace Med.* 1964;10: 990-3.

[27] Collins WE. Performance effects of alcohol intoxication and hangover at ground level and simulated altitude. *Aviat Space Environ. Med.* 1980;51:327-35.

PART THREE: CHRONIC EFFECTS OF ALCOHOL

In: Alcohol-Related Cognitive Disorders   ISBN: 978-1-60741-730-9
Editors: L. Sher, I. Kandel, J. Merrick pp. 235-242   © 2009 Nova Science Publishers, Inc.

Chapter 15

EXECUTIVE FUNCTION AND SOCIAL COGNITION IN ALCOHOLISM

Jennifer Uekermann and Irene Daum

ABSTRACT

Studies on cognitive functions in alcoholism have reported a range of deficits affecting, among other domains, executive functions, and social cognition. The impairment pattern is consistent with the so-called frontal lobe hypothesis, which asserts a specific vulnerability of the prefrontal cortex to the neurotoxic effects of alcohol. This chapter aims to give an overview of the neuropsychological profile relating to executive functions and social cognition in alcoholism by reviewing both patient and functional neuroimaging studies. The implications of such impairments for the therapy of alcoholism will also be addressed.

INTRODUCTION

Alcohol use disorders can be characterized by a consumption of dangerously large quantities of alcohol, despite knowledge of and insight into the adverse effects of such behavior. Chronic alcoholism is associated with functional and structural brain changes, which are thought to underlie the frequently reported cognitive impairments associated with alcoholism. Such deficits have been interpreted in the context of different neuropsychological models [1]. According to the Right Hemisphere Hypothesis, alcoholism results in a dysfunction of the right hemisphere, leading to neuropsychological impairments on tasks which depend on its functional integrity. The Premature Aging Hypothesis postulates that alcoholism is associated with accelerated aging of the brain, yielding cognitive impairments that are usually observed in much older healthy adults. According to the Hypothesis of Mild Generalized Dysfunction, alcoholism leads to a diffuse generalized dysfunction of the brain, with widely variable impairment patterns. None of these models has as yet received convincing empirical support [1]. The current literature focuses on the frontal lobe hypothesis, which asserts a specific vulnerability of the prefrontal cortex (PFC) to the toxic effect of alcohol [2].

As the PFC has long been known to mediate executive functions and recently has also been associated with social cognition, the present review focuses on potential changes in these domains in alcoholism. In the first section, the brain changes associated with alcoholism will be summarized, followed by a critical discussion of executive function impairments that are based on both clinical and functional neuroimaging data in the second section. The third section focuses on changes of social cognition in alcoholism. The chapter will conclude with a discussion of the implications of brain changes and the associated changes in neuropsychological status for the treatment of alcoholism.

THE PREFRONTAL CORTEX:
ANATOMICAL AND FUNCTIONAL CONSIDERATIONS

The prefrontal cortex (PFC) entails approximately 29% of the total cortex and is the single largest brain region in human beings, with afferent and efferent connections to the thalamus, cingulate, limbic, basal ganglia structures as well as all other neocortical regions [3-7]. Prefrontal cortex dysfunction is associated with executive deficits and behavioral changes [8]. Executive functions refer to a range of cognitive processes, which are engaged in superordinate cognitive control and coordination of information processing. Within this context, the attentional model by Norman and Shallice [9] differentiates between two systems: The contention scheduling system is involved in routine situations, in which actions are automatically triggered. The Supervisory Attentional System, on the other hand, is responsible for the execution of behavior in novel situations, in which automatic selection of action is inappropriate and the generation of novel plans and willed actions is necessary.

The behavioral changes after PFC lesions include apathy, perseverative behavior, difficulty in shifting response set, and changes of affect and emotion [2]. In addition, impairments of social cognition deficits relating to perception of affect, impaired theory of mind abilities, and humor-processing deficits are frequently observed as sequelae of PFC dysfunction. Hornak et al [10] reported impairments of emotional prosody and face decoding, as well as socially inappropriate behavior in patients with ventral frontal lobe lesions. These deficits correlated significantly with the severity of emotional changes and behavioral problems. Theory of mind refers to the ability to reason about mental states, to predict and understand other people's behavior based on their mental states [11].

Theory of mind can be assessed by so-called false belief tasks, which assess the ability to understand that an individual can have a false belief. The results from functional neuroimaging and lesion studies indicated that the underlying neuronal network includes the medial prefrontal and temporal cortex [12]. Humor potentially involves expressive abilities for the generation of humorous stimuli and receptive abilities necessary for the comprehension and appreciation of humorous stimuli [13].

The Incongruity Resolution Theory proposes two stages of humor processing [13]. The first stage (incongruity detection) refers to the perception of an incongruent element. The incongruent element is then resolved in the second stage (resolution). Evidence has emerged for a differential contribution of both hemispheres to incongruity detection and resolution, with more recent data emphasizing a more important involvement of the right frontal lobe in humor processing [13].

BRAIN CHANGES IN ALCOHOLISM

According to Mann et al [14] approximately 50% to 70% of alcoholics show signs of brain abnormalities, with cortical changes including volume loss of gray and white matter of the frontal, parietal, and temporal cortex [1]. Alcohol-related volume loss has also been reported for the corpus callosum, cerebellar vermis, hippocampus, mammillary bodies, thalamus, putamen, and caudate [1]. The PFC does, however, appear to be disproportionately affected [2]. The following section therefore focuses on studies of PFC changes in alcoholism.

Post-mortem studies have documented a statistically significant loss of brain tissue in alcoholism (14,15), which could not be attributed to changes in hydration [16,17]. Cortical atrophy was particularly pronounced in the PFC. Post-mortem studies, do, however, often suffer from poor ante-mortem documentation and their results should be interpreted with caution (2). Neuroradiological studies based on computer tomography reported significantly increased ventricular size and cortical atrophy. Cala et al [18] reported cortical atrophy in 73% of their sample, with prominent enlargement of the cortical sulci in frontal and parietal regions. Magnetic resonance imaging studies also yielded grey matter reduction, white matter deficits, and sulcal and ventricular enlargement [2].

Single photon emission computed tomography (SPECT) was used to investigate physiological brain changes in alcoholism. Nicolas et al (19) reported a significant reduction in the regional cerebral blood flow ratio (rCBF) in virtually all regions, with a particularly pronounced reduction in the PFC. Similar patterns of brain changes have been found in studies based on electrophysiology and event-related potentials [2[. The changes in question appear to be partly reversible. The abstinence effects are not completely reversible, however, and abnormalities may still be present after years of abstinence [2].

EXECUTIVE DEFICITS IN ALCOHOLISM

A prominent feature of the neuropsychological profile in alcoholism is the presence of pronounced executive deficits affecting cognitive flexibility, problem solving, verbal- and non-verbal abstraction, and decision making. Executive impairments are also seen for tasks with high ecological validity, such as the Behavioral Assessment of the Dysexecutive Syndrome Battery [20]. Based on the observed impairment patterns, Ihara et al [21] differentiated between four different groups of alcoholics: The first group showed a differential pattern of impaired executive functions and preserved intelligence and memory. The second group included patients with combined executive and memory deficits, but without intellectual impairments. The third group consisted of patients with general intellectual impairments, and the fourth group showed intact cognitive performance. About two-thirds of the patients were assigned to the first two groups. Of particular clinical relevance is the performance of alcoholics on risk-taking tasks, which have shown to be sensitive to ventromedial prefrontal cortex dysfunction. Bowden-Jones et al [22] administered a neuropsychological battery that included a gambling task, in which subjects had to select cards from one of four decks. The decks were arranged in a system in which the cards in two of the decks were associated with higher immediate gains, but also with higher long-term losses. Alcoholics chose significantly more cards from the "bad" decks of the gambling task. The finding that alcoholics made choices governed by immediate gains irrespective of later outcome is relevant for the therapy of alcoholism [5].

The performance of alcoholic patients is influenced by a range of factors, such as the number of detoxifications, gender, family history of alcoholism, and the quantity of consumed alcohol. Planning abilities, vigilance and measures of impulsivity, e.g., were at least partly related to the number of detoxifications [23]. Mann et al [24] observed similar brain shrinkage in female and male alcoholics, despite a shorter ethanol exposition of women. Another important confounding factor may be family history of alcoholism [1]. Executive dysfunction was also found to be associated with the amount of recent alcohol consumption [25]. Variables such as age at disease onset as well as duration of abstinence can also affect the cognitive profile. Early onset alcoholics showed higher levels of impulsive decision making, aggressiveness, and severity of substance-related problems [26]. Johnson-Greene et al [27] studied abstinence effects in alcoholics with evaluation intervals ranging from 10 to 32 months. Patients who managed to remain abstinent showed partial recovery of local cerebral metabolic rates for glucose in frontal regions and improvement of executive functions.

The empirical neuropsychological findings are consistent with the frontal lobe hypothesis, which asserts a disproportionate PFC vulnerability to the toxic effects of alcohol [1]. Combined cognitive and neuro-imaging data offer further support [2].

SOCIAL COGNITION IN ALCOHOLISM

Studies on social cognition in alcoholism have focused on interpersonal problem solving and the interpretation of affective prosody and facial expressions, as well as humor processing. Interpersonal problem solving is an important social skill and can be assessed by the Adaptive Skills Battery [28], involving the presentation of a variety of interpersonal problem situations. A 'competency score' is obtained, which reflects the degree to which responses maximize positive gain and minimize negative outcomes for the respondent. Jones and Lanyon [28] reported positive associations between the competency score and treatment success. The authors did, however, not include a healthy control group. Patterson et al [29] did not find differences between the competency scores of alcoholic patients and healthy controls when asked to give 'the very best response', whereas the alcoholics scored lower when participants were instructed to give their 'typical response'. Interpersonal problem-solving deficits in alcoholics thus seem to be due to their less effective execution of problem-solving skills. The finding that alcoholics are impaired at executing problem-solving skills despite knowledge of the best response may be interpreted in the context of reduced inhibitory abilities, which are frequently observed in alcoholism [3].

Affect perception is an important social skill, which facilitates and supports the interpretation of the communicating partner's intentions. In studies of affect perception, faces and prosody depicting a specific emotion are usually presented, and the subjects are instructed to name the corresponding emotions. Cermak et al [30] investigated the ability to identify the emotional expression of faces in alcoholics and did not find significant differences to controls. In more recent studies, however, identification of emotional facial expressions and prosody was found to be less accurate in alcoholics than in controls [31, 32]. In the Kornreich et al [32] study, recently detoxified alcoholics overestimated the intensity of expressed emotions and mid- to long-term alcoholics showed deficits in decoding anger and disgust. Monnot et al [33] observed significant impairments of affective prosodic compre-hension in alcoholics with and without a probable history of fetal alcohol syndrome. Uekermann et al [34] reported a complex performance pattern of alcoholics, with intact performance on simple tasks such as affect identification, whereas severe impairments were observed if prosody did not match the content of the sentence. Accurate perception of the emotional content of these sentences requires the suppression of the semantic content and thus taps onto inhibitory processes that are reduced in alcoholics. These findings are of particular clinical relevance in light of the study by Kornreich et al [35], who reported significant associations between affect perception deficits and interpersonal social problems.

So far, relatively little is known about social cognition in more complex settings, e.g. within the context of the comprehension of humor. Cermak et al [29] presented cartoons with two alternative endings, and participants were instructed to choose the correct funny ending. When the number of correct funny punch lines was analyzed, alcoholics did not differ from healthy controls. However, alcoholics showed a different pattern of errors. In a recent investigation, Uekermann et al [36] presented joke stems to both alcoholic patients and healthy controls. After reading the joke stem, participants were asked to select the correct funny punch line from an array of four possible endings (the correct punch line, a slapstick alternative, a logical as well as an illogical ending). Whereas the comprehension of the correct punch line requires both stages of the Incongruity Resolution Theory (see above), the comprehension of the slapstick alternative involves incongruity detection only. The logical and illogical endings represent incongruity detection and resolution. In addition, executive functions (working memory, set shifting, and inhibition) and theory of mind abilities were assessed. Theory of mind was screened by three mentalistic questions, which referred to the perspectives of the protagonists in the jokes. The alcoholics selected fewer correct punch lines and a larger number of slapstick and logical alternatives. Based on these findings, Uekermann et al [36] concluded that alcoholics show humor processing deficits, when both stages of humor processing are needed to understand the joke. In addition, regression analyses indicated that the impairments were partly due to executive and theory of mind deficits.

Taken together, alcoholics suffer from a broad range of social cognition deficits, which may contribute to their social problems and which must be considered in rehabilitation settings [5].

IMPLICATIONS FOR TREATMENT

As outlined above, alcoholism is associated with brain changes and problems in a wide range of cognitive domains. Cognitive impairments mainly affect executive function and social cognition, which may in turn influence the treatment and further progression of alcoholism. Within this context, Koob and Le Moal [37] have argued that repeated failures of self-regulation may lead to chronic drug use, which results in progressive dysregulation of the brain reward system. Cognitive deficits affecting attention and executive functions may contribute to the maintenance of drug consumption via loss of control and reduced cognitive flexibility.

With respect to rehabilitation, the fronto-striatal alcohol addiction model by Giancola and Moss [38] is of particular interest. According to this model, alcohol and alcohol-related stimuli are associated with the activation of the ventral striatum and ventral tegmentum, leading to expression of overlearned and stereotypic behaviors, such as alcohol seeking and alcohol intake. Furthermore, the PFC becomes disinhibited by the direct actions of alcohol and by dopaminergic innervation from the ventral tegmentum. These mechanisms lead to deficits in learning and in executing novel adaptive behavior in response to alcohol-related stimuli, thereby contributing to a negative outcome. The relevance of executive functions for the rehabilitation of alcoholics is supported by several studies. Bowden-Jones et al [22] reported that early relapse was associated with choices governed by immediate gains, irrespective of long-term outcome in a decision making task [3]. Performance on executive tasks was a significant predictor of alcohol consumption 3 years after initial assessment [39]. Executive impairments were also found to be associated with higher degree of denial [40].

Impairments of social cognition relating to theory of mind or affect perception may clearly affect social competence and interpersonal problems in personal as well as work contexts, as pointed out by Kornreich et al [32] To our knowledge, there are as yet no investigations of the influence of social cognition impairments on relapse, studies that are clearly needed to further our knowledge about optimal treatment settings.

REFERENCES

[1] Uekermann J, Daum I. The neuropsychology of alcoholism. In: Columbus F, ed. *New research on alcohol abuse and alcoholism*. New York, NY: Nova Science, 2006;1-18.
[2] Moselhy HF, Georgiou G, Kahn A. Frontal lobe changes in alcoholism: A review of the literature. *Alcohol Alcohol* 2001;36(5):357-68.
[3] Nauta WJH. The problem of the frontal lobes: a reinterpretation. *J. Psychiatr Res.* 1971;8(3):167-87.
[4] Nauta WJH. Neural association of the frontal cortex. *Acta Neurobiol. Exp.* 1972;32(2):125-40.
[5] Goldman-Rakic PS, Selemon LD, Schwartz ML. Dual pathways connecting the dorsolateral pre-frontal cortex with hippocampal formation and parahippocampal cortex in rhesus monkey. *Neuroscience* 1984;12(3):719-43.
[6] Fuster JM. *The prefrontal cortex*. New York, NY: Raven Press, 1986.
[7] Stuss DT, Benson DF. *The frontal lobes*. New York, NY: Raven Press, 1989.
[8] Roberts AC, Robbins TW, Weiskrantz L. *The prefrontal cortex. Executive and cognitive funtions*. Oxford, UK: Univ Press, 1988.
[9] Norman DA, Shallice T. Attention to action: willed and automatic control of behaviour. In: Schwartz GE, Shapiro D, eds. *Consciousness and self-regulation*. New York, NY: Plenum, 1986:268-72.

[10] Hornak J, Rolls ET, Wade D. Face and voice expression identification in patients with emotional and behavioral changes following ventral frontal lobe damage. *Neuropsychologia* 1996;34(4):247-61.

[11] Premack D, Woodruff G. Does the chimpanzee have a theory of mind? *Behav. Brain Sci;*1978(4): 515-26.

[12] Singer T. The neuronal basis and ontogeny of empathy and mind reading: review of literature and implications for future research. Neurosci Biobehav Rev 2006;30(6):855-63.

[13] Uekermann J, Channon S, Daum, I. *Towards a cognitive and social neuroscience of humor processing.* Social Cognition, in press.

[14] Mann K, Mundle G, Strayle M, Wakat P. Neuro-imaging in alcoholism: CT and MRI results and clinical correlates. *J. Neural. Transm.* 1995;99(1-3): 145-55.

[15] Harper CG, Kril JJ, Holloway RL. Brain shrinkage in chronic alcoholics: a pathological study. *Br. Med. J.* (Clin Res Ed) 1985;290(6467): 501-4.

[16] Harper C, Kril J, Daly J. Are we drinking our neurones away? *Br. Med. J. (Clin Res Ed)* 1987; 294(6571):534-6.

[17] Harper CG, Kril JJ, Daly JM. Brain shrinkage in alcoholics is not caused by changes in hydration: a pathological study. *J. Neurol. Neurosurg Psychiatry* 1988;51(1):124-7.

[18] Cala LA, Jones B, Mastaglia FL, Wiley B. Brain atrophy and intellectual impairment in heavy drinkers—a clinical, psychometric and computerized tomography study. *Aust NZ J. Med.* 1978;8(2):147-53.

[19] Nicolas JM, Catafau AM, Estruch R, Lomena FJ, Salamero M, Herranz R, et al. Regional cerebral blood flow-SPECT in chronic alcoholism: relation to neuropsychological testing. *J. Nucl. Med.* 1993; 34(9):1452-9.

[20] Wilson BA, Alderman N, Burgess PW, Emslie H, Evans JJ. Behavioral assessment of the dysexecutive syndrome (BADS). Bury St Edmunds, UK: *Thames Valley Test Company*, 1996

[21] Ihara H, Berrios GE, London M. Group and case study of the dysexecutive syndrome in alcoholism without amnesia. *J. Neurol. Neurosurg Psychiatry* 2000;68(6):731-7.

[22] Bowden-Jones H, McPhillips M, Rogers R, Hutton S, Joyce E. Risk-taking on tests sensitive to ventromedial prefrontal cortex dysfunction predicts early relapse in alcohol dependency: a pilot study. *J. Neuropsychiatry Clin. Neurosci.* 2005; 17(3):17-20.

[23] Duka T, Townshend JM, Collier K, Stephens DN. Impairment in cognitive functions after multiple detoxifications in alcoholic inpatients. *Alcohol Clin. Exp. Res.* 2003;27(10):1563-72.

[24] Mann K, Batra A, Gunthner A, Schroth G. Do women develop alcoholic brain damage more readily than men? *Alcohol Clin. Exp. Res.* 1992;16(6):1052-6.

[25] Zinn S, Stein R, Swartzwelder HS. Executive functioning early in abstinence from alcohol. *Alcohol Clin. Exp. Res.* 2004;28(9):1338-46.

[26] Dom G, Hulstijn W, Sabbe B. Differences in impulsivity and sensation seeking between early- and late-onset alcoholics. *Addict. Behav.* 2006;31(2): 298-308.

[27] Johnson-Greene D, Adams KM, Gilman S, Koeppe RA, Junck L, Kluin KJ, et al. Effects of abstinence and relapse upon neuropsychological function and cerebral glucose metabolism in severe chronic alcoholism. *J. Clin. Exp. Neuropsychol* 1997;19(3):378-85.

[28] Jones SL, Lanyon RI. Relationship between adaptive skills and outcome of alcoholism treatment. *J. Stud. Alcohol.* 1981;42(5):521-5.

[29] Patterson BW, Parsons OA, Schaeffer KW, Errico AL. Interpersonal problem solving in alcoholics. *J. Nerv. Ment. Dis* 1988;176(12):707-13.

[30] Cermak LS, Verfaellie M, Letourneau L, Blackford S, Weiss S, Numan B. Verbal and nonverbal right hemisphere processing by chronic alcoholics. *Alcohol Clin. Exp. Res.* 1989;13(5):611-6.

[31] Philippot P, Kornreich C, Blairy S, Baert I, Den Dulk A, Le Bon O, et al. Alcoholics' deficits in the decoding of emotional facial expression. *Alcohol Clin. Exp. Res.* 1999;23(6):1031-8.

[32] Kornreich C, Blairy S, Philippot P, Hess U, Noel X, Streel E, et al. Deficits in recognition of emotional facial expression are still present in alcoholics after mid- to long-term abstinence. *J. Stud. Alcohol.* 2001;62(4):533-42.

[33] Monnot M, Nixon S, Lovallo W, Ross E. Altered emotional perception in alcoholics: deficits in affective prosody comprehension. Alcohol Clin Exp Res 2001;25(3):362-9.

[34] Uekermann J, Daum I, Schlebusch P, Trenckmann U. Processing of affective stimuli in alcoholism. *Cortex* 2005;41(2):189-94.

[35] Kornreich C, Philippot P, Foisy ML, Blairy S, Raynaud E, Dan B, et al. Impaired emotional facial expression recognition is associated with interpersonal problems in alcoholism. *Alcohol Alcohol* 2002;37(4): 394-400.

[36] Uekermann J, Channon S, Winkel K, Schlebusch, P, Daum I. Theory of mind, humor processing and executive functioning in alcoholism. *Addiction* 2007;102(2):232-40.

[37] Koob, GF, Le Moal M. Drug abuse: hedonic homeostatic dysregulation. *Science* 1997;278 (5335):52-8.

[38] Giancola PR, Moss HB. Executive cognitive functioning in alcohol use disorders. *Recent Dev. Alcohol* 1988;14:227-51.

[39] Deckel AW, Hesselbrock V. Behavioral and cognitive measurements predict scores on the MAST: a 3-year prospective study. *Alcohol Clin. Exp. Res.* 1996;20(7):1173-8.

[40] Rinn W, Desai N, Rosenblatt H. Addiction denial and cognitive dysfunction: a preliminary investigation. *J. Clin. Exp. Neuropsychol.* 2002;14(1):52-7.

In: Alcohol-Related Cognitive Disorders   ISBN: 978-1-60741-730-9
Editors: L. Sher, I. Kandel, J. Merrick pp. 243-248   © 2009 Nova Science Publishers, Inc.

Chapter 16

ALCOHOL USE DISORDERS, COGNITIVE IMPAIRMENT AND SUICIDAL BEHAVIOR

Leo Sher

ABSTRACT

Etiological models for alcohol use disorders have traditionally proposed trait and cognitive explanations for initiation, maintenance, and dependence. Numerous studies have shown that heavy drinkers and subjects suffering from alcohol dependence have reduced performance on neurocognitive tests compared with controls. Alcohol dependence is an important risk factor for suicidal behavior. The large population of individuals with alcohol dependence, the relative frequency of suicides and suicide-related behaviors in this population, and the devastating effects of attempted and completed suicides on individuals, families, and society make this an important area for research. Data suggest that neuropsychological dysfunction may play a role in determining risk for suicidal acts. Suicide attempters have been characterized as "cognitively rigid" based on self-ratings and performance on mental flexibility tasks. Depressed subjects with a history of high-lethality suicide attempts exhibited deficits in executive functioning that were independent of deficits associated with depression alone. Alcohol use disorders are associated with both cognitive impairment and suicidal behavior. It is possible that cognitive abnormalities contribute to increased suicidality in individuals with alcohol use disorders. Future studies of the role of cognitive abnormalities in the pathophysiology of suicidal behavior are merited.

INTRODUCTION

The majority of adults in the United States drink alcohol and of these drinkers, a minority has had trouble at some time because of their drinking, while those who do have trouble tend to be young males who drink excessively [1-4]. Problem rates in all ages and ethnic groups, and especially in the young, remain high. The evidence indicates that the percentage of young women with alcohol problems is approaching the percentage of young men with such problems. The morbidity and mortality of alcoholism continue to be a tremendous drain on the human and financial resources of the United States. Morbidity and mortality are greatest among the men and women who are diagnosable as alcohol-dependent at some time in their lives, but are not exclusive to them.

ALCOHOL USE DISORDERS AND COGNITIVE IMPAIRMENT

Traditionally, etiologic models for alcohol use disorders have proposed trait and cognitive explanations for initiation, maintenance, and dependence [5]. Within this framework, temperament and personality models have often focused on trait disinhibition [6], including behavioral undercontrol [7], impulsivity and sensation seeking [8], suggesting that deficits in interrupting ongoing behavior may be central to hazardous drinking. Numerous studies have shown that heavy drinkers and subjects suffering from alcohol dependence have reduced performance on neurocognitive tests, such as the Wisconsin Card Sorting Test, the Stroop Test, Trails A and B test/Trail Making, Tower of Hanoi/London, and the Go No-Go Test compared with controls [9-38]. The effects have been shown to persist after detoxification [12,14,20-23,31-32,34-35,39] and may be based on hereditary predispositions [40-41]. The effects appear to be correlated with years of alcohol use [11,23], although some studies have not found such an effect [19].

Subjects suffering from alcohol dependence have been found to perform like subjects with frontal brain lesions in several investigations [10,15]. Whether the results are general for substance abuse populations is not clear because two investigations found similar effects when comparing subjects dependent on alcohol with subjects dependent on other substances [9-10]. One study, however, has found worse executive functioning among alcohol-dependent subjects [16]. A number of investigations found worse performance among subjects suffering from alcohol dependence, former alcoholics, and heavy social drinkers compared with controls on the standard Stroop Test [10,16,17,22,25,34]) and the Stroop tests containing alcohol-related words [19,27-29,42]. Two studies found that this difference may be specific for the alcohol-related version of the Stroop Test, while alcohol-dependent subjects had normal scores on the standard Stroop Test [28,29]. Another study found that Stroop performance may predict results of detoxification treatment [43]. A recent study found differences in tests scores on the Go No-Go Test between detoxified polysubstance users with alcohol dependence and control subjects [22]. Another study found that subjects with alcohol dependence differ electrophysiologically from control individuals using the Go No-Go Test [12]. In summary, neuropsycho-logical studies of alcohol use disorders overall suggest that individuals with alcohol abuse and dependence are cognitively impaired.

ALCOHOL AND SUICIDE

Alcohol dependence is an important risk factor for suicidal behavior [44-48]. The large population of individuals with alcohol dependence, the relative frequency of suicides and suicide-related behaviors in this population, and the devastating effects of attempted and completed suicides on individuals, families, and society make this an important area for research. Some reports have found that lifetime mortality due to suicide in alcohol dependence is as high as 18% [45]. Murphy and Wetzel [46] reviewed the epidemiologic literature and found that the lifetime risk of suicide among individuals with alcohol dependence treated in outpatient and inpatient settings was 2.2% and 3.4%, respectively. Nonetheless, individuals with alcohol dependence have a 60 to 120 times greater suicide risk than the non-psychiatrically ill population.

High rates of suicide attempts among individuals with alcohol use disorders have also been reported [47,48]. For example, in an urban community in the United States, 24% of subjects with alcohol dependence attempted suicide, as compared with 5% with other psychiatric diagnoses [47]. Forty per cent of a sample of depressed subjects with alcohol dependence who were hospitalized had attempted suicide in the prior week and 70% had attempted suicide at some point in their lives [48]. Depressed subjects with a history of alcohol dependence have higher current suicide ideation scale scores compared with depressed subjects without a history of alcohol dependence [44]. The data indicate that a lifetime diagnosis of alcohol dependence is a major risk factor for attempted or completed suicide.

SUICIDE AND COGNITIVE IMPAIRMENT

Data suggest that neuropsychological dysfunction may play a role in determining risk for suicidal acts. Suicide attempters have been characterized as "cognitively rigid" on the basis of self-ratings and performance on mental flexibility tasks [49-51]. From case studies [52], Rourke et al [53] suggested that a specific nonverbal learning disability could predispose individuals to suicidal behavior. Bartfai et al [54], using standard neuropsychological measures, found poorer performance on measures of fluency (verbal as well as nonverbal) and reasoning in a small sample of recent suicide attempters compared with chronic pain patients and non-patients. Subjects with a history of high-lethality suicide attempts exhibited deficits in executive functioning that were independent of deficits associated with depression alone [55].

CONCLUSION

Alcohol-use disorders are associated with both cognitive impairment and suicidal behavior. Possibly, cognitive abnormalities contribute to increased suicidality in individuals with alcohol-use disorders. Future studies of the role of cognitive abnormalities in the patho-physiology of suicidal behavior are merited.

REFERENCES

[1]   Winokur G, Clayton PJ, eds. *Medical basis of psychiatry*, 2nd ed. Philadelphia, PA: WB Saunders, 1994.

[2]   Sher L, Kandel I, Merrick J, eds. *Alcohol and suicide: Research and clinical perspectives*. Victoria, BC: Int Acad Press, 2007.

[3] US Dept Health Hum Serv. Seventh special report to the US. Congress on alcohol and health. Washington, DC, USA: US Govt Printing Office, DHHS Pub ADM 90-1656, 1990.

[4] Sher L. *Alcohol consumption and suicide*. QJM 2006;99(1):57-61.

[5] Anderson KG, Schweinsburg A, Paulus MP, Brown SA, Tapert S. Examining personality and alcohol expectancies using functional magnetic resonance imaging (fMRI) with adolescents. *J. Stud. Alcohol* 2005;66(3):323-31.

[6] McGue M, Iacono WG, Legrand LN, Malone S, Elkins I. Origins and consequences of age at first drink. I. Associations with substance-use disorders, disinhibitory behavior and psychopathology, and P3 amplitude. *Alcohol Clin. Exp. Res.* 2001;25(8): 1156-65.

[7] Sher KJ, Walitzer KS, Wood PK, Brent EE. Characteristics of children of alcoholics: putative risk factors, substance use and abuse, and psycho-pathology. *J. Abnorm. Psychol.* 1991;100(4):427-48.

[8] Grau E, Ordet G. Personality traits and alcohol consumption in a sample of non-alcoholic women. *Pers. Indiv. Diff.* 1999;27:1057-66.

[9] Beatty WW, Katzung VM, Moreland VJ, Nixon SJ. Neuropsychological performance of recently abstinent alcoholics and cocaine abusers. *Drug Alcohol Depend* 1995;37(3):247-53.

[10] Bechara A, Dolan S, Denburg N, Hindes A, Anderson SW, Nathan PE. Decision-making deficits, linked to a dysfunctional ventromedial prefrontal cortex, revealed in alcohol and stimulant abusers. *Neuropsychologia* 2001;39(4):376-89.

[11] Brokate B, Hildebrandt H, Eling P, Fichtner H, Runge K, Timm C. Frontal lobe dysfunctions in Korsakoff's syndrome and chronic alcoholism: continuity or discontinuity? *Neuropsychology* 2003;17(3):420-8.

[12] Cohen HL, Porjesz B, Begleiter H, Wang W. Neurophysiological correlates of response pro-duction and inhibition in alcoholics. *Alcohol Clin. Exp. Res.* 1997;21(8):1398-406.

[13] Demir B, Ucar G, Ulug B, Ulusoy S, Sevinc I, Batur S. Platelet monoamine oxidase activity in alcoholism subtypes: relationship to personality traits and executive functions. *Alcohol Alcohol* 2002;37(6):597-602.

[14] Fama R, Pfefferbaum A, Sullivan EV. Perceptual learning in detoxified alcoholic men: contributions from explicit memory, executive function, and age. *Alcohol Clin. Exp. Res.* 2004;28(11):1657-65.

[15] George MR, Potts G, Kothman D, Martin L, Mukundan CR. Frontal deficits in alcoholism: an ERP study. *Brain Cogn* 2004;54(3):245-7.

[16] Goldstein RZ, Leskovjan AC, Hoff AL, Hitze-mann R, Bashan F, Khalsa SS, et al. Severity of neuropsychological impairment in cocaine and alcohol addiction: association with metabolism in the prefrontal cortex. *Neuropsychologia* 2004; 42(11):1447-58.

[17] Ihara H, Berrios GE, London M. Group and case study of the dysexecutive syndrome in alcoholism without amnesia. *J. Neurol. Neurosurg. Psychiatry* 2000;68(6):731-7.

[18] Joyce EM, Robbins TW. Frontal lobe function in Korsakoff and non-Korsakoff alcoholics: planning and spatial working memory. *Neuropsychologia* 1991;29(8):709-23.

[19] Lusher J, Chandler C, Ball D. Alcohol dependence and the alcohol Stroop paradigm: evidence and issues. *Drug Alcohol Depend* 2004;75(3):225-31.

[20] Moriyama Y, Mimura M, Kato M, Yoshino A, Hara T, Kashima H, et al. Executive dysfunction and clinical outcome in chronic alcoholics. *Alcohol Clin. Exp. Res.* 2002;26(8):1239-44.

[21] Munro CA, Saxton J, Butters MA. The neuro-psychological consequences of abstinence among older alcoholics: a cross-sectional study. *Alcohol Clin. Exp. Res.* 2000;24(10):1510-6.

[22] Noel X, Van der Linden M, Schmidt N, Sferrazza R, Hanak C, Le Bon O, et al. Supervisory attentional system in nonamnesic alcoholic men. *Arch. Gen. Psychiatry* 2001;58(12):1152-8.

[23] Oscar-Berman M, Kirkley SM, Gansler DA, Couture A. Comparisons of Korsakoff and non-Korsakoff alcoholics on neuropsychological tests of prefrontal brain functioning. *Alcohol Clin. Exp. Res.* 2004;28(4):667-75.

[24] Ratti MT, Bo P, Giardini A, Soragna D. Chronic alcoholism and the frontal lobe: which executive functions are imparied? *Acta Neurol. Scand* 2002; 105(4):276-81.

[25] Rothlind JC, Greenfield TM, Bruce AV, Meyerhoff DJ, Flenniken DL, Lindgren JA, Weiner MW. Heavy alcohol consumption in individuals with HIV infection: effects on neuropsychological performance. *J. Int .Neuropsychol. Soc.* 2005;11(1): 70-83.

[26] Schmidt KS, Gallo JL, Ferri C, Giovannetti T, Sestito N, Libon DJ, Schmidt PS. The neuro-psychological profile of alcohol-related dementia suggests cortical and subcortical pathology. *Dement Geriatr. Cogn. Disord.* 2005;20(5):286-91.

[27] Sharma D, Albery IP, Cook C. Selective attentional bias to alcohol related stimuli in problem drinkers and non-problem drinkers. *Addiction* 2001;96(2):285-95.

[28] Stetter F, Ackermann K, Bizer A, Straube ER, Mann K. Effects of disease-related cues in alcoholic inpatients: results of a controlled "Alcohol Stroop" study. *Alcohol Clin. Exp. Res.* 1995;19(3):593-9.

[29] Stormark KM, Laberg JC, Nordby H, Hugdahl K. Alcoholics' selective attention to alcohol stimuli: automated processing? *J. Stud. Alcohol.* 2000;61(1): 18-23.

[30] Sullivan EV, Mathalon DH, Zipursky RB, Kersteen-Tucker Z, Knight RT, Pfefferbaum A. Factors of the Wisconsin Card Sorting Test as measures of frontal-lobe function in schizophrenia and in chronic alcoholism. *Psychiatry Res.* 1993; 46(2):175-99.

[31] Sullivan EV, Rosenbloom MJ, Pfefferbaum A. Pattern of motor and cognitive deficits in de-toxified alcoholic men. *Alcohol Clin. Exp. Res.* 2000;24(5):611-21.

[32] Sullivan EV, Fama R, Rosenbloom MJ, Pfeffer-baum A. A profile of neuropsychological deficits in alcoholic women. *Neuropsychology* 2002;16(1): 74-83.

[33] Tapert SF, Brown SA. Substance dependence, family history of alcohol dependence and neuro-psychological functioning in adolescence. *Addiction* 2000;95(7):1043-53.

[34] Tedstone D, Coyle K. Cognitive impairments in sober alcoholics: performance on selective and divided attention tasks. *Drug Alcohol Depend* 2004;75(3):277-86.

[35] Uekermann J, Daum I, Schlebusch P, Wiebel B, Trenckmann U. Depression and cognitive func-tioning in alcoholism. *Addiction* 2003;98(11): 1521-9.

[36] Uekermann J, Daum I, Schlebusch P, Trenckmann U. Processing of affective stimuli in alcoholism. *Cortex* 2005;41(2):189-94.

[37] van Gorp WG, Altshuler L, Theberge DC, Wilkins J, Dixon W. Cognitive impairment in euthymic bipolar patients with and without prior alcohol dependence. A preliminary study. *Arch. Gen. Psychiatry* 1998;55(1):41-6.

[38] Zinn S, Stein R, Swartzwelder HS. Executive functioning early in abstinence from alcohol. *Alcohol Clin. Exp. Res.* 2004;28(9):1338-1346.

[39] Smith ME, Oscar-Berman M. Resource-limited information processing in alcoholism. *J. Stud. Alcohol* 1992;53(5):514-8.

[40] Corral M, Holguin SR, Cadaveira F. Neuropsy-chological characteristics of young children from high-density alcoholism families: a three-year follow-up. *J. Stud. Alcohol* 2003;64(2):195-9.

[41] Nigg JT, Glass JM, Wong MM, Poon E, Jester JM, Fitzgerald HE, et al. Neuropsychological executive functioning in children at elevated risk for alcoholism: findings in early adolescence. *J. Abnorm. Psychol.* 2004;113(2):302-14.

[42] Cox WM, Yeates GN, Regan CM. Effects of alcohol cues on cognitive processing in heavy and light drinkers. *Drug Alcohol Depend* 1999;55(1-2):85-9.

[43] Cox WM, Hogan LM, Kristian MR, Race JH. Alcohol attentional bias as a predictor of alcohol abusers' treatment outcome. *Drug Alcohol Depend* 2002;68(3):237-43.

[44] Sher L, Oquendo MA, Conason AH, Brent DA, Gruncbaum MF, Zalsman G, et al. Clinical features of depressed patients with or without a family history of alcoholism. *Acta Psychiatr. Scand* 2005; 112(4):266-71.

[45] Roy A, Linnoila M. Alcoholism and suicide. *Suicide Life Threat Behav.* 1986;16(2):244-73.

[46] Murphy GE, Wetzel RD. The lifetime risk of suicide in alcoholism. *Arch. Gen. Psychiatry* 1990;47(4):383-92.

[47] Weissman MM, Myers JK. Clinical depression in alcoholism. *Am. J. Psychiatry* 1980;137(3):372-3.

[48] Cornelius JR, Salloum IM, Day NL, Thase ME, Mann JJ. Patterns of suicidality and alcohol use in alcoholics with major depression. *Alcohol Clin. Exp. Res.* 1996;20(8):1451-5.

[49] Levenson M, Neuringer C: Problem-solving behavior in suicidal adolescents. *J. Consult Clin. Psychol.* 1971;37:433–6.

[50] Neuringer C: Rigid thinking in suicidal individuals. *J. Consult Psychol.* 1964;28:54–8.

[51] Patsiokas AT, Clum GA, Luscomb RL: Cognitive characteristics of suicide attempters. *J. Consult Clin. Psychol.* 1979;47:478–84.

[52] Bigler E: On the neuropsychology of suicide. *J. Learn Disabil* 1989; 22:181–5.

[53] Rourke BP, Young GC, Leenaars AA: A child-hood learning disability that predisposes those afflicted to adolescent and adult depression and suicide risk. *J. Learn Disabil.* 1989; 22:169–75.

[54] Bartfai A, Winborg I, Nordstrom P, Asberg M: Suicidal behavior and cognitive flexibility: design and verbal fluency after attempted suicide. *Suicide Life Threat Behav* 1990;20:254–65.

[55] Keilp JG, Sackeim HA, Brodsky BS, Oquendo MA, Malone KM, Mann JJ. Neuropsychological dysfunction in depressed suicide attempters. *Am. J. Psychiatry.* 2001;158(5):735-41.

In: Alcohol-Related Cognitive Disorders   ISBN: 978-1-60741-730-9
Editors: L. Sher, I. Kandel, J. Merrick pp. 249-262   © 2009 Nova Science Publishers, Inc.

Chapter 17

ALCOHOLIC KORSAKOFF SYNDROME AND IMPAIRMENT

Matthias Brand

ABSTRACT

Long lasting or excessive alcohol consumption can result in alcoholic Korsakoff syndrome, characterized by severe anterograde and also retrograde memory deficits, as well as impairments in temporal orientation. In addition, further neuropsychological reductions can accompany the syndrome. Executive dysfunctions and emotional abnormalities are commonly reported in patients with Korsakoff's pathology but also seen in non-amnesic subjects with alcohol dependency. In patients with Korsakoff syndrome, the additional deficits mentioned are most commonly less severely pronounced than are amnesic symptoms. For the cognitive decline in patients suffering from this disease, damage to diencephalic and prefrontal brain regions are the most prominent neural correlates. Most likely, lesions within the mammillary bodies and parts of the thalamus are responsible for memory deterioration, whereas prefrontal damage primarily contributes to executive dysfunctions. Still a topic of debate is whether the direct alcoholic neurotoxic effects cause the brain changes in patients with Korsakoff's pathology or whether malnutrition and thiamine deficiency, potentially influenced by a genetic predisposition, are more strongly related to the diencephalic lesions that might be specific for Korsakoff syndrome. In the course of the disease, evidence suggests that cognitive impairments remain more or less stable over time. Therefore, the syndrome can be viewed as a single entity and it does not necessarily result in alcohol-related dementia.

INTRODUCTION

Long-lasting or excessive alcohol consumption or both can result in a syndrome that is characterized by severe memory disorders and other neuropsychological impairments—the alcoholic Korsakoff syndrome (KS). Although in the recent diagnostic inventories—the DSM-IV and DSM-IV-TR [1,2] and the ICD-10 (3)— the condition is referred to as Alcohol-induced persisting amnestic syndrome (DSM-IV-TR) and alcoholic amnesic syndrome (ICD-

10), in clinical routine and in most publications, the term alcoholic Korsakoff syndrome is still used. As described in earlier articles, the main neuropsychological symptoms of KS are anterograde memory deficits, whereas intelligence and general intellectual abilities remain normal [4-6]. In addition, a deterioration of processing temporal information, slight retrograde memory impairments, and a tendency to confabulate were regarded as constituting the cognitive profile of patients with this syndrome.

The main neuropathological correlate of the amnesic condition in patients with KS was assumed to be damage to diencephalic structures, such as lesions within the mammillary bodies and thalamic nuclei [7,8]. More recent studies, however, using either post-mortem analyses or modern imaging techniques, demonstrated that in patients with KS, additional brain changes could be observed beyond the diencephalic damage. Furthermore, several neuropsychological investigations point to a cognitive profile of patients with KS comprising several other neuropsychological reductions beyond the anterograde memory impairments classically associated with the disease.

In this chapter, neuropsychological findings in patients with alcoholic KS are summarized. In the first section, the potential causations of KS and associated brain pathologies are briefly elucidated. Thereafter, it is demonstrated that patients suffer from severe anterograde amnesia that is accompanied by retrograde memory deficits and dysfunctions in other domains, such as emotional processing and executive functioning.

NEUROPATHOLOGY OF THE ALCOHOLIC KS

The causation of KS is not exactly understood so far. Although most patients with the diagnosis of KS have had a long history of alcoholism, the syndrome is also known to occur in the absence of excessive alcohol consumption, i.e. in the course of anorexia or other conditions of malnutrition [9]. In addition, it is well known that alcohol consumption, even very long lasting and extreme alcohol intake, does not necessarily result in the development of Korsakoff's pathology. These circumstances, amongst others, led some researchers to form the hypothesis that malnutrition linked to vitamin B1 (thiamine) deficiency predominantly contributes to the origin of KS. Indeed, in patients suffering from alcoholism, thiamine rates are commonly reduced, although not in all patients. Convergent results point to a potential genetic disposition to an abnormal thiamine absorption or metabolism in individuals who developed the KS [10]. Also postulated is that principally the combination of both thiamine deficits and direct alcohol-associated neurotoxic effects, potentially accompanied by a genetic predisposition for both reduced metabolic rates of thiamine and a higher vulnerability for alcohol effects [11,12], results in the manifestation of KS-specific brain abnormalities [13].

The clinical signs of patients with alcoholic KS are most commonly attributed to a degeneration in the diencephalic regions, such as mammillary bodies and thalamic nuclei (the mediodorsal nucleus or/and the anterior nuclei), and further the cerebellum and the periaqueductal and periventricular grey matter [7,8,14]. Pathologies of additional brain regions are also reported. Such abnormalities include the prefrontal cortex [15,16] and parts of the basal forebrain, i.e., the nucleus basalis [17], as well as various subcortical structures, e.g., the locus coeruleus and the raphé nuclei [18,19]. There is also some indication for a hippocampal involvement in the KS brain pathology [20], although other studies did not find structural alterations but rather only metabolic reductions in KS patients' hippocampal formation [16]. Still a topic of debate is whether brain changes in different cortical and subcortical regions are caused by thiamine deficiency or by direct alcohol-associated toxic effects. Most likely, both causations are responsible for the extensive abnormalities, with thiamine deficiency primarily affecting the mammillary bodies, parts of the thalamus and the hypothalamus, the cerebellum, and parts of the brain stem (see systematic review [12]). Direct alcohol effects preferentially result in frontal lobe damage or dysfunctions, which are also the primary neural correlate of alcoholic dementia in cases of long-term alcoholism and an additional vulnerability for developing dementia per se.

It has also been questioned which brain changes are linked to specific neuropsychological impairments in patients with KS. As described in the following sections, memory deficits are the most prominent neuro-psychological symptoms of the alcoholic KS. Deficits in anterograde (and in parts also retrograde) memory are attributed to the diencephalic pathology, as, for instance, the mammillary bodies and the thalamic nuclei are engaged in neural circuits underlying memory formation and retrieval [21-23]. Additional symptoms, such as executive dysfunctions, are viewed to be linked to prefrontal abnormalities, as these symptoms typically occur in patients with frontal lobe lesions. Accordingly some have argued that in patients with KS, the memory decline is caused by the KS typical thiamine deficiency, whereas executive problems and other cognitive alterations are most likely associated with direct neurotoxic effects of alcohol consumption [24,25].

NEUROPSYCHOLOGICAL FINDINGS

Memory

As outlined above, memory impairment is the core neuropsychological symptom in patients with alcoholic KS. Recent studies showed that both anterograde memory (building new memories based on encoding and consolidation of information into the long-term memory system) and retrograde memory (remembering 'old' memories, meaning retrieval of information stored in the long-term memory system) are reduced. Anterograde deficits, however, are usually more pronounced than the retrograde impairments in most patients with KS [26]. Nonetheless, one has to keep in mind that the brain damage develops gradually in patients with KS. Therefore, a clear distinction between information stored in long-term memory before the brain changes and those learned after brain damaging has started is very difficult.

The anterograde memory disturbances are well described for both verbal and figural material [27-29], although earlier studies described more pronounced deficits in the verbal than in the figural modality [30]. An example for figural memory deficits can be found in figure 1 showing performance in copying a complex figure (the Rey-Osterrieth figure [31]) almost perfectly. In the delayed recall condition 30 minutes after copying the figure, however, the patient remembered the cross, only. This result is typical in patients with KS. Other examples for figural memory deficits in patients with KS are disturbances in processing object locations [32] and other visuo-spatial deficits [33].

As in healthy individuals, however, performance in free-recall conditions is inferior to that in recognition [34,35]. In verbal learning and memory paradigms—for example learning a word list and recalling the items after a delay of 15 or 30 minutes—patients with KS are severely impaired. In the study by Brand et al [36], the patients with KS performed comparably to patients with "Alzheimer's disease in the delayed recall condition in a verbal selective reminding task (the Memo test [37])"

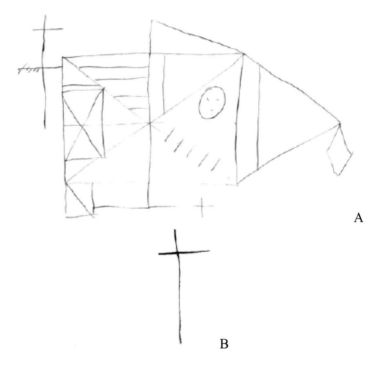

A

B

Figure 1. Copy (A) of the Rey-Osterrieth-Figure by a male patient with alcoholic KS. The patient copied the figure almost perfectly with only slight reductions (one line is missing) indicating normal visuo-constructive abilities. After a delay of 30 minutes, the patient was asked to draw the figure by heart (B). He only remembered the cross but no other details or the outline of the figure. This result demonstrates severe anterograde memory deficits in the figural domain.

Out of the ten words learned during five learning trials, KS patients freely recalled only one word (median; range 0-6), while patients with Alzheimer's disease recalled zero words (range 0-4) (note that healthy subjects on average remembered seven words). Similar results of clearly reduced verbal anterograde memory performance in laboratory tasks were also obtained in other studies (e.g., 26, 30, 38).

Retrograde memory deficiencies comprise both the recall of autobiographical-episodic events as well as semantic information [39, 40]. One example for compromised semantic memory in KS patients is their reduced performance in tasks assessing memory for famous events or famous people [41] or in temporal ordering of famous events [42]. Semantic memory impairments can also be found in tasks assessing general knowledge (i.e. in tasks measuring verbal intelligence, such as the WAIS-R [43]), in which patients with KS perform inferior to healthy individuals (e.g., in the study by Brand et al. [44]). However, general knowledge was less severely affected in KS patients compared to patients with Alzheimer's disease [36].

One neuropsychological symptom that is classically associated with alcoholic KS is a tendency to confabulate, implying that patients produce disproportionately false memories, either spontaneously or provoked (for a definition and review of confabulations see (45,46)). Although Bonhoeffer [4] already pointed out that KS patients were "confabulators", only a few studies are investigating confabulations and false memories in this syndrome (47). In a recent study, Borsutzky et al [48] provoked confabulations in KS patients using a new task (consisting of questions normally rejected by healthy subjects, e.g. "What did you do on March/13 in 1985"). The results revealed that KS patients produced significantly more false memories than did the healthy comparison subjects in all dimensions (autobiographical-episodic, autobiographical-semantic, general semantic memory). The rate of produced confabulations was correlated with executive functions, emphasizing that false memories are linked to prefrontal cortex damage, as previously described in other patient populations.

The results concerning short-term and working memory in patients with KS are disparate. Whereas some studies found deficient performance on verbal or visuo-spatial tasks, others showed normal levels of short-term and working memory [44,49-52]. In addition, whether KS patients have impairments in other memory systems, such as priming [53,54] or procedural memory [55] is also still unclear.

Beyond the prominent memory deficits and other neuropsychological symptoms (see sections below), several reports indicate abnormalities in emotional processing in patients with KS [56-58]. These reports are in line with clinical observations that often describe such patients as apathetic and emotionally detached, showing little spontaneous affective behavior [59,60]. Consequently, whether patients with KS show declined benefit from emotional connotation of information during encoding compared with healthy individuals who normally remember emotional stimuli superiorly in contrast to neutral material has been questioned [61]. The findings regarding emotional memory in KS patients are controversial. Oscar-Berman et al [57] reported emotion-specific reduced memory performance for faces (but note that memory for the emotional faces was not compared directly with memory for neutral material). Other studies found specific rather than global emotion effects on memory, i.e., a better memory performance for sexual but not for aggressive content [62]. The emotion-specific memory effect might also be restricted to direct recall conditions in patients with KS [35]. As in the previous study by Brand et al [44], however, which found changes in affective judgments in patients with KS in a simple judgment task (evaluating whether a single word has a negative, neutral or positive meaning), we recently investigated both affective judgments and implicit memory for the material evaluated afore in both verbal (nouns) and figural (pictures) dimension [63]. The results showed that patients had difficulties in affective judgments in either domain due to problems in classifying neutral stimuli correctly. This finding means that the patients were almost unimpaired in evaluating the emotional items as either positive or negative, but they also classified the neutral words and pictures as positive or negative. The memory performance (recognition paradigm) was inferior to that of the healthy subjects but did not differ between emotional and neutral items. Accordingly, the facilitating effect of emotionality on memory performance previously described in healthy individuals (see above) was absent in patients with KS. In summary, the studies mentioned, although they are disparate in detail, emphasize that patients with KS have deficits in emotional processing that can negatively influence memory performance, at least in a way so that KS patients do not profit from the emotionality of material to be encoded and retrieved.

Executive and Other Cognitive Functions

Executive dysfunctions, meaning reductions in problem solving abilities, cognitive flexibility, set shifting, task and goal monitoring and other higher order cognitions and meta-cognitions [64], were not regarded as a symptom typically occurring in patients with KS for a long time. In recent studies, however, executive functions were increasingly investigated in patients with KS and also in subjects with alcohol dependency without having KS typical brain pathology. This investigation was the consequence of results indicating that structural and functional frontal lobe alterations can emerge in both alcohol-dependent individuals without and with KS. Indeed, nowadays good evidence is available for reductions in executive functioning in KS patients. Deficits are typically found in classical executive tests, such as in the Wisconsin Card Sorting Test, Tower of Hanoi, Trail Making Test, Word-Color-Interference Test, or in tasks measuring verbal fluency [36,38,44,65]. The task descriptions can be found in [66] and [67].

The results on deficits in complex cognitive tasks in KS patients can be confounded by other neuropsychological impairments, primarily the severe amnesic symptoms, and vice versa, as consistently described across studies. An example is cognitive estimation, a function typically associated with frontal lobe integrity [68] but more recently viewed as being also strongly linked to semantic memory [36]. The ability to estimate the length or the weight of an object or the time needed for a specific action co-varies with general knowledge as revealed in the study mentioned above. For KS patients, cognitive estimations are difficult, especially guessing time-intervals, which is in line with the proposed deficits in time orientation as a cardinal symptom of the syndrome [4]. In the temporal dimension, the KS patients' estimates were even more frequently erroneous and bizarre than those of the subjects with Alzheimer's disease [36].

In addition, KS patients are impaired in other complex functions, which are most likely dependent upon executive functioning, such as decision making. Recently, we have shown that in a decision-making task with explicit rules for gains and losses as well as obvious and stable winning probabilities, the Game of Dice Task (measuring decisions under risk conditions), patients with KS showed performance inferior to that of healthy comparison subjects [69]. In the 18 trials of the Dice Task, the patients chose the risky alternatives significantly more often, leading to a negative balance in the long run. The frequency of risky decisions was correlated with performance in the modified Wisconsin Card Sorting Test assessing categorization and cognitive flexibility. Memory performance was unrelated to decision making.

Nevertheless, as subjects with alcohol addiction without having signs of the KS are also frequently found to have decreased executive functioning, whether the frontal lobe dysfunctions in patients with KS appear in the course of the KS by itself or whether they are the consequence of long-term alcoholism without a direct link to the KS pathology is questionable. In the study by Brokate et al [38], memory and executive functions were investigated both in patients with KS and in neurologically intact alcoholic subjects and contrasted with performance of a healthy control group. The results revealed that KS patients were impaired in both anterograde memory and executive functions, whereas the alcohol-addicted subjects without KS showed decreased performance in executive functions only. A similar comparison was reported by Hildebrandt et al [70] contrasting working memory and response shifting as well as inhibition in alcoholics and KS patients, controlled for duration of dependency and other basic variables. Summarizing the results mentioned, one might have the impression that executive functions do not differentiate between patients with and without KS, whereas memory reductions are genuine for the KS. Actually, severe anterograde memory deficits are not typically shown in subjects with a history of alcohol addiction not suffering from KS. Evidence has also been presented for a stronger impairment in executive functions in KS patients compared with alcoholic subjects without KS (i.e., in verbal fluency and rules detection [38]). In the same way, we recently compared the performances of KS patients and alcoholic subjects on the Dice Task, mentioned above, and revealed that the performance of subjects with alcohol dependency without KS was inferior to that of healthy individuals but superior to that of patients with KS (71, manuscript in preparation). Other tasks, such as the Wisconsin Card Sorting Test or Trail-Making-Test, did not differentiate substantially between the two patient groups. Figure 2 demonstrates the number of risky decisions in the Game of Dice Task.

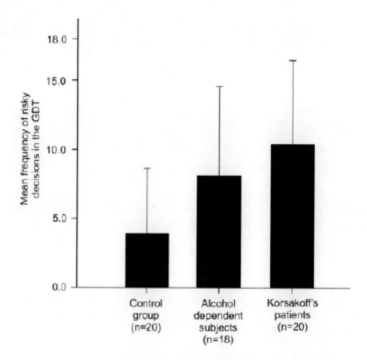

Figure 2. Mean frequency of risky decisions in the Game of Dice Task (GDT) in subjects with alcohol dependency and patients with KS compared with healthy individuals. Both patient groups differed significantly from the control group. The patients with KS selected more risky than non-risky alternatives (mean number of risky decisions about 10 of 18 decisions), whereas alcoholic subjects chose approximately 8 times the risky alternatives.

In summary, both alcoholic patients with and without KS show reduced executive functioning and the deficits are task-dependently either similar or stronger in patients with KS. Nonetheless, one has to differentiate between clinically impaired performance and test results that are significantly inferior to a control group but within a normal range, meaning a performance that is within one standard deviation of the average of a normal population. For instance, in the studies by Brand et al [36,44], the KS patients performed significantly lower than the control group did, but the mean scores of the patients were at the edge discriminating between clinically deficient and normal performance. This finding indicates that some KS subjects obviously had considerable executive dysfunctions whereas others had a low but more or less normal functioning.

By contrast, memory impairments were clinically relevant (outside of at least one standard deviation from the scores of a normal population) in all patients. These disparate findings concerning clear memory disturbances and—at the same time—'merely' significant reductions in executive functioning compared with a control group in most studies emphasize the view of KS as a syndrome dominated by learning and memory deterior-ations which can be accompanied by some additional, but more secondary symptoms.

This conclusion is also exemplarily visualized in figure 3 showing a typical profile of neuropsychological functioning in a patient with KS.

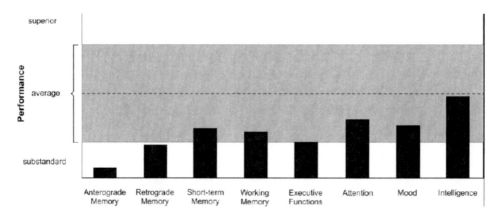

Figure 3. A typical neuropsychological profile of a patient with alcoholic KS. While anterograde memory performance (verbal and figural domain combined) is most strongly impaired, other memory or cognitive functions are less severely affected, though they are also within the clinically impaired or at least within the lower range of normal performance.

THE COURSE OF COGNITIVE SYMPTOMS

Still a topic of debate is whether cognitive decline in patients with KS is progressive, resulting in alcohol-related dementia or whether dysfunctions are reversible or at least stable over time. Although some studies reported recovery from the chronic phase of KS in more than 75% of patients (6), other studies found a recovery rate of zero (7). Also discussed controversially is whether excessive alcohol consumption generally leads to a higher vulnerability for cognitive decline or dementia in older age, even in subjects not developing KS.

Addressing the question of progression in patients with KS, Fujiwara et al [72] assessed performance on neuropsychological tasks (examining verbal and visual short- and long-term memory, general knowledge working memory, executive functions, language, and visual-spatial abilities) in 20 detoxified chronic KS inpatients at one point in time (T1) and two years later (T2). During the time interval between both test sessions, all patients were permanent residents within socio-therapeutic clinics. At both T1 and T2, the performance of KS patients on most neuropsychological tasks was reduced compared with normal subjects. Anterograde memory functions were most severely affected, congruent with the neuropsychological profile described in the previous paragraphs.

In addition, executive dysfunctions frequently occurred, whereas intelligence was normal in all patients. The comparison between the two test sessions within the KS group revealed no significant decline in any of the investigated functions. By contrast, visual long-term memory, general knowledge, and verbal fluency slightly improved after two years, although remaining within the pathological range. In summary, in this sample of detoxified patients with KS, on average no evidence was found of accelerated cognitive decline and no indication for the onset of dementia over two years. Nonetheless, Fujiwara et al calculated performance changes between T1 and T2 per patient by subtracting individual z-total scores (the z-total score indicates an overall test performance on a standardized level) of T2 from z-total scores of T1. Thereafter, they divided the group of 20 patients into three subgroups: those subjects with most extensive cognitive decline over the two years (six patients), those with more or less stable functioning (eight patients), and patients who improved (six patients). A comparison of the two "extreme" groups revealed only a few specific characteristics that differed between these two subgroups. The differences are illustrated in figure 4.

Although the results appear as indicating that the KS is variable in symptom severity and progression, one has to keep in mind that all patients had severe anterograde memory deficits at both test sessions but no patient developed clear signs of dementia (measured by a dementia screening).Thus, the extreme groups comparison solely demonstrates that within a pathological range of cognitive functioning symptoms can slightly vary across patients.

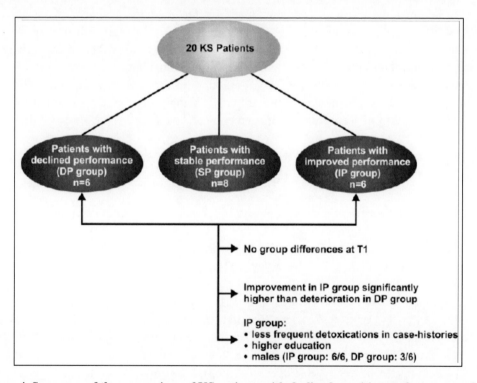

Figure 4. Summary of the comparison of KS patients with declined cognitive performance and those with improved overall cognitive functioning, described in the study by Fujiwara et al [72].

However, all patients had the KS typical cognitive profile at both examinations. In conclusion, results of previous reports and the recent study mentioned indicate that the KS can be viewed as a single entity and that patients with KS do not categorically develop alcohol related dementia.

CONCLUSION

The KS is linked to severe memory impairments comprising primarily anterograde amnesic symptoms and, to a lesser degree, retrograde deficits. Beyond the memory deterioration, executive functions and emotional processing are also reduced compared with normal healthy individuals. Brain changes that include diencephalic and—as a long-term consequence—alcohol-induced frontal lobe damage are most likely the main neural correlates of the cognitive decline of the patients. One has to keep in mind, however, that both frontal damage and associated cognitive dysfunctions are not genuinely restricted to the KS specific pathology as subjects with long lasting alcoholism but without having the clinical signs of KS also suffer from executive reductions and (functional) alterations of the prefrontal cortex. Nevertheless, the symptoms mentioned seem to be generally stronger in patients with KS when compared with alcoholic patients without KS. Given that neuropsychological functions are intercorrelated, whether the stronger executive deficits in KS are attributable directly to the KS or whether they are more secondary symptoms which result from the alcohol-associated frontal dysfunctions and aggravated by the memory decline remains unclear. Nonetheless, the symptomatology in KS patients seems to be stable rather than progressive. If any, changes over time are rather in the positive direction meaning that specific cognitive functions in patients with KS can slightly improve, although they still remain within a pathological range. Accordingly, the KS does not necessarily result in alcohol-related dementia. Future research should further address the topic of symptom specificity in KS patients in contrast to subjects with alcohol addiction and those with alcohol related dementia.

REFERENCES

[1]   Am Psychiatr Assoc. *Diagnostic and statistical manual of mental disorders* (DSM-IV), 4th ed. Washington, DC: APA, 1994.

[2]   First MB, Tasman A. DSM-IV-TRTM mental disorders. *Diagnosis, etiology and treatment.* New York, NY: John Wiley, 2004.

[3]   World Health Organization. International statistical classification of diseases and health related problems, ICD-10. Geneva, CH: WHO, 1994.

[4]   Bonhoeffer K. Der Korsakowsche Symptomenkomplex in seinen Beziehungen zu den verschiedenen Krankheitsformen. *Allg Zeitschr Psychiatrie* 1904;61:744-52. [German]

[5]   Korsakoff SS. Disturbance of psychic function in alcoholic paralysis and its relation to the disturbance of the psychic sphere in multiple neuritis of non-alcoholic origin. In: Victor M, Adams RD, Collins GH, eds. *The Wernicke-Korsakoff Syndrome*, 1971. Oxford, UK: Blackwell, 1887.

[6]   Victor M, Adams RD, Collins GH. *The Wernicke-Korsakoff Syndrome*, Second ed. Philadelphia, PA: FA Davis, 1989.

[7]   Malamud N, Skillicorn SA. Relationship between the Wernicke and Korsakoff syndrome. *Arch. Neurol. Psychiatry* 1956;76:585-96.

[8]   Mair WG, Warrington EK, Weiskrantz L. Memory disorder in Korsakoff's psychosis: a neuropathological and neuropsychological investigation of two cases. *Brain* 1979;102:749-83.

[9]   Becker JT, Furman JMR, Panisset M, Smith C. Characteristics of the memory loss of a patient with Wernicke-Korsakoff's syndrome without alcoholism. *Neuropsychologia* 1990;28:171-9.

[10]   Heap LC, Pratt OE, Ward RJ, Waller S, Thomson AD, Shaw GK, Peters TJ. Individual susceptibility to Wernicke-Korsakoff syndrome and alcoholism-induced cognitive deficit: impaired thiamine utilization found in alcoholics and alcohol abusers. *Psychiatr Genet* 2002;12:217-24.

[11]   Blass JP, Gibson GE. Abnormality of a thiamine-requiring enzyme in patients with Wernicke-Korsakoff syndrome. *N Engl. J. Med.* 1977;297: 1367-70.

[12]   Martin PR, Singleton CK, Hiller-Sturmhofel S. The role of thiamine deficiency in alcoholic brain disease. *Alcohol. Res. Health* 2003;27:134-42.

[13]   Lishman WA. Alcohol and the brain. *Br. J. Psychiatry* 1990;156:635-44.

[14]   Cravioto H, Korein J, Silberman J. Wernicke's encephalopathy. *Arch. Neurol.* 1961;4:54-63.

[15]   Kril JJ, Halliday GM, Svoboda MD, Cartwright H. The cerebral cortex is damaged in chronic alcoholics. *Neuroscience* 1997;79:983-98.

[16]   Reed LJ, Lasserson D, Marsden P, Stanhope N, Stevens T, Bello F, Kingsley D, Colchester A, Kopelman MD. FDG-PET findings in the Wernicke-Korsakoff syndrome. *Cortex* 2003;39: 1027-45.

[17]   Cullen KM, Halliday GM, Caine D, Kril JJ. The nucleus basalis (Ch4) in the alcoholic Wernicke-Korsakoff syndrome: Reduced cell number in both amnesic and non-amnesic patients. *J. Neurol. Neurosurg. Psychiatry* 1997;63:315-20.

[18]   Halliday GM, Ellis J, Harper C. The locus coeruleus and memory: A study of chronic alcoholics with and without the memory impairment of Korsakoff's psychosis. *Brain Res* 1992;598:33-7.

[19]   Halliday GM, Ellis J, Heard R, Caine D, Harper C. Brainstem serotonergic neurons in chronic alcoholics with and without the memory impairment of Korsakoff's psychosis. *J. Neuropathol. Exp. Neurol.* 1993;52:567-79.

[20]   Visser PJ, Krabbendam L, Verhey FRJ, Hofman PAM, Verhoeven WMA, Tuinier S, Wester A, Van Den Berg YWMM, Goessens LFM, Van Der Werf YD, Jolles J. Brain correlates of memory dysfunction in alcoholic Korsakoff's syndrome. *J. Neurol. Neurosurg Psychiatry* 1999;67:774-8.

[21]   Markowitsch HJ. The anatomical bases of memory. In: Gazzaniga MS, ed. *The new cognitive neurosciences*. 2nd ed. Cambridge, MA, USA: MIT Press, 2000:781-95.

[22]   Markowitsch HJ. Which brain regions are critically involved in retrieval of old episodic memory? *Brain Res. Brain Res. Rev.* 1995;21:117-27.

[23]   Brand M, Markowitsch HJ. The principle of bottleneck structures. In: Kluwe RH, Lüer G, Rösler F, eds. *Principles of learning and memory*. Basel, CH: Birkhäuser, 2003:171-84.

[24] Tarter RE. Brain damage associated with chronic alcoholism. *Dis. Nerv. Syst.* 1975;36:185-7.

[25] Noel X, Van der Linden M, Schmidt N, Sferrazza R, Hanak C, Le Bon O, De Mol J, et al. Supervisory attentional system in nonamnesic alcoholic men. *Arch. Gen. Psychiatry* 2001;58:1152-8.

[26] Fama R, Marsh L, Sullivan EV. Dissociation of remote and anterograde memory impairment and neural correlates in alcoholic Korsakoff syndrome. *J. Int. Neuropsychol. Soc.* 2004;10:427-41.

[27] Holdstock JS, Mayes AR, Cezayirli E, Aggleton JP, Roberts N. A comparsion of egocentric and allocentric spatial memory in medial temporal lobe and Korsakoff amnesics. *Cortex* 1999;35: 479-501.

[28] Mayes AR, Meudell PR, MacDonald C. Disproportionate intentional spatial-memory impairments in amnesia. *Neuropsychologia* 1991;29:771-84.

[29] Kixmiller JS, Verfaellie MM, Mather MM, Cermak LS. Role of perceptual and organizational factors in amnesics' recall of the Rey-Osterrieth complex figure: A comparsion of three amnesic groups. *J. Clin. Exp. Neuropsychol.* 2000;22:198-207.

[30] Butters N, Lewis R, Cermak LS, Goodglass H. Material-specific memory deficits in alcoholic Korsakoff patients. *Neuropsychologia* 1973;11: 291-9.

[31] Osterrieth PA. Le test de copie d'une figure complex: Contribution à l'étude de la perception et de la mémoire. *Arch. Psychologie* 1944;30:286-56. [French]

[32] Kessels RPC, Postma A, Wester AJ, de Haan EHF. Memory for object locations in Korsakoff's amnesia. *Cortex* 2000;36:47-57.

[33] van Asselen M, Kessels RP, Wester AJ, Postma A. Spatial working memory and contextual cueing in patients with Korsakoff amnesia. *J. Clin. Exp. Neuropsychol.* 2005;27:645-55.

[34] Kessler J, Irle E, Markowitsch HJ. Korsakoff and alcoholic subjects are severely impaired in animal tasks of associative memory. *Neuropsychologia* 1986;24:671-80.

[35] Markowitsch HJ, Kessler J, Denzler P. Recognition memory and psychophysiological responses to stimuli with neutral or emotional content: a study of Korsakoff patients and recently detoxified and longterm abstinent alcoholics. *Int. J. Neurosci* 1986;29:1-35.

[36] Brand M, Kalbe E, Fujiwara E, Huber M, Markowitsch HJ. Cognitive estimation in patients with probable Alzheimer's disease and alcoholic Korsakoff patients. *Neuropsychologia* 2003;41: 575-84.

[37] Schaaf A, Kessler J, Grond M, Fink G. Memo Test. *Ein verbaler Gedächtnistest nach der Methode des selektiven Erinnerns.* Weinheim: Beltz Test Verlag, 1992. [German]

[38] Brokate B, Hildebrandt H, Eling P, Fichtner H, Runge K, Timm C. Frontal lobe dysfunctions in Korsakoff's syndrome and chronic alcoholism: continuity or discontinuity? *Neuropsychology* 2003;17:420-8.

[39] Kopelman MD. Remote and autobiographical memory, temporal context memory, and frontal atrophy in Korsakoff and Alzheimer patients. *Neuropsychologia* 1989;27:437-60.

[40] Kopelman MD, Stanhope N, Kingsley D. Retrograde amnesia in patients with diencephalic, temporal lobe or frontal lesions. *Neuropsychologia* 1999;37:939-58.

[41] Mayes AR, Daum I, Markowitsch HJ, Sauter B. The relationship between retrograde and anterograde amnesia in patients with typical global amnesia. *Cortex* 1997;33:197-217.

[42] Shimamura AP, Janowsky JS, Squire L. Memory for the temporal order of events in patients with frontal lobe lesions and amnesic patients. *Neuropsychologia* 1990;28:803-13.

[43] Wechsler D. *Wechsler adult intelligence scale-revised.* San Antonio, TX: Psychol Corp, 1981.

[44] Brand M, Fujiwara E, Kalbe E, Steingass H-P, Kessler J, Markowitsch HJ. Cognitive estimation and affective judgments in alcoholic Korsakoff patients. *J. Clin. Exp. Neuropsychol.* 2003;25:324-34.

[45] Chiaramelli E, Ghetti S. What are confabulators' memories made of? A study of subjective and objective measures of recollection in confabulation. *Neuropsychologia* 2007;45:1489-1500.

[46] Schnider A. Spontaneous confabulation, reality monitoring, and the limbic system—a review. *Brain Res. Brain Res. Rev.* 2001;36:150-60.

[47] Benson DF, Djenderedjian A, Miller BL, Pachana NA, Chang L, Itti L, et al. Neural basis of confab-ulation. *Neurology* 1996;46:1239-43.

[48] Borsutzky S, Fujiwara E, Brand M, Markowitsch HJ. *Confabulations in patients with alcoholic Korsakoff's syndrome.* In preparation.

[49] Cermak LS, Butters N. The role of interference and encoding in the short-term memory deficits of Korsakoff patients. *Neuropsychologia* 1972;10: 89-95.

[50] Kopelman MD. Non-verbal, short-term forgetting in the alcoholic Korsakoff syndrome and Alzheimer type dementia. *Neuropsychologia* 1991;2 9:737-47.

[51] Kopelman MD. The Korsakoff syndrome. *Br. J. Psychiatry* 1995;166:154-73.

[52] Joyce EM, Robbins TW. Frontal lobe function in Korsakoff and non-Korsakoff alcoholics: Planning and spatial working memory. *Neuropsychologia* 1991;29:709-23.

[53] Beauregard M, Chertkow H, Gold D, Karama S, Benhamou J, Babins L, et al. Word priming with brief multiple presentation technique: preservation in amnesia. *Neuropsychologia* 1997;35:611-22.

[54] Brunfaut E, d´Ydewalle G. A comparison of implicit memory tasks in Korsakoff and alcoholic patients. *Neuropsychologia* 1996;34:1143-50.

[55] Swinnen SP, Puttemans V, Lamote S. Procedural memory in Korsakoff's disease under different movement feedback conditions. *Behav. Brain Res.* 2005;159:127-33.

[56] Snitz BE, Hellinger A, Daum I. Impaired processing of affective prosody in Korsakoff's syndrome. *Cortex* 2002;38:797-803.

[57] Oscar-Berman M, Hancock M, Mildworf B, Hutner N, Altman Weber D. Emotional perception and memory in alcoholism and aging. *Alcohol Clin. Exp. Res.* 1990;14:383-93.

[58] Montagne B, Kessels RP, Wester AJ, de Haan EH. Processing of emotional facial expressions in Korsakoff's syndrome. *Cortex* 2006;12:313-24.

[59] Rapaport D. *Emotions and memory.* New York, NY: Science Editions, 1961.

[60] Talland GA. *Deranged memory.* San Diego, CA: Academic Press, 1965.

[61] LaBar KS, Cabeza R. Cognitive neuroscience of emotional memory. *Nat. Rev. Neurosci.* 2006;7:54-64.

[62] Davidoff DA, Butters N, Gerstman LJ, Zurif E, Paul IH, Mattis S. Affective/motivational factors in the recall of prose passages by alcoholic Korsakoff patients. *Alcohol* 1984;1:63-9.

[63] Labudda K, Todorovski S, Markowitsch HJ, Brand M. Judgment and memory performance for emotional stimuli in patients with alcoholic Korsakoff syndrome. *J. Clin. Exp. Neuropsychol.* 2008;30:224-35.

[64] Smith EE, Jonides J. Storage and executive processes in the frontal lobes. *Science* 1999;283: 1657-61.

[65] Krabbendam L, Visser PJ, Derix MMA, Verhey F, Hofman P, Verhoeven W, Tuinier S, Jolles J. Normal cognitive performance in patients with chronic alcoholism in contrast to patients with Korsakoff's syndrome. *J. Neuropsychiatry Clin. Neurosci.* 2000;12:44-50.

[66] Lezak MD, Howieson DB, Loring DW. *Neuropsychological assessment*, Fourth ed. New York, NY: Oxford Univ Press, 2004.

[67] Strauss E, Sherman EMS, Spreen O. *A compendium of neuropsychological tests: administration, norms, and commentary*, Third ed. New York, NY: Oxford Univ Press, 2006.

[68] Shallice T, Evans ME. The involvement of the frontal lobes in cognitive estimation. *Cortex* 1978; 14:294-303.

[69] Brand M, Fujiwara E, Borsutzky S, Kalbe E, Kessler J, Markowitsch HJ. Decision-making deficits of Korsakoff patients in a new gambling task with explicit rules: associations with executive functions. *Neuropsychology* 2005;19: 267-77.

[70] Hildebrandt H, Brokate B, Eling P, Lanz M. Response shifting and inhibition, but not working memory, are impaired after long-term heavy alcohol consumption. *Neuropsychology* 2004;18: 203-11.

[71] Brand M, Adler N, Markowitsch HJ. Decision-making and executive functions in patients with alcoholic Korsakoff's syndrome and alcohol dependent patients without Korsakoff's pathology. In preparation.

[72] Fujiwara E, Brand M, Borsutzky S, Steingass H-P, Markowitsch HJ. Cognitive performance of detoxified alcoholic Korsakoff syndrome patients remains stable over two years. *J. Clin. Exp. Neuropsychol.* 2007 (Epub ahead of print).

In: Alcohol-Related Cognitive Disorders   ISBN: 978-1-60741-730-9
Editors: L. Sher, I. Kandel, J. Merrick pp. 263-275   © 2009 Nova Science Publishers, Inc.

Chapter 18

ALCOHOLISM AND DEMENTIA

Elisabeth Kapaki, George P. Paraskevas, Ilia Theotoka and Ioannis Liappas

ABSTRACT

Alcoholism may result in impaired cognition and dementia. The increased risk of dementia in older individuals interferes with the differential diagnosis, especially when an elderly patient with a long history of alcohol abuse is the case. The aim of the chapter is to evaluate the diagnostic value of the putative cerebrospinal fluid (CSF) biomarkers tau (τ), β-amyloid 1–42 (Aβ42) and their ratio in differentiating alcohol related dementia (ARD) from others of vascular or degenerative aetiology. Double-sandwich ELISAs (Innotest htau antigen and β-Amyloid (1–42), Innogenetics) were used to quantify the above markers in a total of 151 patients and 82 controls. Patient groups comprised: 24 ARD, 17 vascular dementia, 11 dementia with Lewy bodies, 23 frontotemporal dementia and 76 Alzheimer's disease (AD) patients. Tau protein succeessfully differentiated ARD from AD with 88% specificity and 86% sensitivity. Aβ42 alone had a specificity of 86% and a sensitivity of 70%, while tau/Aβ42 ratio was better than τ alone with corresponding values 100% and 91% respectively. For the discrimination of ARD from other dementias the diagnostic value of the above markers is substantially lower. In conclusion, the combined use of CSF τ and Aβ42 seems to be a useful tool in the differential diagnosis of ARD from AD, while in other primary dementias only a positive result may be useful.

INTRODUCTION

Heavy and chronic alcohol abuse and dependence can lead to various neuropsychiatric symptoms, including cognitive decline ranging from isolated amnesia to fully developed dementia [1,2]. Beyond the confusional state occurring with acute intoxication or withdrawal, alcohol abuse is responsible for several subacute or chronic disorders attributable not to alcohol per se but to some other factor(s) engendered by alcoholism [3]. The mechanisms of indirect toxicity involve (a) malabsorption and/or malnutrition resulting in vitamin deficiency; (b) liver failure resulting in increased NH_3, decreased protein biosynthesis, and/or clotting deficiency; (c) disorders in lipid and carbohydrate metabolism, and (d) disorders of water and electrolytes [4]. According to Victor [5], many cases with cognitive decline can be attributed to certain well-established secondary alcohol-related disorders, such as the Wernicke-Korsakoff syndrome, acquired hepatocerebral degeneration, pellagrous encephalopathy, Marchiafava-Bignami disease, and some other rare conditions [5]. More or less, these syndromes are characterized by distinctive pathology and are linked to established pathogenesis.

However, cognitive impairment and dementia may be present in the absence of the above, attributed directly to ethanol's toxicity in the brain. Indication of such direct toxicity comes from studies in cerebellum, where alcoholism has been shown to damage neurons of the superior vermis containing the GABA A receptors, whereas ethanol decreases the firing rate of Purkinje cells through a GABA A receptor-related mechanism [6,7]. Ethanol, administered to rats for 20 months, induced significant changes in the status of glutathione, primarily in the cerebellum and hippocampus, where a decrease in reduced glutathione (GSH) and the GSH/oxidized glutathione ratio was found, thus mediating free radical damage [8].

In the cerebrum, evidence of neuronal and/or glial loss has been found in the superior frontal cortex, the hypothalamus, the hippocampus, and the amygdala of uncomplicated alcoholics [9,10]. Ethanol induces DNA damage and apoptosis in the alcoholic brain, mainly in the hippocampus and the superior frontal cortex. These involve primarily the glial cells but may involve neurons as well [11]. Ethanol also causes degeneration of the cholinergic system, known to play an important role in learning and memory [12].

Alcohol and the Risk for Dementia

The risk of dementia in alcohol abuse has been reported to follow a J- or U-shaped curve [13]. Aldehyde dehydrogenase polymorphisms may increase the risk for Alzheimer's disease (AD) especially in ApoE ε4 c carriers [14]. Concomitant ethanol-induced oxidative stress, excitotoxicity, mitochondrial dysfunction, and apoptosis may potentiate vascular mechanisms and/or reduce symptomatic threshold [15]. Subsequently questions arise as to whether alcohol is a causative factor for dementia or a risk factor for other types of dementia or may be both.

The term alcoholic dementia, formerly used to describe cognitive impairment in alcohol-dependent subjects, has cast doubt on its existence due to the absence of clinical, neuropathological and radiological criteria. Jacques and Stevenson [16] suggested that brain damage resulting from alcohol abuse may be best seen as a spectrum of disorders merging into each other and overlapping. A broader definition, such as alcohol related dementia (ARD) has been introduced to encompass the spectrum of alcohol-related cognitive disorders. Clinical criteria have also been proposed [17].

ARDs, especially those seen in older individuals, share a number of similar features with other dementias, especially Alzheimer Disease (AD), the most common cause of dementia in the elderly [18]. Memory and learning are impaired early in the course of both syndromes. Heavy alcohol consumption often results in shrinkage of the brain [19], enlargement of the ventricles and widened sulci, evident in CT or MRI scans [20], which are indistinguishable from the atrophy observed during a neurodegenerative process. Other dementias also share common clinical characteristics with ARD. A fronto-subcortical syndrome characterizes frontotemporal dementia (FTD), vascular dementia (VD) and ARD. Additionally, alcohol abuse may be a symptom of FTD. Psychiatric features are common in ARD and dementia with Lewy bodies (DLB) [21].

The increased risk of other types of dementia, mainly AD, in older individuals often presents a dilemma for the clinician in the differential diagnosis, especially when dealing with elderly patients with a long and heavy history of alcohol abuse. Since alcohol effects on cognition and on the brain may be reversible in contrast to other neurodegenerative dementias, the significance of the early differentiation is obvious [19,22].

CSF Biomarkers

Recently the cerebrospinal fluid (CSF) biomarkers tau protein and β-amyloid 1–42 (Aβ42) have received much attention as diagnostic markers for AD. They are considered to have a role in the ante-mortem diagnosis because they reflect the principal neurochemical and pathologic features of the disease [23,24].

Tau is a phosphoprotein and its normal function is to promote polymerization and stability of microtubules [25]. Total tau (τ) is clearly increased in the CSF of AD patients, even at the early stages [26]. Its sensitivity and specificity for the discrimination from normal aging have been consistently high, with mean values of all studies 81% and 90% respectively [27-29]. However, τ levels are also increased in other conditions, without tau-related pathology, rendering CSF τ levels a more general marker of neuronal/ axonal damage [30,31].

The amyloid (Aβ) deposition, mainly consisting of 39-43 residue peptides, appears early in the evolution of AD. Aβ peptides terminating in amino acids 40 and 42 are the major forms produced; the latter being highly amyloidogenic [32]. CSF levels of Aβ42 have been found decreased in AD, but also in other dementias (Creutzfeldt-Jakob disease and DLB), thus rendering this marker also non-specific [31,33]. Both biomarkers have been recently recognized by the EFNS task force, as an adjunct for dementia diagnosis in cases of diagnostic doubt [34].

The aim of our study was to determine the levels and to evaluate the diagnostic value (in terms of sensitivity and specificity) of CSF τ , Aβ42, and their combination, in the form of τ/Aβ42 ratio, in cognitively impaired patients with chronic alcohol dependence and patients with other dementias.

OUR STUDY

The aim of our study was to determine the levels and to evaluate the diagnostic value (in terms of sensitivity and specificity) of CSF τ , Aβ42, and their combination, in the form of τ/Aβ42 ratio, in cognitively impaired patients with chronic alcohol dependence and patients with other dementias.

A total of 151 patients and 82 controls of Caucasian origin were included in the study. Patients were divided into well characterized groups as follows:

- The chronic alcohol-dependent subjects (n=24) fulfilled the DSM-IV diagnostic criteria for alcohol abuse/dependence [35] as well as the criteria of Oslin et al [17] for ARD. These patients were admitted at the specialized Drug and Alcohol Addiction Clinic of the Athens University Psychiatric Clinic at Eginition Hospital for alcohol detoxification. Participation in the project was on a voluntary basis. Subjects included in the study had to fulfil the following criteria: age > 40, absence of serious physical illness or another pre- or coexisting major psychiatric disorder on the DSM-IV axis I and absence of other drug abuse. Evaluation of alcohol abuse was made by the Pattern of Abuse tool [36], the section on alcoholism of Composite International Diagnostic Interview [37] and the Diagnostic Interview Schedule [38]. The mean duration of alcohol abuse (SD) was 18.3 (8.9) years (range 4-33 years).

- The probable vascular dementia group (VD, n=17) diagnosed according to the NINDS-AIREN criteria [39]. In VD, only two patient had multiple infarcts; all the remaining patients had multiple, sometimes confluent lacunes and/or progressive leucoaraiosis.
- The group with probable dementia with Lewy bodies (DLB, n=11) was diagnosed according to consensus guidelines [40].
- The frontotemporal dementia group (FTD, n=23) was diagnosed according to the criteria of Neary et al. [41].
- The probable Alzheimer's disease group (AD, n=76) was diagnosed according to the NINCDS-ADRDA criteria [42].

All patients with primary dementias were recruited from the Department of Neurology of the Athens National University. In addition to clinical criteria, extensive neuropsychological examination and 1-2 years follow up was required to ensure correct diagnosis.

The control group (CTRL) consisted of 82 mentally intact and otherwise healthy elderly individuals, who underwent hernia repair or other orthopedic surgery under spinal anesthesia; all were free of any history, symptoms, signs or routine biochemical findings suggestive of neurological, malignant or systemic disease. The Mini Mental State Examination (MMSE) was used prior to surgery [43], since it has been found to be a standardized screening and staging tool for dementia [44]. Clinical and demographic data for both patients and controls are shown in table 1.

Assessments

All patient groups completed a full battery of neuropsychological tests. For the group of alcohol-dependent subjects these tests were administered sixty days after admission to the hospital, in order to avoid possible interference from the tranquilizers administered.

Tests administered included the MMSE, the Syndrome Short-Test (SKT; which assesses attention, naming, immediate and delayed recall, recognition memory and cognitive rigidity), the Clock Test (which assesses visuoconstructive ability), the Verbal Fluency Test (Letter and Category; which evaluates verbal and executive function) and the Digit Span Forward and Backward (WAIS-R; which evaluates attention, immediate recall and working memory).

Sample Collection and Biochemical Measurements

Lumbar puncture was performed at 9–11 AM, after overnight fasting, using a standard 21 or 22 G Quincke type needle. CSF samples were centrifuged immediately and stored in polypropylene tubes at –70oC until analysis. Bloody or cloudy samples were discarded. CSF τ and Aβ42 levels were measured in duplicate by double sandwich ELISA using the "Innotest htau antigen" and the "Innotest β-Amyloid (1–42)" kits respectively (Innogenetics, Gent, Belgium), according to the manufacturer's instructions. Freeze-thawing of specimens was avoided. Both τ and Aβ42 were run as a routine neurochemical analysis in our clinic. The intra and inter-assay variabilities for both tests were < 10%.

Statistical Analysis

All variables were checked for normality and for the homogeneity of variances by the Shapiro-Wilk's and Leven's tests respectively. As regards CSF biomarker levels, significant deviations from the normal distribution were found and variances were heterogeneous. However, logarithmic transformation restored the above violations and permitted the use of 2-way analysis of covariance (ANCOVA) with diagnostic group and sex as factors and age and MMSE as covariates, followed by post-hoc Tukey's honest significant difference tests. The effects of age, age of onset, disease duration and MMSE score were also tested separately in each group by the Spearman correlation coefficient. One-way ANOVA and χ^2-test were also used as appropriate. The level of statistical significance was set at 0.05.

OUR FINDINGS

Results are summarized in table 1 and figure 1. As expected, significant differences in age and sex were observed among groups.

Table 1. Clinical and biochemical data of the studied groups

	CTRL	ARD	VD	DLB	FTD	AD	P level
n (m/f)	82 (50/32)	24 (22/2)	17 (11/6)	11 (7/4)	23 (12/11)	76 (27/49)	0.00006
Age (y)	68 ± 10	65 ± 12	72 ± 8	66 ± 6	58 ± 10	66 ± 10	<0.0001
Duration (y)		3.1 ± 1.9	2.4 ± 3.1	2.9 ± 1.5	3.3 ± 2.9	3.4 ± 2.7	NS
MMSE	29 [28–30]	20 [15–26]	19 [13–25]	18 [5–25]	20[4–26]	17 [2–24]	0.0001
CSF τ (pg/ml)	181 (120–250)	225 (163–288)	208 (170–242)	168 (129–334)	372 (256–490)	591 (457–972)	<0.000001
CSF Aβ42 (pg/ml)	637 (454–806)	782 (568–875)	563 (402–714)	382 (268–446)	654 (452–786)	389 (314–480)	0.0009
CSF τ/Aβ42	0.28 (0.20–0.38)	0.28 (0.20–0.35)	0.35 (0.28–0.48)	0.34 (0.18–0.60)	0.49 (0.39–0.75)	1.71 (0.98–2.45)	<0.000001

Data are presented as mean ± SD, median [range] or median (25th – 75th quartile). m = males, f = females, NS = non-significant. CSF = cerebrospinal fluid; ARD = alcohol related dementia; VD = vascular dementia; DLB = dementia with Lewy bodies; FTD = frontotemporal dementia; AD = Alzheimer's disease; CTRL = control.

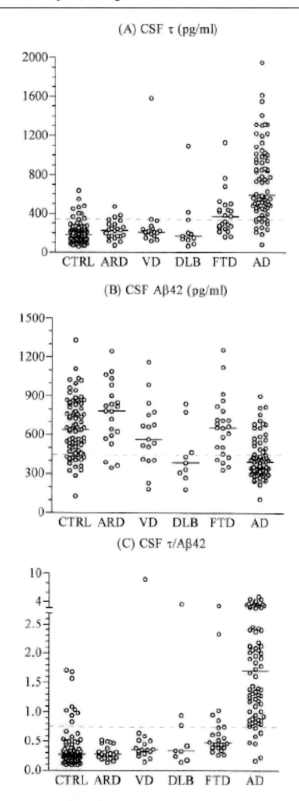

Figure 1. Scatterplot of CSF tau and Aβ2 levels and their ratio in the studied groups. Horizontal bars indicate median values and horizontal broken lines indicate cut-off levels.

The FTD patients were younger, whereas female sex predominated in AD, and male sex was overrepresented in VD and ARD. The MMSE score was significantly lower in all groups as compared with the controls, but patient groups did not differ among each other.

For CSF τ, Aβ42, and τ/Aβ42 ratio, 2-way ANCOVA revealed a significant effect by group, but not by sex, whereas age and MMSE did not affect the models significantly. Post-hoc Tuckey's tests revealed that CSF τ levels in ARD, VD, and DLB did not differ from those of CTRL, whereas in AD, τ levels were significantly higher than those of ARD, CTRL, VD, and DLB (P< 0.0001) and FTD (P< 0.001). In FTD, τ levels were higher as compared with CTRL and ARD (P< .0001).

The levels of CSF Aβ42 in ARD, FTD, and VD did not differ significantly from those of CTRL, whereas in AD they were significantly lower than those of ARD, CTRL (P< .0001), FTD (P< .001) and VD (P=.05). In DLB, they were also significantly lower as compared with ARD, CTRL (P =.02), and FTD (P = .05), but they did not differ as compared with AD. The τ/Aβ42 ratio in ARD, VD, and DLB did not differ as compared with CTRL, whereas in AD the ratio was higher than ARD, CTRL, VD, FTD (P< .0001), and DLB (P< .001). In FTD, the ratio was also higher as compared with CTRL (P< .001) and ARD (P< .0001).

To calculate the diagnostic sensitivity and specificity of the biomarkers studied, cut off levels of τ, Aβ42 and τ/Aβ42 were set at 340 pg/ml, 445 pg/ml, and 0.75 respectively, based on previous studies of our laboratory (28, 30, 31). Using these cut-off values, we estimated the specificities and sensitivities among groups (see table 2).

Table 2. Sensitivity (Sn) and specificity (Sp) of CSF biomarkers

Biomarker	Sn for AD	Sn for FTD	Sn for DLB	Sp from ARD	Sp from CTRL
CSF					
τ >340 pg/ml	86%	52%	-	88%	89%
CSF					
Ab42					
< 445 pg/ml	70%	-	67%	86%	80%
CSF					
τ/Aβ42 > 0.75	91%	26%	33%	100%	89%

CSF = cerebrospinal fluid ARD = alcohol related dementia; DLB = dementia with Lewy bodies; FTD = frontotemporal dementia; AD = Alzheimer's disease; CTRL = control,

With specificity approaching 90%, τ alone achieved 86% sensitivity for the discrimination between AD and either ARD or CTRL. Keeping a specificity of = 80%, Aβ42 alone was 70% sensitive. On the contrary, the τ/Aβ42 ratio, at levels of specificity approaching or exceeding 90%, achieved sensitivity >90%. For the discrimination between ARD or CTRL and FTD, τ alone, at the same levels of specificity identified only 52% of the FTD patients, while the ratio was not helpful (26%). For the discrimination between ARD or CTRL and DLB, and at the same levels of specificity, Aβ42 alone achieved 67% sensitivity, whereas the ratio was inadequate.

DISCUSSION

The aim of the present study was to evaluate the diagnostic potential of the CSF biomarkers τ protein, Aβ42 peptide, and their combination in the form of a ratio in clinically well-defined groups of elderly ARD patients vs. patients with vascular or degenerative dementias.

The studied groups had comparable MMSE scores and age with the exception of FTD patients as for age, which is in accordance with epidemiology of this disorder, being usually of presenile onset. With regard to sex, males were over-represented in VD and ARD groups. Saunders et al [1] found that dementia was 4.6 times more likely to occur in men aged > 65 who had a lifetime history of heavy drinking [1]. In the opposite, females were over-represented in AD, in accordance with disease predilection to female sex. However, age, sex, disease duration, age of disease onset, and MMSE score had no effect on biomarker levels, neither in the patient nor in the control groups, indicating that the diagnostic value of these biomarkers is generally unaffected by the above factors. In agreement with previous reports, the present study confirmed τ and τ / Aβ42 ratio increase in AD as compared with the CTRL, ARD, VD, and DLB groups. The results for τ are also in accordance with the results of Morikawa et al [45], who reported τ levels within the normal range in demented and non demented alcoholics as compared with AD patients and controls. Calculated sensitivities and specificities for given cut-off values as previously reported by our group [27,28,46] are shown in table 2. According to the results, the sensitivity and specificity for τ alone is high (both > 86%) when the 340 pg/ml is used as the optimal cut-off level for the differential diagnosis of ARD vs. AD. Aβ42 levels in ARD were in the range of the control group, with sensitivity and specificity lower than that of τ alone (70% and 86%, respectively) when the cut-off value of 445 pg/ml was used. The τ/Aβ42 ratio was clearly superior to Aβ42 alone and slightly superior to τ alone for the discrimination of these disorders. At excellent levels of specificity (approaching 100%), achieved an excellent sensitivity as well (> 90%).

However, for the discrimination between ARD and FTD, τ alone, at the same levels of specificity identified only half of the FTD patients, whereas the ratio was not helpful. The FTD patients presented with increased t levels, although this increase was not in the magnitude observed in AD. Tau is known to be involved in FTD pathology [47] and CSF τ levels have been reported increased [48].

The Aβ42 levels were decreased in the CSF of patients with DLB in accordance with the results of Kanemaru et al [33], and this finding may be of value in certain rare cases for the discrimination between ARD and DLB. However, at high levels of specificity (86%), Aβ42 alone achieved a moderate sensitivity (67%), whereas the ratio was inadequate.

With regard to VD, normal levels of the studied biomarkers were found. Vascular dementia is known to be heterogeneous in its pathogenesis [39], and different authors may study different subpopulations of VD. It has been suggested that patients with lacunar infarcts [49] and patients with progressive "leukoaraiosis", which tend to have "pure" vascular disease [50] present with normal t levels (51). Since most of our VD patients had lacunar infarcts, our results are compatible with this notion. Vascular factors may contribute to the pathogenesis of dementia in patients with alcohol abuse, through ischemic and/or hemorrhagic mechanisms, easily identified in neuroimaging. However, significant cortical or subcortical infarctions or subdural hematomas, cast doubt on the diagnosis of ARD [17].

Previous studies demonstrated that heavy alcohol consumption is a major contributing factor in the emergence of dementia in more than 20% of patients diagnosed as having dementia, especially when older populations are included [2,22]. An increased prevalence of dementia has been reported in older as compared with younger drinkers [52]. Alzheimer disease is the main disease in the differential diagnosis, accounting for about 50% to 60% of all causes of dementia in most Western populations [53]. In the last decade, the ante-mortem diagnostic accuracy of dementia has risen to a high degree, due to the better understanding of the clinical picture of dementias and the use of widely accepted criteria. However, clinical and differential diagnosis is not always easy. It is generally accepted that in mild cases, especially when being examined in primary care settings [54], in the presenium [55] and in the presence of confounding factors, such as alcohol abuse, diagnostic uncertainty considerably increases, especially when according to the NINCDS-ADRDA criteria, the case is defined as possible. In this case, according to the results of Galasko et al [56], the probability for postmortem verification of AD may drop from 92% for probable to 77% for possible AD.

The results of our study must be seen as directed toward the verification or exclusion of AD or other "tauopathic" dementia, in a given clinical question (e.g. AD vs. ARD) through the combination of high τ and low Aβ42 which is highly specific for AD, whereas the reverse combination is highly specific for the absence of AD. The results do not aim in confirming ARD because normal τ levels can be found in other dementing disorders (e.g. depression, dementia with Lewy bodies, or vascular dementia) that sometimes can interfere with ARD differential diagnosis [24,33,49]. The same holds true for FTD or DLB. An increased τ or a decreased Aβ42 in analogous clinical questions favors an FTD or a DLB diagnosis, respectively.

A limitation of the present study is that the diagnosis is clinical, lacking pathological confirmation. Unfortunately postmortem verification of diagnosis in the field of biomarker research is generally lacking [57].

CONCLUSIONS

In conclusion, according to the above data we recommend the determination of τ, Aβ42 and their ratio in the CSF in elderly patients with dementia and a history of alcohol consumption, provided that there is no contraindication for lumbar puncture and the patient or relatives have consented. Both τ and the τ / Aβ42 ratio fulfil the Reagan Research Institute criteria for useful biomarkers in the differential diagnosis of ARD vs AD, but the ratio seems better than τ alone [58].

REFERENCES

[1]   Saunders PA, Copeland JR, Dewey ME, Davidson IA, McWilliam C, Sharma V, Sullivan C. Heavy drinking as a risk factor for depression and dementia in elderly men. Findings from the Liver-pool longitudinal community study. *Br. J. Psychiatry* 1991;159: 213–6.

[2]   Smith DM, Atkinson RM. Alcoholism and dementia. *Int. J. Addictions* 1995;30:1843–69.

[3]   Parsons OA, Nixon SJ. Neurobehavioral sequelae of alcoholism. *Neurologic clinics* 1993;11:205–18.

[4]   Harper C, Butterworth R. Nutritional and metabolic disorders. In: Graham DI, Lantos PL, eds. *Greenfield's neuropathology*, Sixth ed. London, UK: Arnold, 1997:600–55.

[5]   Victor M. Alcoholic dementia. *Can. J. Neurol. Sci.* 1994;21:88–99.

[6]   Olsen RW, Liang J, Cagetti E, Spigelman I. Plasticity of GABAA receptors in brains of rats treated with chronic intermittent ethanol. *Neurochem. Res.* 2005;30(12):1579–88.

[7]   Ming Z, Criswell HE, Yu G, Breese GR. Competing presynaptic and postsynaptic effects of ethanol on cerebellar purkinje neurons. *Alcohol Clin. Exp. Res.* 2006;30(8):1400–7.

[8]   Calabrese V, Scapagnini G, Latteri S, Colombrita C, Ravagna A, Catalano C, et al. Long-term ethanol administration enhances age-dependent modulation of redox state in different brain regions in the rat: protection by acetyl carnitinc. *Int. J. Tissue React* 2002;24(3):97–104.

[9]   Korbo L. Glial cell loss in the hippocampus of alcoholics. *Alc. Clin. Exp. Res.* 1999;23:164–8.

[10]   Brun A, Andersson J. Frontal dysfunction and frontal cortical synapse loss in alcoholism. The main cause of alcoholic dementia? *Dement Geriatr. Cogn. Disord.* 2001;12:289–94.

[11]   Ikegami Y, Goodenough S, Inoue Y, Dodd PR, Wilce PA, Matsumoto I. Increased TUNEL positive cells in human alcoholic brains. *Neurosci. Lett.* 2003; 349(3):201–5.

[12]   Arendt T. The cholinergic deafferentation of the cerebral cortex induced by chronic consumption of alcohol: Reversal by cholinergic drugs and transplantation. In: Hunt WA, Nixon SJ, eds. Alcohol-induced brain damage. Rockville, MD: US Dept Health *Human Serv,* 1993:431–60.

[13]   Mukamal KJ, Kuller LH, Fitzpatrick AL, Longs-treth WT Jr, Mittleman MA, Siscovick DS. Prospective study of alcohol consumption and risk of dementia in older adults. *JAMA* 2003;289(11): 1405–13.

[14]   Kamino K, Nagasaka K, Imagawa M, Yamamoto H, Yoneda H, Ueki A et al. Deficiency in mito-chondrial aldehyde dehydrogenase increases the risk for late-onset Alzheimer's disease in the Japanese population. *Biochem. Biophys. Res. Commun* 2000; 273(1):192–6.

[15]   Chen CP, Kuhn P, Chaturvedi K, Boyadjieva N, Sarkar DK. Ethanol induces apoptotic death of developing beta-endorphin neurons via suppression of cyclic adenosine monophosphate production and activation of transforming growth factor-beta1-linked apoptotic signaling. *Mol. Pharmacol.* 2006;69(3):706–17.

[16]   Jacques A, Stevenson G. Korsakoff's syndrome and other chronic alcohol related brain damage. Stirling: *Dementia Serv. Dev. Centre*, 2000.

[17]   Oslin D, Atkinson RM, Smith DM, Hendrie H. Alcohol related dementia: Proposed Clinical Criteria. *Int. J. Geriatr. Psychiatry* 1998;13:203–12.

[18]   Friedland RP. Alzheimer's disease: Clinical features and differential diagnosis. *Neurology* 1993;43 (Suppl 4): S45–S51.

[19]   Kril JJ, Halliday GM. Brain shrinkage in alcoholics: A decade on and what have we learned? *Prog. Neurobiol.* 1999;58:381–7.

[20] Jernigan TL, Butters N, DiTraglia G, Schafer K, Smith T, Irwin M, Grant I, Schuckit M, Cermak LS. Reduced cerebral grey matter observed in alcoholics using magnetic resonance imaging. *Alcohol Clin. Exp. Res.* 1991;15:418–27.

[21] Knopman DS. An overview of common non-Alzheimer dementias. *Clin. Geriatr. Med.* 2001; 17(2):281–301.

[22] Carlen PL, Wilkinson DA. Reversibility of alcohol- related brain damage: Clinical and experimental observations. *Acta Med. Scand.* 1987;717(Suppl): 19–26.

[23] Trojanowski JQ, Clark CM, Arai H, Lee VM. Elevated levels of tau in cerebrospinal fluid: implications for the antemortem diagnosis in Alzheimer's disease. *J. Alzheimers Dis.* 1999;1(4-5):297–305.

[24] Andreasen N, Minthon L, Davidsson P, Van-mechelen E, Vanderstichele H et al. Evaluation of CSF-tau and CSF-Abeta42 as diagnostic markers for Alzheimer disease in clinical practice. *Arch. Neurol.* 2001;58(3):373–9.

[25] Kosik KS, Greenberg SM. Tau protein and Alzheimer's disease. In: Terry RD, Katzman R, Bick KL, eds. *Alzheimer's disease.* New York, NY: Raven, 1994:335–44.

[26] Kurz A, Riemenschneider M, Buch K, Willoch F, Bartenstein P, Muller U et al. Tau protein in cerebrospinal fluid is significantly increased at the earliest stage of Alzheimer's disease. *Alzheimer Dis. Assoc. Disord* 1998;12(4):372–7.

[27] Blennow K, Hampel H. CSF markers for incipient Alzheimer's disease. *Lancet Neurol.* 2003;2:605–13.

[28] Kapaki E, Paraskevas GP, Zalonis I, Zournas C. CSF tau protein and b-amyloid (1-42) in Alzheimer's disease diagnosis: discrimination from normal ageing and other dementias in the Greck population. *Eur. J. Neurol.* 2003;10:119–28.

[29] Sobów T, Flirski M, Liberski PP. Amyloid-beta and tau proteins as biochemical markers of Alzheimer's disease. *Acta Neurobiol. Exp.* 2004; 64:53–70.

[30] Kapaki E, Paraskevas GP, Michalopoulou M, Kilidireas K. CSF Tau is increased in multiple sclerosis. *Eur. Neurol.* 2000;43:228–32.

[31] Kapaki E, Kilidireas K. Paraskevas GP, Michal-opoulou M, Patsouris E. Highly increased CSF tau protein and decreased ß-amyloid (1-42) in sporadic CJD: a discrimination from Alzheimer's disease? *J. Neurol. Neurosurg. Psychiatry* 2001;71: 401–3.

[32] Small DH, McLean CA. Alzheimer's disease and the Amyloid ß protein: What is the role of Amyloid? *J. Neurochem.* 1999;73:443–9.

[33] Kanemaru K, Kameda N, Yamanouchi H. Decreased CSF amyloid b42 and normal tau levels in dementia with Lewy bodies. *Neurology* 2000; 54:1875–6.

[34] Waldemar G, Dubois B, Emre M, Georges J, McKeith IG, Rossor M et al. EFNS. Recom-mendations for the diagnosis and management of Alzheimer's disease and other disorders associated with dementia: EFNS guideline. *Eur. J. Neurol.* 2007;14(1):e1–26.

[35] American Psychiatric Association. Diagnostic and statistical manual of mental disorders, 4th ed. Washington, DC: APA, 1994.

[36] Hughes PH, Venulet J, Khant U, Medina Mora ME, Navaratnam V et al. *Core data for epidemio-logical studies on nonmedical drug use.* Geneva, CH: WHO, 1980;56:1–100.

[37] World Health Organization. Composite inter-national diagnostic interview-CIDI, Core Version 1.0. Geneva, CH: WHO, Div Ment Health, 1990.

[38] Wells JC, Tien AY, Garrison R, Eaton WW. Risk factors for the incidence of social phobia as determined by the Diagnostic Interview Schedule in a population-based study. *Acta Psychiatr. Scand.* 1994;90:84–90.

[39] Román GC, Tatemichi TK, Erkinjuntti T, Cummings JL, Masdeu JC, Garcia JH et al. Vascular dementia: diagnostic criteria for research studies. Report of the NINDS-AIREN International Workshop. *Neurology* 1993;43(2):250–60.

[40] McKeith IG, McKeith IG, Dickson DW, Lowe J, Emre M, O'Brien JT et al. Consortium on DLB. Diagnosis and management of dementia with Lewy bodies: third report of the DLB Consortium. *Neurology* 2005;65(12):1863–72.

[41] Neary D, Snowden JS, Gustafson L, Passant U, Stuss D, Black S et al. Frontotemporal lobar degeneration: a consensus on clinical diagnostic criteria. *Neurology* 1998;51(6):1546–54.

[42] McKhann G, Drachman D, Folstein M, Katzman R, Price D, Stadlan EM. Clinical diagnosis of Alzheimer's disease: report of the NINCDS-ADRDA work group under the auspices of the Department of Health and Human Services Task Force on Alzheimer's disease. *Neurology* 1984; 34(7):939–44.

[43] Folstein M, Folstein S, McHugh PR. Mini-Mental State: a practical method for grading the cognitive state of patients for the clinician. *J. Psychiatr. Res.* 1975;12:189–98.

[44] Tombaugh TN, McIntyre NJ. The mini-mental stage examination: A comprehensive review. *J. Am. Geriatr. Soc.* 1992;40:992.

[45] Morikawa Y, Arai H, Matsushita S, Kato M, Higuchi S, Miura M et al. Cerebrospianl fluid tau protein levels in demented and nondemented alcoholics. *Alcohol Clin. Exp. Res.* 1999;23(4): 575–7.

[46] Kapaki E, Liappas I, Paraskevas GP, Theotoka I, Rabavilas A. The diagnostic value of tau protein, beta-amyloid (1-42) and their ratio for the discrimination of alcohol-related cognitive dis-orders from Alzheimer's disease in the early stages. *Int. J. Geriatr Psychiatry* 2005;20(8):722–9.

[47] Spillantini MG, Goedert M. Tau protein pathology in neurodegenerative diseases. *Trends Neurosc.i* 1998; 21: 428–33.

[48] Paraskevas GP, Kapaki E, Liappas I, Theotoka I, Mamali I, Zournas C, Lykouras L. The diagnostic value of cerebrospinal fluid tau protein in dementing and nondementing neuropsychiatric disorders. *J. Geriatr. Psychiatry Neurol.* 2005;18(3): 163–73.

[49] Mori H, Hosoda K, Matsubara E, Nakamoto T, Furiya Y, Endoh R et al. Tau in cerebrospinal fluids: establishment of the sandwich ELISA with antibody specific to the repeat sequence in tau. *Neurosci Lett.* 1995;186(2-3):181–3.

[50] Tarvonen-Schröoder S, Räihä I, Kurki T, Rajala T, Sourander L. Clinical characteristics of rapidly progressive leuko-araiosis. *Acta Neurol. Scand* 1995; 91(5):399–404.

[51] Nagga K, Gottfries J, Blennow K, Marcusson J. Cerebrospinal fluid phospho-tau, total tau and beta-amyloid(1-42) in the differentiation between Alzheimer's disease and vascular dementia. *Dement. Geriatr. Cogn. Disord* 2002;14:183–90.

[52] Blow F, Cook FL, Booth B et al. Age-related psychiatric comorbidities and level of function in alcohol veterans seeking outpatient treatment. *Hosp. Community Psychiatry* 1992;43:990–5.

[53] Jellinger K, Danielczyk W, Fischer P, Gabriel E. Clinicopathological analysis of dementia disorders in the elderly. *J. Neurol. Sci.* 1990; 95:239–58.

[54] Mendez M, Mastri AR, Sung JH, Frey WH. Clinically diagnosed Alzheimer's disease: neuro-pathologic findings in 650 cases. *Alzheimer Dis. Assoc. Disord.* 1992;6:35–43.

[55] Risse SC, Raskind MA, Nochlin D, Sumi SM, Lampe TH, Bird TD et al. Neuropathological findings in patients with clinical diagnoses of probable Alzheimer's disease. *Am. J. Psychiatry* 1990;147(20):168–71.

[56] Galasko D, Hansen LA, Katzman R, Wiederholt W, Masliah E, Terry R et al. Clinical-neuropatho-logical correlations in Alzheimer's disease and related dementias. *Arch. Neurol.* 1994;51(9):888–95.

[57] Clark CM, Xie S, Chittams J, Clark CM, Xie S, Chittams J et al. Cerebrospinal fluid tau and beta-amyloid: how well do these biomarkers reflect autopsy-confirmed dementia diagnoses? *Arch. Neurol.* 2003;60(12):1696–1702.

[58] The Ronald and Nancy Reagan Research Institute of the Alzheimer's Association and the National Institute of Aging Working Group. Concensus Report of the Working Group on: "Molecular and Biochemical Markers of Alzheimer's disease". *Neurobiol. Aging* 1998;19:109–16.

In: Alcohol-Related Cognitive Disorders
Editors: L. Sher, I. Kandel, J. Merrick pp. 277-290

ISBN: 978-1-60741-730-9
© 2009 Nova Science Publishers, Inc.

Chapter 19

MODERATE ALCOHOL CONSUMPTION: IS IT HEALTHY?

Graham J. McDougall Jr, Heather Becker, Carol L. Delville, Phillip W. Vaughan and Taylor W. Acee

ABSTRACT

We examined the relationships between alcohol use, cognitive and affective variables, and the potential differential benefits of training for older adults drinkers and non-drinkers who participated in a randomized trial implemented between 2001-2006. Participants, who were living independently in the community, were randomly assigned to either twelve hours of memory training or health promotion classes. Outcomes included depression, health, cognition, verbal, visual, memory, and performance-based IADLs. The sample was 79% female, 17% Hispanic and 12% African-American. The typical participant had an average age of 75 years with 13 years of education. In the memory intervention group, there were 135 individuals (63 drinkers, 72 non-drinkers). In the health promotion condition, there were 129 individuals (58 drinkers and 71 non-drinkers). At baseline, drinkers scored higher on cognition, verbal memory, and lower on depression than non-drinkers. Alcohol use was positively related to physical health at baseline as measured by the Physical Component Summary Score of the Medical Outcomes Health Scale (SF-36).

We found significant effects for the time*drinking*treatment group interaction in the repeated measures ANCOVA for the Mini Mental Status Examination, the Hopkins Verbal Learning Test, and the SF-36 Mental Health sub-scale. The time*drinking*group interactions were not statistically significant for any of the other outcomes. This study demonstrated that older adults benefited from targeted psychosocial interventions on affective, cognitive and functional outcomes.

In addition, the SeniorWISE study provides empirical support to the research evidence emphasizing the health benefits of moderate alcohol consumption in older adults.

INTRODUCTION

The recommended 2003 Healthy Eating Pyramid released by the United States Department of Agriculture now includes the moderate daily consumption of alcohol, unless contraindicated, as a 'brick' within the healthy choices [1]. This change in the food pyramid was influenced by studies that documented the preventive cognitive and physical health benefits of moderate alcohol consumption [2-4].

Depending upon the setting and quantity of consumption, moderate alcohol use among adults over age 65 has been reported to be between 23% and 31% [5-6]. Older adults are more likely to engage in the moderate regular use of alcohol rather than in binge or problem drinking [7-8]. Older adult drinkers including almost equal numbers of Hispanic and non-Hispanic white men and women obtained better cognitive test scores than did those participants who abstained [9]. Women who consumed moderate amounts of alcohol had higher levels of cognitive function than non-drinkers and were less likely to develop cognitive impairment over a follow-up period of 24 to 48 months [10-11].

The findings from numerous health intervention studies have demonstrated that such health-related activity as exercise, mental stimulation, and social engagement may prevent disability and improve health and function [12-13]. The Advanced Cognitive Training for Independent and Vital Elderly (ACTIVE) trials demonstrated that mental stimulation through targeted cognitive training improves cognitive abilities and prevents the cognitive decline that would have occurred in older adults without dementia, with the gains being maintained for five years [14]. McDougall and his associates [15] found that including content on stress inoculation, health promotion, memory self-efficacy, and memory strategy in a psychosocial intervention study assisted community dwelling elderly to maintain their cognitive function over 2 years, and the intervention was of most benefit to the minority elders with low literacy. Alcohol consumption, however, does not uniformly protect older adults and may lead to mental health problems, cognitive impairment, and dementia [16-17].

Depression and problems with alcohol vary by gender. In women the depression tends to precede alcohol use, whereas in men alcohol use typically precedes depression [18]. A subsequent study failed to confirm this finding, however [19] for females; depressive symptoms predicted subsequent alcohol problems over 3 and 4 years, but not at seven years; whereas no evidence was found for such a relation in males.

Elders admitted to a psychiatric facility with a dual diagnosis of depression and substance abuse were 6 times more likely to make a suicide attempt before admission, and this increased risk of suicide continues through 85 years of age [20]. Gazmararian and associates reported that 8.8% of moderate drinkers experienced depressive symptoms, whereas 15% of non-drinkers and 18.5% of heavy drinkers reported depression [21]. The results of that study were supported 6 years later by Kirchner and associates [5] who identified an incidence of depression as 15% in older adults that drank moderately compared with non-drinkers (21%), or heavy drinkers (25%).

In the present secondary analysis, we examined the relations between alcohol use and cognitive performance, instrumental activities, depression, and health in a group of nondemented older adults. Furthermore, because only two intervention studies focused on the differential benefits of a psychosocial intervention, we were interested in the possible differential benefits of memory and health training between drinkers and non-drinkers over time [22-23].

OUR STUDY

A Phase III randomized clinical trial tested two inter-ventions—memory training versus health promotion. In the community, the study was advertised as SeniorWISE (Wisdom Is Simply Exploration). Participants received 12 hours of classroom learning content and met twice a week for 1.5 hours each; lectures were delivered with PowerPoint presentations. Individuals were post tested withintwo weeks after completing the classes.

Interventions

Health Promotion

The health intervention emphasized successful aging based on three focus groups conducted in the community with older adults. The topics included exercise, spirituality and health, alternative medicine, weight management, getting the most from your doctor visit, caring for the caretaker, healing foods, drug interactions, osteoporosis, maintaining relationships, health myths, consumer fraud, nutrition, leisure activities, writing family stories, health monitoring tests for home use and buying drugs in foreign countries.

Memory Training

The memory-training curriculum emphasized stress and relaxation, memory strategies for everyday activities, confidence building, and problems and expectations related to aging memory. Based on self-efficacy theory, performance accomplishments, practice, homework assignments, encouragement, and persuasion were woven into the classroom lectures by the facilitator, a septuagenarian licensed counselling psychologist.

Participants in Our Study

A total of 346 independent adults were recruited from a metropolitan area in Central Texas via print and TV media, as well as by direct recruitment at city-run senior activity centers, churches, health fairs and festivals. A total of 81 individuals were excluded, 21 did not meet inclusion criteria, 38 declined, and 22 were couples, of which the female spouse was excluded from the testing so that adequate numbers of males would be represented in the sample. The final sample (N=264) was 71% Non-Hispanic White, 17% Hispanic, and 11% African American. The average age was 75 years. The majority of the participants were female (77%). Table 1 describes the demographics of the participants in each group.

Randomization to the memory or health intervention occurred within each of nine different community sites and consisted of 11 groups. One hundred thirty-five individuals were assigned to the memory and 130 were assigned to the health groups. Each intervention was delivered in a small group format. No group was smaller than four individuals or larger than 15; however we strove for an average group composed of 12 individuals. The memory intervention and health promotion group did not differ significantly at baseline on either the study variables or the demographics.

Table 1. Demographic characteristics of drinkers and non-drinkers in health and cognitive intervention groups

	Health Intervention (n=130) Mean (SD)		Cognitive Intervention (n= 135) Mean (SD)	
	Nondrinker (n=71)	Drinker (n=58)	Nondrinker (n=72)	Drinker (n=63)
Age (years)	74.87 (6.36)	74.67 (6.1)	75.18 (5.95)	74.13 (5.48)
Education	12.68 (3.81)	15.22 (3.12)	13.03 (4.35)	13.8 (3.29)
Numbers (%)				
Gender				
Females	58 (82)	41 (71)	60 (83)	45 (71)
Males	13 (18)	17 (29)	12 (17)	18 (29)
Race				
White	39 (55)	53 (91)	39 (54)	57 (90)
Black	13 (18)	2 (3)	14 (19)	1 (2)
Other	19 (27)	3 (5)	19 (26)	5 (8)
Ethnicity				
Hispanic	19 (27)	3 (5)	19 (26)	5 (8)
Non-Hispanic	52 (73)	55 (95)	53 (74)	58 (92)
Marital Status				
Married	16 (23)	21 (36)	19 (26)	26 (41)
Never Married	2 (3)	1 (2)	2 (3)	3 (5)
Divorced	16 (23)	10 (17)	12 (17)	13 (21)
Widowed	37 (52)	26 (45)	38 (53)	20 (32)

We evaluated sensory loss and visual and hearing acuity with an in-person eligibility screening by evaluator observation and by a self-report checklist developed for this study. Other eligibility criteria included age ($\geq$ 65 years), ability to speak and understand English, and reliable transportation.Diagnoses such as Alzheimer's disease or other dementia, Hodgkin's disease, neuroblastoma, or cancer of the liver, lung, or brain were considered exclusionary criteria. Participants were also screened with the Mini-Mental State Examination (MMSE) with scores > 23, and were also required to pass Trails A and/or Trails B at or above the 10th percentile for their age group.

Variables in Our Study

Alcohol Consumption

On the health questionnaire, we asked participants to self-report whether they drank alcohol with a Yes/No response to the interviewer. If they answered in the affirmative, then we asked them to state how many drinks they consumed in a given period of time, usually a day, a week, or a month. We did not offer the participants any prompts to indicate comparisons among the types or quantities of alcohol, such as beer, wine, spirits, etc.

Cognition

Cognitive function was evaluated with the Mini Mental State Exam, a screening instrument with a range of possible scores between 0 and 30. Generally, a score between 23 and 30 classifies an individual into the nonimpaired range. We included individuals with scores greater than or equal to 23, although eight minority participants were admitted with MMSE scores ≥ 20.

Verbal Memory

Verbal memory performance was tested with the Hopkins Verbal Learning Test-Revised (HVLT-R), which assesses immediate recall, delayed recall, and recognition memory. The Delayed Recall Subscale, was used for this analyses.

Visual Memory

Visual memory performance was deter-mined with the Brief Visuospatial Memory Test-Revised (BVMT-R), in which the individual is asked to repro-duce a series of geometric designs.

Everyday Memory

The Rivermead Everyday Behavioral Memory test bridges laboratory-based measures of memory and assessments obtained by self-report and observation. The standardized profile score (SPS) has a possible range from 0-24.

Instrumental Activities

The Direct Assessment of Functional Status (DAFS) measured performance in the instrumental activities of daily living. The DAFS included specific tasks such as addressing a letter, writing a check, balancing the check register, identifying and calculating money, making change from a grocery purchase, reading a prescription label and dialing the pharmacy to order a refill, dialing a telephone number, and remembering a grocery list given orally given and reading from the book. The DAFS has demonstrated high interrater and test-retest reliabilities for both patients presenting to a memory disorder clinic (English and Spanish speaking) and for normal controls.

Depression

The Centers for Epidemiologic Studies Scale (CES-D) evaluated depressive symptoms. Somatic complaints are emphasized on this measure to which individuals respond on a 4-point Likert scale.

Health

The Medical Outcomes Study Health Scale. (SF-36) was our measure of health status from the individual's point of view. Individuals respond to 36 items on a 5-point Likert scale ranging from poor to excellent and from much worse too much better. In addition to the eight health subscales, we have also included the Physical and Mental component summary scales [24].

Statistical Analysis of Our Data

For each dependent variable of interest, we sought to answer two major questions. First, we wanted to know how alcohol use might be associated with participants' baseline scores on outcomes related to affect, cognition, memory, instrumental activities, and mental and physical health. To answer this question, we regressed each outcome of interest at baseline on age, education, ethnicity (with separate dummy variables indicating Black or Hispanic status), and alcohol use. Alcohol use was coded as a dichotomous variable (drinker = 1, non-drinker = 0). Some of the results were previously reported for men and women separately, but here we present similar analyses with both genders combined [25-26].

Second, we wanted to determine the differential benefits, if any, of memory training for drinkers vs. non-drinkers over time (i.e., from baseline to post-classes). This research question was investigated by conducting separate repeated measures ANCOVAs for each dependent variable from baseline to post-classes, controlling for age, education, and ethnicity (again with separate dummy variables indicating Black or Hispanic status). Alcohol use (drinker = 1, nondrinker = 0) and treatment (memory group = 1, health group = 0) were between subjects factors, providing tests involving the interaction of these two factors with time (i.e., baseline and post-class). The test of the interaction between time, alcohol use, and treatment was of primary concern because it indicated whether there might be differential benefits of training from baseline to post-classes.

RESULTS

The analytic sample consisted of 265 randomized participants at baseline and 249 at post-test. In the memory intervention group, 135 individuals (63 drinkers, 72 non-drinkers) participated. In the health promotion condition, 129 individuals (58 drinkers and 71 non-drinkers) participated (see table 1). Ninety-four percent of participants completed the memory treatment, and 87% completed the health intervention (six or more of the eight training sessions). Consequently, the analyses of differential benefits of training described below exclude the 16 individuals who did not have post-intervention scores.

Drinking and Baseline Performance

Of the sixty male participants, 35 (58%) reported some degree of alcohol consumption; of the 182 females, 43% acknowledged drinking alcohol. Drinkers in both the health-intervention and cognitive-intervention groups were more likely to be married, male, and non-Hispanic whites. Whereas the average age was similar across the groups, those who drank had a higher education level. The means and standard deviations for study variables are shown in table 2-5.

Table 2. Means and standard deviations for outcome measures for groups and drinking status. Health intervention

| | Health Intervention Mean (SD) | | | |
| | Time 1 | | Time 2 | |
	Non-drink (n= 71)	Drink (n= 58)	Non-drink (n=70)	Drink (n= 53)
Instrumental Activities	79.87 (7.17)	83.69 (3.36)	80.59 (7.10)	84.79 (3.30)
Depression	11.11 (7.30)	7.56 (5.78)	11.09 (8.28)	8.52 (6.32)
Cognition	27.10 (2.44)	28.62 (1.62)	26.84 (2.74)	28.66 (1.47)
Memory Everyday	16.89 (4.99)	19.52 (3.37)	17.39 (5.06)	20.15 (3.51)
Verbal	42.8 (10.88)	51.50 (9.75)	42.47 (11.28)	53.38 (9.81)
Visual	39.48 (14.69)	46.47 (14.19)	37.39 (13.44)	46.15 (12.99)

Table 3. Means and standard deviations for outcome measures for groups and drinking status. Memory intervention

| Memory Intervention Mean (SD) | | | |
| Time 1 | | Time 2 | |
Non-drink (n= 72)	Drink (n= 63)	Non-drink (n= 66)	Drink (n=60)
81.45 (4.84)	83.41 (4.01)	81.81 (5.19)	84.63 (3.75)
10.74 (6.70)	7.29 (6.28)	9.56 (6.72)	7.85 (7.13)
27.47 (2.22)	28.59 (1.63)	27.81 (2.08)	28.78 (1.32)
18.08 (3.97)	19.70 (3.07)	19.12 (3.78)	20.43 (2.79)
45.05 (11.61)	51.86 (9.94)	47.24 (11.33)	52.62 (8.11)
40.07 (13.57)	45.43 (13.30)	39.36 (13.72)	52.62 (8.11)

Table 4. Means and standard deviations for outcome measures for groups and drinking status. Health scales

| | Health Intervention Mean (SD) | | | |
| | Time 1 | | Time 2 | |
	Non-drink (n= 71)	Drink (n= 58)	Non-drink (n=70)	Drink (n= 53)
Physical Function	58.40 (26.51)	71.35 (24.93)	60.92 (24.02)	71.92 (21.05)
Role-Physical	59.04 (43.52)	71.93 (36.31)	53.52 (40.55)	74.04 (35.34)
Bodily Pain	70.15 (25.39)	75.55 (21.63)	64.56 (24.24)	71.74 (23.16)
General Health	64.46 (19.65)	76.88 (16.65)	62.70 (17.92)	76.02 (16.43)
Vitality	59.93 (19.20)	68.97 (16.48)	59.21 (20.97)	66.51 (16.60)
Social Function	83.45 (21.83)	89.01 (16.40)	81.84 (22.71)	86.06 (18.13)
Role Emotional	77.46 (35.08)	86.55 (26.62)	67.20 (40.38)	82.69 (29.88)
Mental Health	79.09 (16.22)	83.66 (12.36)	75.88 (17.33)	82.79 (12.71)
Physical Component Score	40.90 (11.38)	45.81 (10.51)	40.71 (9.77)	45.71 (9.03)
Mental Component Score	54.15 (8.92)	56.24 (7.57)	51.87 (10.52)	54.86 (7.91)

Drinkers generally outscored non-drinkers except on the CES-D, where a high score indicates more depressive symptoms. Many of these differences on the SF-36 tended to be more pronounced at baseline than following the intervention, particularly in the memory group.

Table 5. Means and standard deviations for outcome measures for groups and drinking status. Health scales-health intervention

Memory Intervention Mean (SD)			
Time 1		Time 2	
Non-drink (n= 72)	Drink (n= 63)	Non-drink (n= 66)	Drink (n=60)
81.45 (4.84)	83.41 (4.01)	81.81 (5.19)	84.63 (3.75)
10.74 (6.70)	7.29 (6.28)	9.56 (6.72)	7.85 (7.13)
27.47 (2.22)	28.59 (1.63)	27.81 (2.08)	28.78 (1.32)
18.08 (3.97)	19.70 (3.07)	19.12 (3.78)	20.43 (2.79)
45.05 (11.61)	51.86 (9.94)	47.24 (11.33)	52.62 (8.11)
40.07 (13.57)	45.43 (13.30)	39.36 (13.72)	52.62 (8.11)
62.10 (29.60)	72.12 (24.06)	62.95 (27.60)	73.22 (21.45)
64.93 (37.92)	81.35 (29.09)	67.05 (36.99)	71.61 (38.69)
68.79 (23.37)	73.16 (22.08)	74.42 (23.42)	72.23 (20.05)
68.79 (20.96)	78.65 (17.11)	69.31 (21.35)	79.29 (16.40)
64.86 (16.36)	71.51 (16.84)	64.23 (19.71)	66.50 (18.94)
88.37 (19.83)	93.25 (13.99)	87.12 (18.60)	86.25 (19.76)
77.00 (36.77)	86.24 (25.14)	76.26 (35.45)	79.66 (33.91)
82.06 (14.00)	85.52 (11.73)	82.29 (13.80)	80.27 (17.98)
42.17 (11.14)	46.72 (9.18)	43.23 (10.15)	46.82 (9.17)
55.51 (7.88)	57.16 (6.61)	54.91 (7.91)	53.74 (9.49)

Memory Performance Measures

Table 6 presents standardized regression coefficients for each dependent variable of interest at baseline, and these beta weights provide effect estimates for predictors in each equation. Note that including age, education, ethnicity, gender, and marital status variables as predictors along with alcohol usage is the same as controlling for these variables. Self-reported alcohol use was a statistically significant, positive predictor of performance on the cognition (MMSE) and verbal memory (HVLT). Drinkers would be expected to score approximately 0.62 points higher than non-drinkers on the MMSE and 5.19 points higher on the HVLT (p<.05 and p < .01, respectively). Though not statistically significant, alcohol was also a positive predictor of scores for visual memory (BVMT), everyday memory (Rivermead SPS score), and instrumental activities (DAFS).

Table 6. Standard regression coefficients to predict outcome measures at baseline

	Cognition	Memory Everyday	Verbal	Visual	Instrumental Activities	Depression
	ß	ß	ß	ß	ß	ß
Age	−.03	−.21†	−.05	−.23†	−.16†	.07
Education	.42†	.25†	.26†	.24†	.36†	−.14
Hispanic	−.10	−.21†	−.08	−.20†	−.02†	−.04
Black	−.23†	−.29†	−.27†	−.28†	−.26†	.06
Male	−.16†	−.06	−.30†	−.17†	−.08	−.04
Married	.04	.01	.33	.06	−.07	−.11
Drinker	.14*	.06	.23†	.04	.09	−.21†

	Health: SF-36					
	General Health	Physical Function	Role Physical	Vitality	Pain	Social Function
	ß	ß	ß	ß	ß	ß
Age	−.07	−.14*	−.16*	−.18†	−.13*	−.02
Education	.05	.16	.07	.04	.01	.06
Hispanic	−.04	.11	.11	.15	.03	.07
Black	−.15*	−.01	0	.13*	−.12	−.03
Male	−.01	−.07	−.02	−.07	−.07	−.01
Married	.06	.14*	.03	.07	.08	.01
Drinker	.23†	.19†	.20†	.27†	.07	.13

	Role Emotional	Mental Health	Physical Component Score	Mental Component Score
	ß	ß	ß	ß
Age	−.11	−.02	−.16†	−.26
Education	.1	.15*	.07	0.08
Hispanic	.04	−.06	.09	−.01
Black	−.14*	.03	−.05	−.01
Male	.11	.03	−.08	.08
Married	.07	.11	.09	.05
Drinker	.06	.08	.21†	.07

*p < .05, †p < .01; Cognition=Mini Mental State Examination; Everyday Memory = Standard profile score (Rivermead Behavioral Memory Test); Verbal Memory = Delayed recall T score (Hopkins Verbal Learning Test-Rev); Visual Memory = Delayed recall T score (Brief Visuospatial Memory Test Rev); Instrumental Activities = Direct Assessment of Functional Status; Depression = Center for Epidemiological Diseases-Depression.

Depressive Symptoms

Self-reported alcohol consumption was a statistically significant, negative predictor of scores for depression (p<.01). Drinkers would be expected to score approximately 2.80 points lower than nondrinkers on this measure of depression, net of the covariates in the model. Twenty-three percent of non-drinkers, compared with 12% of drinkers scored 16 or above on the CESD, the cut-point for depressive symptomatology.

Physical and Mental Health

Alcohol use was positively related to participants' physical health at baseline as measured by the SF-36 Physical Component Summary Score (p < .01). Drinkers would be expected to score 4.56 points higher than non-drinkers. Alcohol use was positively related to participant's mental health as measured by the SF-36 Mental Component Summary Score, but this was not statistically significant (p = .33).

Possible Differential Benefits of Training

We found statistical significance for the time*drinking*treatment group effect in the repeated measures ANCOVA for only three variables: the MMSE, the HVLT, and the SF-36 Mental Health sub-scale. Graphs of these interactions over time are shown in figure 1. While the pattern varies somewhat across these three outcomes, non-drinkers in the health intervention tended to score lowest. On the two memory outcome measures, non-drinkers in the memory condition are gaining, but do not quite catch up with the drinkers in this group. The drinkers in the memory intervention decreased their SF-36 Mental Health scores more than the other groups from baseline to end of classes.

DISCUSSION

In national samples, 23% to 31% of older adults have reported consuming moderate amounts of alcohol [5-6], and this result often depends on the type of recruitment site. Of the participants in the SeniorWISE study, 43% of females and 58% of male participants reported drinking moderate amounts of alcohol. Older adults are more likely to engage in moderate regular use of alcohol rather than binge or problem drinking, and the majority of our sample reported similar use patterns [6-7]. The majority (65%) of the non-drinker women in Senior WISE were minorities. As previous research has suggested that Hispanic respondents may underreport drinking, this subgroup may not adequately represent their cohort.

When controlling for age, gender, education, marital status, and race/ethnicity, drinking status was a statistically significant predictor in half the 16 baseline analyses. In all cases, drinkers outperformed non-drinkers. Although few of the interactions between drinking status and intervention group were statistically significant across time, it appears as though the abstainers in the memory group are catching up to the drinkers as a result of the memory intervention, whereas in general, drinkers in the health group seem to benefit more than abstainers in the health group, either in terms of gaining or not declining.

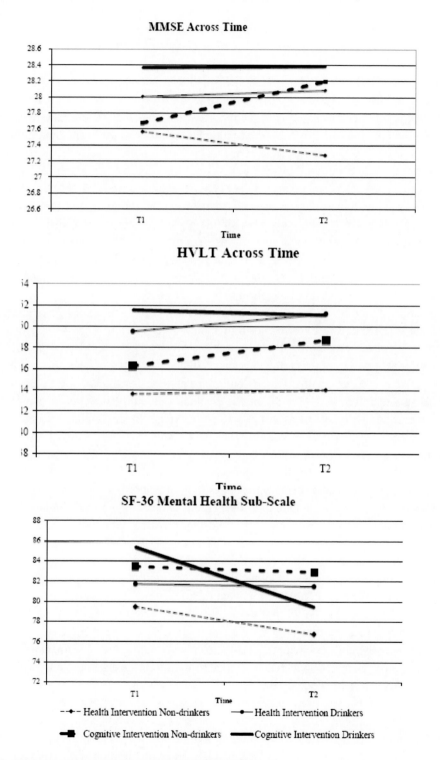

Figure 1. Change over time by group and drinking status.

The SeniorWISE participants scored higher on all subscales of the SF-36 compared with the other community-based elderly [2,24]. However, we should note that previous studies have included clinic samples, whereas our participants were recruited from the community and were living independently. Our findings on health are supported by large-scale national and international samples of older adults whose alcohol consumption was in the moderate range [9-11].

Nationally, 9% to 15%% of moderate drinkers experienced depressive symptoms [5,21]. Among SeniorWISE drinkers, 12% had CES-D scores above 16, the cut-off for depressive symptomatology. Other investigators have reported that abstainers and heavy drinkers were more likely than moderate drinkers to identify symptoms of depression and anxiety [6, 24]. In the current study, 23% of the non-drinkers had CES-D scores above 16.

A major strength of our study was the inclusion of a triethnic sample of minority elderly with 21 (10%) African-Americans, 34 (17%), Hispanics, and 77 (29%) males. The convenience sample was highly motivated to take action for their self-reported memory concerns. Alcohol use was reported with a simple question that was part of the larger health questionnaire, and because an interviewer was administering this measure, there may have been responses that were socially desirable. The participants in this study were a robust group of older adult volunteers with an average age of 75 years with 13 years of education, with many individuals working and volunteering in the community.

A major strength of the SeniorWISE study was the comprehensive cognitive and memory testing battery implemented over twenty-four month study period. Each testing might have taken between two to three hours. Even though previous studies included large samples and longitudinal designs, cognitive function was evaluated in two of the four studies with screening instruments, either the MMSE or the Telephone Instrument for Cognitive Status (TICS) for a general measure of cognition, whereas this study included a comprehensive battery of neuropsychological measures [10-11]. We extend this research by utilizing multiple memory measures, including everyday, verbal, and visual. We noted that the two memory performance measures in which drinkers scored significantly higher than nondrinkers involve the auditory presentation of stimuli. Future research should investigate why drinking status might be more related to some memory measures than to others.

The results of our study could help to deepen our understanding of the value of moderate alcohol consumption for older adults. We found that the affective, cognitive, and functional outcomes did not differ and were therefore not intervention-specific. Neither the drinkers nor the non-drinkers, regardless of their assignment to the health group or to the memory group, tended to improve based on their baseline alcohol consumption. Two studies of community-residing older adults that found differential benefits of training were available for comparison. Losada and colleagues [23] found that the family caregiver group that was taught cognitive behavioral skills rather than problem-solving skills to deal with a relative having dementia reported less stress and behavioral problems. Katula et al [22] demonstrated that a psychological empowerment inter-vention added to traditional strength training had a positive influence on social cognitive outcomes.

Our study extends the empirical support that psychosocial interventions targeted to older adults have demonstrated—namely, that outcomes focused on health promotion, mental stimulation, social engage-ment, and leisure enjoyment may prevent cognitive decline, improve health, and prevent functional decline [12-13,22]. In addition, the SeniorWISE study provides empirical support to the cognitive aging literature, emphasizing the health benefits of moderate alcohol consumption in older adults.

ACKNOWLEDGMENTS

The study was supported by Grant R01 AG15384 from the National Institutes on Aging.

REFERENCES

[1]   Willett W, Stampfer M. Rebuilding the Food Pyramid. *Sci. Am.* 2003; 288(1):64.

[2]   Blow FC. The spectrum of alcohol interventions for older adults. In: Lisansky Gromberg ES Hededus AM, Zucker RA, eds. *Alcohol problems and aging*. Bethesda, MD: US Dept Human Serv, 1998: 373-96.

[3]   McGuire L, Ajani U, Ford E. Cognitive functioning in late life: the impact of moderate alcohol consumption. *Ann. Epidemiol.* 2007; 17(2):93-9.

[4]   Mukamal K, Kuller L, Fitzpatrick A, Longstreth W, Mittleman M, Siscovick D. Prospective study of alcohol consumption and risk of dementia in older adults. *JAMA* 2003;289(11):1405-13.

[5]   Kirchner J, Zubritsky C, Cody M, Coakley E, Chen H, Ware J, et al. Alcohol consumption among older adults in primary care. *J. Gen. Intern. Med* 2007;22(1):92-7.

[6]   Resnick B, Perry D, Applebaum G, Armstrong L, Cotterman M, Dillman S, et al. The impact of alcohol use in community-dwelling older adults. *J. Community Health Nurs* 2003;20(3):135-45.

[7]   Wiscott R, Kopera-Fry K, Bogovic A. Binge drinking in later life: Comparing young-old and old-old social drinkers. *Psychol. Addict. Behav.* 2002;16(3):252-5.

[8]   Blow FC, Walton MA, Barry KL, Coyne JC Mudd SA, Copeland. The relationship between alcohol problems and health functioning of older adults in primary care settings. *J. Am. Geriat Soc.* 2000;48(7):769-74.

[9]   Lindeman R, Wayne S, Baumgartner R, Garry P. Cognitive function in drinkers compared to abstainers in the New Mexico Elder Health Survey. *J. Gerontol. A Bio. Sci. Med. Sci.* 2005;60A(8):1065-70.

[10]   Espeland M, Gu L, Masaki K, Langer R, Coker L, Stefanick M, et al. Association between reported alcohol intake and cognition: results from the Women's Health Initiative Memory Study. *Am. J. Epidemiol.* 2005;161(3):228-38.

[11]   Stampfer M, Kang J, Chen J, Cherry R, Grodstein F. Effects of moderate alcohol consumption on cognitive function in women. *New Engl. J. Med.* 2005;352(3):245-53.

[12]   Cattan M, White M, Bond J, Learmouth A. Preventing social isolation and loneliness among older people: a systematic review of health promotion interventions. *Ageing Soc* 2005; 25(1):41-67.

[13]   Phelan E, Williams B, Penninx B, LoGerfo J, Leveille S. Activities of daily living function and disability in older adults in a randomized trial of the health enhancement program. *J. Gerontol. A Bio. Sci. Med. Sci.* 2004;59(8):838-43.

[14] Willis S, Tennstedt S, Marsiske M, Ball K, Elias J, Koepke K, et al. Long-term effects of cognitive training on everyday functional outcomes in older adults. *JAMA* 2006;296(23):2805-14.

[15] McDougall GJ, Becker H, Pituch K, Vaughn PW, Acee TW, Delville CL. The SeniorWISE study: Cognitive training with a triethnic sample of community-residing older adults. *Nur. Res.* (under review).

[16] Anttila T, Helkala EL, Viitanen M, Kareholt I, Fratiglioni L, Winblad B, et al. Alcohol drinking in middle age and subsequent risk of mild cognitive impairment and dementia in old age: a prospective population based study. *BMJ* 2004; 329(7465):539.

[17] Lang I, Guralnik J, Wallace R, Melzer D. What level of alcohol consumption is hazardous for older people? Functioning and mortality in U.S. and English national cohorts. *J. Am. Geriatr. Soc.* 2007;55(1): 49-5.

[18] Helzer JE, Pryzbeck TR. The co-occurrence of alcoholism with other psychiatric disorders in the general population and its impact on treatment. *J. Stud. Alcohol.* 1988;49:219-24.

[19] Moscato B, Russell M, Zielezny M, Bromet E, Egri G, Mudar P, et al. Gender differences in the relation between depressive symptoms and alcohol problems: a longitudinal perspective. *Am. J. Epidemiol.* 1997;146(11):966-74.

[20] Blow F, Brockmann L, Barry K. Role of alcohol in late-life suicide. *Alcohol. Clin. Exp. Res.* 2004; 28(5 Suppl):48S-56S.

[21] Gazmararian J, Baker D, Parker R, Blazer D. A multivariate analysis of factors associated with depression: evaluating the role of health literacy as a potential contributor. *Arch. Intern Med.* 2000; 160(21): 3307-14.

[22] Katula J, Sipe M, Rejeski W, Focht B. Strength training in older adults: an empowering inter-vention. *Med. Sci. Sport Exer.* 2006; 38(1):106-11.

[23] Losada Baltar A, Izal Fernández de Trocóniz M, Montorio Cerrato I, Márquez González M, Pérez Rojo G. [Differential efficacy of two psychoedu-cational interventions for dementia family caregivers]. *Revista De Neurologia* 2004;38(8):701-8.

[24] Ware JE, Kosinski M, Dewey JE. How to score version 2 of the SF-36 health survey. Lincoln RI: QualityMetric Inc, 2000.

[25] Zimmerman T, McDougall G, Becker H. Older women's cognitive and affective response to moderate drinking. *International J. Geriatr. Psychiat* 2004;19(11):1095-1110.

[26] McDougall GJ, Becker H, Arheart KL. Older adults in the SeniorWISE study at-risk for mild cognitive impairment. Arch. Psychiat. Nurs. 2006; 20(3):126-34.

In: Alcohol-Related Cognitive Disorders   ISBN: 978-1-60741-730-9
Editors: L. Sher, I. Kandel, J. Merrick pp. 291-298   © 2009 Nova Science Publishers, Inc.

Chapter 20

EFFECT OF ALCOHOL ON COGNITIVE FUNCTION

Elisabeth M. Weiss and Josef Marksteiner

ABSTRACT

The aim of this chapter is to discuss how acute and chronic alcohol consumption affects on cognitive functions. In general, greater deficits in executive functions compared with other cognitive functions have been reported in patients suffering from alcohol addiction with deficits in problem solving, abstraction, planning, organizing and working memory. The acute effects of alcohol cause a decline in explicit memory processes. Alcohol impairs memory formation, at least in part, by disrupting activity in the hippocampus. Persisting neuropsychological deficits after cessation of alcohol consumption may lead to alcohol amnestic disorder and dementia associated with alcoholism. Considerable inconsistencies in neuropsychological study results will be discussed referring to variations in methodological designs such as amount of alcohol assumed or length of alcohol abuse. Despite advances in human neuroimaging techniques, detecting clear relations between brain structures and specific cognitive functions has so far been difficult.

INTRODUCTION

Cognitive functions in alcoholism have been investigated extensively in the last years. Without any doubt chronic extensive alcohol drinking leads to distinct cognitive deficits that may lead to permanent cognitive impairment and in the most severe forms, to alcohol-related dementia. These cognitive deficits can arise through the direct toxic effects of alcohol or withdrawal, associated deficiency of vitamins like thiamine, or via cirrhosis of the liver. Only little attention has been paid to date to the question as to how acute and chronic alcohol withdrawal and abstinence affect cognitive functions. Early recovery of the brain through abstinence does not simply reflect rehydration, but particularly the white matter seems to possess genuine capabilities for regrowth [1]. More large scale epidemiologic studies of the potential recovery of neuro-cognitive function in patients suffering from alcohol dependence after long abstinence are warranted.

COGNITION

Frontal Executive Functions

The frontal lobe hypothesis of alcoholism asserts a specific vulnerability of the prefrontal cortex and their connections with other brain regions to the toxic effects of alcohol, supported by findings of neuroimaging studies, neurophysiologic studies, and neuropsychological studies (for a review see [2]. In general, greater deficits in executive functions compared with other cognitive functions have been reported. Therefore, frontal executive deficits are most constantly found, such as deficits in problem solving, abstraction, planning, organizing, and working memory. Additionally, reduced visuospatial functions and slowed processing of information, learning, and memory impairments have been reported [3-5], and a recent study demonstrated that alcoholic patients are using more costly learning strategies, which are nonetheless less efficient [6]. In alcohol-dependent persons, executive dysfunction is among the cognitive impairments that can persist after abstinence. Even more obvious, early in abstinence, both normal and alcohol-dependent groups differ on abstract reasoning, memory discrimination, and effectiveness on timed tasks [7].

Memory Functions

Acute alcohol intoxication disrupts memory acquisition in humans and laboratory animals. Ethanol is known to inhibit long-term potentiation, a putative cellular substrate of memory. Alcohol interferes with establishing long-term potentiation, and this impairment begins at concentrations equivalent to those produced by con-suming just one or two standard drinks [8, 9]. The ability to learn new information is impaired under the influence of alcohol. As the alcohol dose increases, the resulting memory impairments can become much more profound, sometimes culminating in blackout periods [10]. A recent report that cognitive tasks performed by an individual are not similarly affected by rising and declining blood alcohol concentrations suggests that one cerebral hemisphere may be more affected [11]. In healthy subjects, the acute effects of alcohol leads to a decline in explicit memory processes but not in implicit memory processes [12]. The ability to acquire new memories seems to be the phase of the memory process that is affected the most by alcohol consumption. Acute effects of ethanol (0.6 g/kg) have been found on the acquisition of both semantic and figural memory in a sample of young adults from 21 to 29 years [13].

Acheson and colleagues [13] observed that intoxicated subjects could recall items on word lists immediately after the lists were presented but were impaired when asked to recall the items 20 minutes later. Working memory can be relatively preserved because after long-term heavy alcohol consumption, response shifting and inhibition is impaired but not working memory [14]. Non-amnesic patients suffering from alcohol dependence have difficulty in strategically accessing event-specific autobiographical knowledge, which might result from changes in frontal lobe function [15].

Patients with Korsakoff syndrome (see also chapter 17) often have profound deficits in their explicit memory or ability to recall recent events. Patients suffering from alcoholic Korsakoff syndrome have marked remote memory impairment together with characteristic profound anterograde memory deficits. The severity of the remote memory deficit in these patients is not associated with the severity of anterograde memory deficit [16]. Examination of brain structure-function relations in patients suffering from Korsakoff syndrome revealed that photo naming of remote historical information was related to posterior cortical white matter volumes but not hippocampal volumes [16]. A recent study has reported that patients with Korsakoff syndrome retain the ability to learn information that is presented visually, even without a conscious recollection of that learning indicating that implicit memory is at least partially intact [17].

INCONSISTENCY IN NEUROPSYCHOLOGICAL FINDINGS

The neuropsychological findings also differ in the literature, however, ranging from more subtle problems related to impaired executive functions [18-19] to severe amnesia. Such inconsistencies in study results may be due to variations in methodological designs, such as the age of participants, gender, amount of alcohol assumed, length of alcohol abuse, associated medical problems etc. Nevertheless, the approach to explain the discrepancies in test results by including different subgroups of alcoholics that are defined based on one or more of these influencing variables still yielded inconsistent study results. For example, age seemed to be an important modifying variable, with older alcoholic individuals showing more severe cognitive deficits and less recovery of function in early abstinence. Alcohol may accelerate normal aging or cause premature aging of the brain. The premature aging hypothesis evolved from observations of similar cognitive profiles and changes in brain structures in alcoholics and older non-alcoholics [20]. Nevertheless, the hypothesis of pre-mature aging in alcoholics could not be confirmed in other neuropsychological studies [21-22]. Discounting the potential effect of sex differences in alcohol and age-alcohol interactions may account in part for these discrepancies in study results. Other studies aiming at factors causing or influencing the cognitive functions, such as duration of alcohol use, recent alcohol quantity or days of sobriety, could not find a significant association between lifetime alcohol consumption or the total amount of alcohol consumed and cognitive deterioration. Despite the mixed results found in the literature, we can conclude that the brain damage associated with long-term alcoholism can be extensive and that a wide range of variability in the severity and pattern of cognitive impairments exists.

Neuropsychological Differences Due to Gender Differences

Neuropsychological deficits, most notably in executive, visuospatial, and functions of gait and balance, are detectable in alcoholic men even after a month of sobriety. Less well established are the severity and profile of persisting deficits in alcoholic women. In alcoholic women, longer sobriety was associated with larger white matter volumes. Alcoholic men and women show different brain morphological deficits, relative to same sex comparison subjects.

However, age and alcoholism interact in both sexes, placing all older alcoholics at particular risk for the negative sequelae of alcoholism [23]. Women typically start to drink later in life, consume alcohol less frequently and in smaller amounts than men [24-25], and metabolize alcohol differently than men [26-27]. Yet, alcohol dependence seems to develop faster in women than in men [28-30] and sex differences have also been reported in the onset of adverse consequences of alcoholism [31-32]. Furthermore recent studies could demonstrate that brain atrophy also develops faster in women than in men [33-34], and some evidence has been found that female patients have a higher risk for co-morbid psychiatric disorders, such as anxiety and depression—for review see [35-36]. Because of these drinking and pharmacokinetic differences, one hypothesis is that women are especially vulnerable to the toxic effects of alcohol [37-38] leading to comparable cognitive deficits despite less alcohol intake compared with men. No significant associations have been reported between higher levels of drinking (15.0 to 30.0 g per day) and the risk of cognitive impairment or decline in women with moderate alcohol consumption [39], no significant differences in risks according to the beverage, and no interaction with the apolipoprotein E genotype.

The sex differences in cognitive function that appear to be influenced by alcohol consumption are for spatial visualization but not for episodic memory. Whereas men with as few as three drinks per day begin to show cognitive impairment in visuospatial ability, higher performance by women on episodic memory tasks was consistent across all levels of alcohol consumption [40].

SEVERE NEUROPSYCHOLOGICAL DEFICITS—ALCOHOL RELATED DEMENTIA

The diverse signs of severe brain dysfunction that persist after the cessation of alcohol consumption have been conceptualized in terms of two organic mental disorders—alcohol amnestic disorder and dementia associated with alcoholism [41]. Dementia associated with alcoholism consists of global loss of intellectual abilities with impairment in memory function, together with disturbances of abstract thinking, judgment, other higher cortical functions, or personality change without an impairment of consciousness. Oslin et al [42] have proposed validated specific criteria for probable alcohol-related dementia. Recent evidence of a distinct neuropsychological profile for alcohol-related dementia patients includes impairment on both executive control and memory tests. This pattern of performance suggests that long-term alcohol abuse, in comparison with Alzheimer disease or vascular dementia, may be associated with both cortical and subcortical neuro-pathology [42]. Subcortical lesions due to nutritional deficiency have been suggested to be characteristic of Korsakoff syndrome, whereas alcoholic dementia is associated more with cortical changes [43].

Recently however, it has been recognized that these two disorders are not mutually exclusive and that some features of each often coexist in the same patient. Some evidence indicates that a genetic abnormality may predispose certain people to Korsakoff syndrome in the presence of excessive alcohol use and malnutrition [44]. A body of literature suggests a gradual progression of neurocognitive symptoms or a substantial time period of subclinical symptoms in patients with Wernicke-Korsakoff syndrome [45]. Despite the distinctions in terminology between Wernicke-Korsakoff and non-Korsakoff patients within the neuropsychological literature, this distinction may not be justified because many neuropathologists do not make such a differentiation because of the widespread neuropathological changes in alcoholics, regardless of a clinical diagnosis of Wernicke-Korsakoff syndrome [45].

CORRELATION BETWEEN NEUROIMAGING AND NEUROPSYCHOLOGY

In alcohol research, detecting relations between brain structures and specific cognitive functions has so far been difficult. Research conducted using animal models supports the hypothesis that alcohol impairs memory formation, at least in part, by disrupting activity in the hippocampus [46]. Neuroimaging has mainly focused on cortical areas and might not have detected all the brain areas affected by alcohol, as for example brain stem structures. Several neuroimaging studies have recently described global and regional brain atrophy in alcohol dependent patients in both cross-sectional and longitudinal imaging studies [47-49]. The regional reduction of grey matter volumes may result from alcohol induced neuronal loss, whereas global brain shrinkage might be caused by loss of white matter [50]. Voxel-based morphometry based on magnetic resonance imaging suggests the involvement of anterior thalamus, posterior hippocampus, insular cortex and periventricular white matter in alcohol-associated brain damage [51]. In this study, we also found a substantial volume reduction in middle frontal gyrus and precentral gyrus, whereas no changes were detected in other frontal regions. These findings are in line with previous reports on decreased glucose metabolic rates in middle frontal regions in alcohol addicted patients [52] and a reduction of GABAA/benzodiazepine receptors in superior medial parts of the frontal lobes [53]. Executive functions are typically disrupted by lesions of the prefrontal cortex, whereas balance and postural stability are disrupted by lesions of the cerebellum; yet, the cerebellum may also be important for cognitive functions [54]. The characteristic memory deficit of Korsakoff syndrome involves hippocampal and diencephalic pathology [55]. A causal relationship between alcohol consumption and brain regional atrophy and cognition still demands further extensive research.

CONCLUSION

Both acute and chronic alcohol consumption has an impact on cognition. Executive functions are proportionally more severely affected than other cognitive domains. Some evidence suggests that gender has an influence on the individual neuropsychological profile. Future functional studies will further decipher the relation between cognition and brain areas affected by alcohol.

REFERENCES

[1]   Bartsch AJ, Homola G, Biller A, Smith SM, Weijers HG, Wiesbeck GA, et al. Manifestations of early brain recovery associated with abstinence from alcoholism. *Brain* 2007;130:36-47.

[2]   Moselhy HF, Georgiou G, Kahn A. Frontal lobe changes in alcoholism: a review of the literature. *Alcohol Alcohol* 2001;36:357-68.

[3]   Mann K, Gunther A, Stetter F, Ackermann K. Rapid recovery from cognitive deficits in abstinent alcoholics: a controlled test-retest study. *Alcohol Alcohol* 1999;34:567-74.

[4]   Nixon SJ, Tivis RD, Jenkins MR, Parsons OA. Effects of cues on memory in alcoholics and controls. *Alcohol Clin. Exp. Res.* 1998;22:1065-9.

[5]   Parsons OA, Nixon SJ. Cognitive functioning in sober social drinkers: a review of the research since 1986. *J. Stud. Alcohol* 1998;59:180-90.

[6]   Pitel AL, Witkowski T, Vabret F, Guillery-Girard B, Desgranges B, Eustache F, et al. Effect of episodic and working memory impairments on semantic and cognitive procedural learning at alcohol treatment entry. *Alcohol Clin. Exp. Res.* 2007;31:238-48.

[7]   Zinn S, Stein R, Swartzwelder HS. Executive functioning early in abstinence from alcohol. *Alcohol Clin. Exp. Res.* 2004;28:1338-46.

[8]   Pyapali GK, Turner DA, Wilson WA, Swartzwelder HS. Age and dose-dependent effects of ethanol on the induction of hippocampal long-term potentiation. *Alcohol* 1999;19:107-11.

[9]   Schummers J, Bentz S, Browning MD. Ethanol's inhibition of LTP may not be mediated solely via direct effects on the NMDA receptor. *Alcohol Clin. Exp. Res.* 1997;21:404-8.

[10]   Goodwin DW. Alcohol amnesia. *Addiction* 1995;90:315-7.

[11]   Schweizer TA, Vogel-Sprott M, Danckert J, Roy EA, Skakum A, Broderick CE. Neuropsycholo-gical profile of acute alcohol intoxication during ascending and descending blood alcohol concen-trations. *Neuropsychopharmacology* 2006;31:1301-9.

[12]   Lister RG, Gorenstein C, Fisher-Flowers D, Wein-gartner HJ, Eckardt MJ. Dissociation of the acute effects of alcohol on implicit and explicit memory processes. *Neuropsychologia* 1991;29:1205-12.

[13]   Acheson SK, Stein RM, Swartzwelder HS. Impairment of semantic and figural memory by acute ethanol: age-dependent effects. *Alcohol Clin. Exp. Res.* 1998;22:1437-42.

[14]   Hildebrandt H, Brokate B, Eling P, Lanz M. Response shifting and inhibition, but not working memory, are impaired after long-term heavy alcohol consumption. *Neuropsychology* 2004;18:203-11.

[15]   D'Argembeau A, Van der LM, Verbanck P, Noel X. Autobiographical memory in non-amnesic alcohol-dependent patients. *Psychol. Med.* 2006;36: 1707-15.

[16]   Fama R, Marsh L, Sullivan EV. Dissociation of remote and anterograde memory impairment and neural correlates in alcoholic Korsakoff syndrome. *J. Int. Neuropsychol Soc.* 2004;10:427-41.

[17]   Fama R, Pfefferbaum A, Sullivan EV. Visuoper-ceptual learning in alcoholic Korsakoff syndrome. *Alcohol Clin. Exp. Res.* 2006;30:680-7.

[18]   Moriyama Y, Mimura M, Kato M, Yoshino A, Hara T, Kashima H, et al. Executive dysfunction and clinical outcome in chronic alcohol-ics. *Alcohol Clin. Exp. Res.* 2002;26:1239-44.

[19]   Noel X, Van der LM, Schmidt N, Sferrazza R, Hanak C, Le Bon O, et al. Supervisory attentional system in nonamnesic alcoholic men. *Arch. Gen. Psychiatry* 2001;58:1152-8.

[20]   Ryan C, Butters N. Alcohol consumption and pre-mature aging. A critical review. *Recent Dev. Alcohol* 1984;2:223-50.

[21] Sullivan EV, Fama R, Rosenbloom MJ, Pfeffer-baum A. A profile of neuropsychological deficits in alcoholic women. *Neuropsychology* 2002;16: 74-83.

[22] Sullivan EV, Rosenbloom MJ, Pfefferbaum A. Pattern of motor and cognitive deficits in detoxified alcoholic men. *Alcohol Clin. Exp. Res.* 2000;24:611-21.

[23] Pfefferbaum A, Rosenbloom M, Deshmukh A, Sullivan E. Sex differences in the effects of alcohol on brain structure. *Am. J. Psychiatry* 2001;158:188-97.

[24] Elias PK, Elias MF, D'Agostino RB, Silbershatz H, Wolf PA. Alcohol consumption and cognitive performance in the Framingham Heart Study. *Am. J. Epidemiol.* 1999;150:580-9.

[25] Kessler RC, McGonagle KA, Zhao S, Nelson CB, Hughes M, Eshleman S, et al. Lifetime and 12-month prevalence of DSM-III-R psychiatric dis-orders in the United States. Results from the National Comorbidity Survey. *Arch. Gen. Psychiatry* 1994;51:8-19.

[26] Li TK, Beard JD, Orr WE, Kwo PY, Ramchan-dani VA, Thomasson HR. Variation in ethanol pharmacokinetics and perceived gender and ethnic differences in alcohol elimination. *Alcohol Clin. Exp. Res.* 2000;24:415-6.

[27] Lieber CS. Ethnic and gender differences in ethanol metabolism. *Alcohol Clin. Exp. Res.* 2000; 24:417-8.

[28] Mann K, Batra A, Gunthner A, Schroth G. Do women develop alcoholic brain damage more readily than men? *Alcohol Clin. Exp. Res.* 1992; 16:1052-6.

[29] Randall CL, Roberts JS, Del Boca FK, Carroll KM, Connors GJ, Mattson ME. Telescoping of landmark events associated with drinking: a gender com-parison. *J. Stud Alcohol* 1999;60:252-60.

[30] Schuckit MA, Daeppen JB, Tipp JE, Hesselbrock M, Bucholz KK. The clinical course of alcohol-related problems in alcohol dependent and nonalcohol dependent drinking women and men. *J. Stud. Alcohol* 1998;59:581-90.

[31] Fernandez-Sola J, Estruch R, Nicolas JM, Pare JC, Sacanella E, Antunez E, et al. Comparison of alcoholic cardiomyopathy in women versus men. *Am. J. Cardiol.* 1997;80:481-5.

[32] Hesselbrock MN, Meyer RE, Keener JJ. Psychopathology in hospitalized alcoholics. *Arch. Gen. Psychiatry* 1985;42:1050-5.

[33] Hommer D, Momenan R, Kaiser E, Rawlings R. Evidence for a gender-related effect of alcoholism on brain volumes. *Am. J. Psychiatry* 2001;158:198-204.

[34] Mann K, Ackermann K, Croissant B, Mundle G, Nakovics H, Diehl A. Neuroimaging of gender differences in alcohol dependence: are women more vulnerable? *Alcohol Clin. Exp. Res.* 2005; 29:896-901.

[35] Brady KT, Randall CL. Gender differences in substance use disorders. *Psychiatr. Clin. North Am.* 1999;22:241-52.

[36] Davidson KM, Ritson EB. The relationship between alcohol dependence and depression. *Alcohol Alcohol* 1993;28:147-55.

[37] Glenn SW, Parsons OA, Sinha R, Stevens L. The effects of repeated withdrawals from alcohol on the memory of male and female alcoholics. *Alcohol Alcohol* 1988;23:337-42.

[38] Hochla NA, Parsons OA. Premature aging in female alcoholics. A neuropsychological study. *J. Nerv. Ment. Dis.* 1982;170:241-5.

[39] Stampfer MJ, Kang JH, Chen J, Cherry R, Grodstein F. Effects of moderate alcohol con-sumption on cognitive function in women. *N. Engl. J. Med.* 2005;352:245-53.

[40] Yonker JE, Nilsson LG, Herlitz A, Anthenelli RM. Sex differences in spatial visualization and episodic memory as a function of alcohol consumption. *Alcohol Alcohol* 2005;40:201-7.

[41] Lishman WA. Cerebral disorder in alcoholism: syndromes of impairment. *Brain* 1981;104:1-20.

[42] Oslin DW, Cary MS. Alcohol-related dementia: validation of diagnostic criteria. *Am. J. Geriatr. Psychiatry* 2003;11:441-7.

[43] Victor M, Laureno R. Neurologic complications of alcohol abuse: epidemiologic aspects. *Adv. Neurol.* 1978;19:603-17.

[44] Singleton CK, Martin PR. Molecular mechanisms of thiamine utilization. *Curr. Mol. Med.* 2001; 1: 197-207.

[45] Bowden SC. Separating cognitive impairment in neurologically asymptomatic alcoholism from Wernicke-Korsakoff syndrome: is the neuropsy-chological distinction justified? *Psychol Bull* 1990;107:355-66.

[46] White AM, Matthews DB, Best PJ. Ethanol, memory, and hippocampal function: a review of recent findings. *Hippocampus* 2000;10:88-93.

[47] Mann K, Agartz I, Harper C, Shoaf S, Rawlings RR, Momenan R, et al. Neuroimaging in alcoholism: ethanol and brain damage. *Alcohol Clin. Exp. Res.* 2001; 25:104S-9S.

[48] Pfefferbaum A, Sullivan EV, Mathalon DH, Lim KO. Frontal lobe volume loss observed with magnetic resonance imaging in older chronic alcoholics. *Alcohol Clin. Exp. Res.* 1997;21:521-9.

[49] Sullivan EV, Rosenbloom M, Serventi KL, Pfefferbaum A. Effects of age and sex on volumes of the thalamus, pons, and cortex. *Neurobiol Aging* 2004;25:185-92.

[50] Harper C. The neuropathology of alcohol-specific brain damage, or does alcohol damage the brain? *J. Neuropathol Exp. Neurol.* 1998;57:101-10.

[51] Mechtcheriakov S, Brenneis C, Egger K, Koppelstaetter F, Schocke M, Marksteiner J. A wide-spread distinct pattern of cerebral atrophy in patients with alcohol addiction revealed by voxelbased morphometry. *J. Neurol. Neurosurg. Psychiatry* 2007;78(6):610-4.

[52] Adams KM, Gilman S, Koeppe RA, Kluin KJ, Brunberg JA, Dede D, et al. Neuropsychological deficits are correlated with frontal hypometabolism in positron emission tomography studies of older alcoholic patients. *Alcohol Clin. Exp. Res.* 1993;17:205-10.

[53] Gilman S, Koeppe RA, Adams K, Johnson-Greene D, Junck L, Kluin KJ, et al. Positron emission tomographic studies of cerebral benzodiazepine-receptor binding in chronic alcoholics. *Ann. Neurol.* 1996;40:163-71.

[54] Sullivan EV, Harding AJ, Pentney R, Dlugos C, Martin PR, Parks MH, et al. Disruption of frontocerebellar circuitry and function in alcoholism. *Alcohol Clin. Exp. Res.* 2003;27:301-9.

[55] Sullivan EV, Marsh L. Hippocampal volume deficits in alcoholic Korsakoff's syndrome. *Neurology* 2003; 61:1716-9.

In: Alcohol-Related Cognitive Disorders   ISBN: 978-1-60741-730-9
Editors: L. Sher, I. Kandel, J. Merrick pp. 299-317   © 2009 Nova Science Publishers, Inc.

Chapter 21

ALCOHOL AND HUMAN IMMUNODEFICIENCY VIRUS (HIV) INFECTION

Ramani S. Durvasula

ABSTRACT

Both human immunodeficiency virus (HIV) and alcohol use contribute to neuropsychological (NP) impairment, and a relatively large proportion of HIV seropositive individuals have histories of heavy alcohol use. Evidence from neuropathological, and both structural and functional neuroimaging studies have supported the direct central nervous system effects of both HIV and alcohol. HIV preferentially affects frontal regions of the brain as well as subcortical structures including the basal ganglia, while alcohol has been shown to result in cortical atrophy and cerebellar and frontal damage. These central nervous system changes are clinically manifested through psychomotor slowing, memory impairments, slowed reaction time, and executive dysfunction in persons with HIV. Alcohol use and abuse are associated with similar deficits as well as dysfunction in domains including visuoperception. While some studies have observed a synergistic effect between alcohol and HIV on NP performance, particularly reaction time, this has not been consistent. Whether HIV and alcohol exert purely independent, additive or interactive NP effects remains unresolved, and this may in part be due to methodological issues inherent in the measurement of alcohol use, comorbidities such as substance use, and other co-factors, such as socioeconomic status and neurologic history. The picture of NP decline due to HIV continues to evolve in the era of highly active antiretroviral therapy (HAART), and it is still unclear whether such changes will mitigate the impact of alcohol on NP functioning in persons with HIV.

INTRODUCTION

Alcohol use and abuse play numerous roles in the transmission, pathogenesis, and clinical manifestations of human immunodeficiency virus (HIV) infection. Mounting evidence points to the role of alcohol as a contributor to sexual risk behaviors, and in those infected with HIV, alcohol can have direct and indirect effects on host susceptibility, viral replication, and immunosuppression [1]. Alcohol use has been shown to be associated with increased susceptibility to infectious diseases including sepsis and tuberculosis (TB) and can deleteriously impact nutritional status, which in turn, can heighten the vulnerability to opportunistic infections and other acquired immune deficiency syndrome (AIDS)-related complications [1]. The rates of alcohol use in HIV-infected populations and in those at highest risk for HIV (e.g. men who have sex with men [MSM], injection drug users) are higher than expected, and new infections are rematerializing in cohorts having higher rates of drug and alcohol use and riskier lifestyles [1-3]. Within cohorts of alcohol abusers, the rates of HIV are higher than for the general population [4]. In a sample of HIV-seropositive men and women recruited into an ongoing study of psychiatric disorder and health behaviors, 6% had a current diagnosis of alcohol abuse/ dependence however and 55% had a lifetime history of either alcohol abuse or dependence [5]. Alcohol use can serve as a risk factor for HIV transmission as intoxication may diminish the likelihood of engaging in safer sexual practices like condom use.

Alcohol abuse can lead to increased systemic immune dysfunction in HIV-seropositive individuals via immune suppression [6]. Wang and Watson [7] reviewed animal and human studies and concluded that in animals, alcohol can serve as a cofactor in the development of AIDS. In humans, however, such findings are not yet conclusive. Even when controlling for adherence to highly active anti-retroviral therapy (HAART), HIV-seropositive individuals with alcohol abuse histories have lower CD4+ T-cell counts and higher HIV RNA levels do than non-drinkers [8]. Such differences could be attribu-table to faster disease progression, faster therapeutic efficacy of HAART in HIV-seropositive alcohol abusers, or some combination of these conditions.

HIV and Neuropsychological Performance

The direct and deleterious effects of HIV infection on the central nervous system (CNS) have been documented by numerous sources [9-10]. Early studies of neuropathological change in persons with AIDS revealed that nearly 75% evidenced some CNS damage [11]. Magnetic resonance imaging (MRI) reveals mild atrophy in asymptomatic HIV-seropositive individuals, although in those with HIV associated dementia or with more advanced illness, brain volume loss in white matter, temporal regions, basal ganglia, posterior cortex, and caudate are observed. Magnetic resonance spectro-scopy (MRS) reveals lower n-acetyl-aspartate levels, particularly in frontal white matter, in persons with HIV-related cognitive impairment. Taken together, neuroimaging and neuropathological studies reveal that HIV preferentially affects the basal ganglia, white matter, and cortex.

HIV-associated neuropsychological (NP) dysfunc-tion is exerted via two general mechanisms: (a) immunocompromise engendered by HIV renders the patient more vulnerable to opportunistic infections of the CNS, such as toxoplasmosis; (b) HIV exerts direct effects on the CNS with accompanying symptomatology ranging from mild neurocognitive dysfunction to full dementia. Generally, the severity of the NP deficits observed in HIV increases with disease progression and typically, greater NP impairment is observed in persons with AIDS when compared with those who are HIV-seropositive but asymptomatic or who are seronegative.

The American Academy of Neurology (AAN) AIDS Task Force, in conjunction with other scientific advisory groups, including the World Heath Organization (WHO), developed consensus nomenclature for research purposes. The AAN distinguishes the subtypes of HIV-related neurobehavioral disorders based on severity. HIV-associated dementia complex (HADC), and HIV-associated minor cognitive-motor disorder (MCMD) can be viewed on a continuum, and both are characterized by psychomotor and motor slowing, memory decrements, increased reaction time, deficits in information processing, attentional impairments, and by executive dysfunction, with the symptomatology observed in HIV-associated dementia being more severe and pronounced than that observed in HIV-associated cognitive motor disorder. In addition, in HADC, the NP impairment results in greater disruption in social and occupational function. The onset of dementia is usually a poor prognostic sign in HIV disease and is often predictive of approaching mortality. A third category labeled subsyndromic neuro-cognitive compromise or asymptomatic neurocognitive impairment can be used to describe the subtle cognitive irregularities that do not adversely impact functioning. Each of the three variants becomes more prevalent with greater disease progression. However, a fourth classification or stage recently has been included—NP deficits. This stage is categorized as pre-asymptomatic NP impairment with some abnormality or change in one cognitive ability area [12].

The HADC is rare among medically asymptomatic (CDC Stage A) individuals, but may be seen in 5% to 10% of those with AIDS (13). The MCMD is more prevalent among persons with more advanced disease (CDC Stages B and C), but can be seen in a subset of asymptomatic individuals. Such qualifiers as probable and possible are also used to express the degree of diagnostic certainty. A diagnosis of HADC or HAM is sufficient for a diagnosis of AIDS.

The American Psychiatric Association included dementia due to HIV disease in the 4th edition of the Diagnostic and Statistical Manual of Mental Disorders (DSM) (14). Unfortunately, the DSM-IV criteria for this syndrome are modeled after the criteria for Alzheimer's disease and place a heavy emphasis on cortical abnormalities, such as apraxia and aphasia, symptoma-tology that is typically inconsistent with the charac-teristic NP sequelae of HIV infection. Most clinicians and researchers who work with HIV-infected patients prefer the AAN diagnostic criteria because they better capture the varying severity of HIV-associated cognitive impairment, and the subsequent subdivisions of the clinical conditions (e.g. HADC, MCMD) are more useful. In addition, the AAN criteria address better the subcortical nature of the disorder through the inclusion of such diagnostic criteria as attentional impairment and cognitive slowing—key symptomatology that is not included in the DSM-IV criteria.

Among HIV-infected persons, NP complications that are not a direct consequence of the virus can arise. Medical co-morbidities (e.g. hepatitis C), secondary opportunistic infections of the CNS, and other neurological conditions (e.g. stroke, seizure disorder) can have a deleterious impact on NP performance in persons with HIV, and such complications are more common among HIV-seropositive than in HIV-seronegative individuals. Studies of NP performance in HIV use varied inclusion/exclusion criteria, and how well such studies screen or account for these co-factors is unclear. To definitively diagnose cognitive dysfunction as HIV-associated, one must be confident that the acquired change in cognitive functioning following infection cannot be explained by other causes.

Alcohol Use and Neuropsychological Performance

Neuropathological studies reveal that at autopsy, the brains of chronic alcoholics are smaller and evidence greater atrophy [11]. Two basic types of cortical damage from alcohol use are observed—neuronal loss in the frontal cortex and global neuronal shrinkage—and white matter reduction is observed as well [15]. Specific regions of neuronal loss include the superior frontal association cortex, hypothalamus, and cerebellum, and dendritic shrinkage has been documented [15]. Reductions in thalamic volume have been observed in chronic alcoholics, with white matter abnormalities in other subcortical structures, including the cerebellar vermis, mammilary bodies, hippocampus, and corpus callosum [15].

The thiamine deficiency observed in chronic alcoholics can lead to the severe cognitive impairment observed in Wernicke-Korsakoff syndrome, and can also contribute to myelin loss. Structural neuroimaging in chronic alcoholics has revealed white matter volume reduction, cortical loss in the frontal lobe, thinning of the corpus callosum, loss of temporal lobe white matter, hippocampal volume loss, and cerebellar changes (see Pfefferbaum et al [16] for review). Longitudinal studies have shown a recovery of cortical white matter volume following abstinence [17]. Proton MRS in alcoholics has shown reduced N-acetylaspartate (NAA) in both frontal and cerebellar regions as compared with controls [18]. Such MRS changes have also been observed following periods of abstinence, with increased NAA/Choline (Cho) (likely decreased Cho) following abstinence [19].

Magnetic resonance spectroscopy imaging (MRSI) was used to examine alcoholism and HIV and both were found to act interactively to have an impact on brain metabolism. An examination of NAA, creatine (Cr), and Cho in the parieto-occipital cortex revealed that only those with both HIV and alcoholism showed significant effects, with nearly one standard deviation deficits on NAA and Cr, deficits that were independent of the effects of HAART. Neither HIV nor alcohol operated inde-pendently to result in metabolic abnormalities [20].

Diffusion tenor imaging (DTI) is a newer imaging technique that provides quantitative data on the co-herence, orientation, and connectivity of white matter bundles and microstructure—for an excellent review of this and other imaging techniques please refer to Pfefferbaum et al (2002) [16]. The few studies employing this technique with alcohol abusers have found changes in white matter tracts and support the hypothesis that such disruption in white matter microstructure may be a contributor to attentional and working memory disturbances in alcoholism.

The adverse NP consequences of alcohol abuse and dependence are well documented, and congruent with the neuropathological findings of cortical (particularly frontal) and cerebellar damage. Mild to moderate NP deficits have been observed in individuals with histories of alcohol dependence [21]. Deficits are typically observed in attention, visuospatial functioning, executive functioning, and in learning and memory [22]. Even after a period of abstinence, deficits in problem solving, short-term memory, visuospatial functioning, and motor skills persist [23]. Studies that combined imaging techniques with NP testing have described differences in functional activation in alcoholics when performing working memory tasks, which may speak to a re-organization of brain systems due to alcohol use [16]. Similar findings were obtained by Tapert et al [24], who described reduced frontal activation during a working memory task in alcoholics.

Using a twist on the Stroop paradigm, Schulte et al [25] found that the HIV-positive/alcoholism-positive group evidenced greater impairment in the processing of conflicted inputs and in attentional allocation, findings that are consistent with fronto-parietal disruption. Such impairments were more pronounced in the combined HIV/alcoholism group than conferred by either HIV or alcoholism alone. A wide spectrum of effects as a function of alcohol abuse has been reported, with effects on memory ranging from temporary short-term memory deficits in social drinkers to an anterograde amnestic syndrome in chronic alcohol abusers [26]. A recent study examining memory deficits and executive function observed that among recently detoxified alcohol abusers, episodic memory deficits are more prevalent than among control subjects, and that such deficits are not solely attributable to executive dysfunction [27]. Electrophysiological evidence of working memory deficits in alcohol abusers has also been provided. Using event-related potential (ERP) techniques, researchers have found that alcoholics make more errors and have longer response times when compared with controls [28].

Studies that have examined the combined abuse of alcohol and drugs on cognitive functioning have yielded mixed results. In general, and particularly in HIV infected cohorts, alcohol and drug use are commonly confounded, making it difficult to draw definitive conclusions about the contribution of either in isolation. In a study comparing the performance of alcoholics and poly-substance abusers, cocaine abusers with concurrent alcohol abuse performed more poorly on measures of learning and recall relative to alcoholics without concomitant cocaine abuse. Beatty, Blanco, Hames and Nixon [29] examined spatial cognition in alcohol abusers both with and without concurrent abuse of other substances, and found that both polysubstance abusers (alcohol plus drugs) and alcohol abusers evidenced deficits in visuospatial perception, construction, and learning and memory.

The results of that study suggest that drug abuse may not confer additional risk for NP dysfunction above and beyond that attributable to alcohol abuse or may do so only in a subset of heavy drinkers.

Numerous studies to date have investigated the synergistic effects of psychoactive drugs and HIV on disease progression and NP functioning [30]. Such studies, which have largely examined the independent and interactive effects of heroin and cocaine abuse on NP functioning, have yielded mixed results, and most studies were conducted with injection drug users. Basso and Bornstein [31] examined the interactive effects of past non-injection drug abuse and HIV. As expected, the investigators obtained the main effects for HIV, with an AIDS diagnosis being associated with poorer NP performance, yet they found no effects for a history of drug abuse on executive function or working memory. To date, few studies have focused on whether HIV and alcohol consumption operate synergistically to produce more marked cognitive impairment in HIV-infected samples. This oversight is noteworthy, given the relatively high rates of alcohol abuse and alcohol dependence among HIV positive individuals.

Alcohol, HIV and Neuropsychological Function

Given the independent contributions of alcohol and HIV to NP decline, the potential for additive or multiplicative effects of alcohol and HIV on NP performance warrants further examination. Several convergent lines of neuro-pathological, structural, metabolic, and NP evidence indicate that HIV and alcohol have both shared and separate effects on the CNS. Alcohol use preferentially affects frontal and parietal regions, as well as white matter, basal ganglia, and cerebellum, whereas HIV has a greater affinity for periventricular and supraventricular white matter, and basal ganglia, with evidence also pointing to HIV effects on frontal and parietal regions [11]. As such, HIV-seropositive persons having current and/or past histories of chronic alcohol use or abuse are most likely to evidence damage and the associated NP deficits on central white matter, sub-cortical structures, and frontal cortex [11]. A magnetic resonance spectroscopy (MRS) study of 15 alcohol abusing HIV-seropositive men and 23 HIV-seronegative controls revealed an interactive effect of alcohol and HIV on N-acetylaspartate (NAA) and creatine (Cr), with the HIV-positive alcohol-positive group revealing significant deficits in both NAA and Cr, but no independent effect of alcohol or HIV alone, and no beneficial effect of HAART.

The precise mechanism by which HIV enters the CNS is not clear, although evidence of the ability of HIV to penetrate the blood brain barrier (BBB) has been reported. As such, examining the factors that can diminish the integrity of the BBB could reveal mechanisms by which neurotoxic agents like alcohol could exert additional CNS effects in persons infected with HIV. Bryant [1] describes several studies that highlight the multiple putative mechanisms by which alcohol can magnify the CNS effects of HIV, including the effects of alcohol on the blood brain barrier, augmented expression of pro-inflammatory cytokines, effects of membrane permeability, and viral replication.

Electrophysiological studies examining chronic alcohol abuse and HIV infection on the frontal cortex using the auditory P3A evoked potential revealed that HIV infection and active chronic alcohol abuse results in a lengthening of the P3A latency in a novel non-target condition, and that alcohol abuse worsens the P3A latency effect of HIV disease [32]. The results suggest deleterious effects of alcohol on the functioning of the frontal cortex. In another study, auditory and spatial P3A latency increased with the progression of HIV-associated cognitive impairments in the auditory and spatial modalities, respectively, and P3A latency indicated an additive effect of comorbid alcohol abuse and HIV infection [33]. In HIV-seropositive persons who were light drinkers or who abstained from alcohol use, P3A latency delays occurred primarily in subjects with more advanced disease, whereas in HIV-sero-positive chronic heavy drinkers, P3A latency delays occurred even in asymptomatic seropositive subjects.

Meyerhoff et al [18] described the effects of HIV and chronic alcohol abuse on brain phosphorous metabolites and reported cumulative decreases in white matter concentrations of phosphodiester and phospho-creatine in HIV-seropositive alcoholics compared with HIV-seronegative light/non-drinkers and HIV-seronegative alcoholics. In addition, the authors reported relatively lower concentrations of gray matter phospho-diester in alcoholics with AIDS compared with HIV-seronegative nondrinkers.

The chronic use of alcohol in persons with HIV can augment metabolic injury in the CNS. Animal studies examining the controlled administration of ethanol in simian immunodeficiency virus (SIV)-infected rhesus monkeys reveal an interactive effect of alcohol and the immunodeficiency virus, with decreased accuracy of responding in an acquisition/learning task in SIV-infected monkeys that were administered ethanol [34]. Taken together, both metabolic and electrophysiological studies, as well as animal studies of alcohol and HIV on CNS function suggest cumulative effects. In addition, the impact of normal aging must also be considered, particularly because the HIV-infected populations are getting older with the benefit of HAART. To this end, it is likely that areas of the brain and the associated NP domains that are affected by the confluence of HIV, alcohol and aging (e.g. frontal regions, subcortical structures) will show the greatest deterioration in HIV-seropositive alcohol abusers [16].

The NP studies of the effects of alcohol use and HIV have described both independent and interactive effects. In a study conducted during the pre-HAART era, examination of 497 African American men revealed an interactive effect between HIV and alcohol use on NP functioning [35]. The results revealed that HIV seropositive persons who reported the heaviest levels of alcohol consumption during the 12 month period before the assessment evidenced the slowest performance on measures of psychomotor speed, motor speed, and computerized reaction time—domains that are prefer-entially affected by both HIV and alcohol use. In addition, the main effects for HIV serostatus (with HIV seropositive individuals performing worse) were obtained on a computerized measure of reaction time, yet, no main effects of alcohol use were obtained. Unfortunately, no diagnostic measures of alcohol abuse/dependence were available for this cohort, nor were lifetime measures of alcohol use. In addition, the scale used to measure alcohol use was relatively crude (average number of drinks per week). Nonetheless, the findings support the likelihood that alcohol and HIV operate synergistically to have a deleterious impact on NP function.

Another study examining a subset of men from the same cohort (N = 237), which focused on cocaine use and NP function, found no independent or interactive impact of cocaine use on NP performance [30]. The NP studies of HIV infected cohorts raise some important methodological issues because ascertaining an HIV-seropositive cohort comprising persons who endorse ONLY alcohol use is very difficult, and considering the impact of other neurotoxic drugs of abuse, such as cocaine and methamphetamine, can snarl the ability to accurately target the true independent effects of alcohol. It is likely that our findings for alcohol may have been augmented by the presence of heavy cocaine use in a subset of persons in the sample. Future studies that will undertake far more careful assessment of use AND abuse of alcohol and other drugs of abuse are needed to understand better these complex issues.

Rothlind et al [36] examined a sample of 268 HIV-seronegative and HIV-seronegative adults. The groups were stratified by serostatus and level of drinking (light/ non drinkers and heavy drinkers (more than 100 drinks per month). The authors further subdivided the heavy drinkers into those who drank more than six drinks per day. Although Rothlind did not obtain results suggestive of a synergistic effect between alcohol use and HIV on neurocognition, contrasts comparing HIV-seropositive heavy drinkers and HIV-seronegative light drinkers revealed the most pronounced differences on measures of working memory, visual attention, and motor and psychomotor speed. In addition, the investigators observed greater effects of alcohol on executive function and motor balance and of HIV on processing speed. Their findings suggest that in general, the co-presence of alcohol and HIV is associated with poorer NP performance than is either factor singularly. Regardless of the level of alcohol consumption, better NP function was observed in HIV seropositive persons receiving HAART and among those with a lower viral load. A strength of their study lies in their attempt to understand the impact of NP function and alcohol use on medication adherence, and the authors observed that executive functioning as well as heavy alcohol use are associated with adherence.

The interactive effects of alcohol and HIV on a test of psychomotor speed, which also provided indices of sustained attention, associative learning, and incidental learning, have also been described. Sassoon et al [37] examined 44 alcohol dependent HIV-seronegative subjects, 43 HIV seropositive subjects (no alcohol dependence), 55 alcohol dependent HIV seropositive subjects, and 49 normal controls. Although the authors found no main effect for alcohol dependence or HIV serostatus, they found a greater likelihood of impaired performance on psychomotor speed in the alcohol-dependent HIV-seropositive group.

Green, Saveanu and Bornstein [38] examined a smaller sample (N = 80) of HIV-seropositive and HIV-seronegative men, which was relatively homogenous with respect to past alcohol use histories. Their sample comprised men who were engaged in stable, light-moderate levels of current alcohol use. In contrast to the findings obtained by Durvasula et al [35], Green and coworkers obtained independent effects of HIV and a previous history of alcohol abuse, but no interaction. As expected, main effects for alcohol were observed on measures of verbal reasoning, auditory processing, reaction time, verbal IQ and a summary index of NP impairment, whereas the main effects for HIV were noted on measures of learning and memory and motor speed. Green et al suggest that even in current light-moderate users of alcohol, a history of past alcohol abuse may engender a vulnerability that exacerbates the NP effects of HIV. The authors raise the idea of HIV acting as a "second disease state"— that although chronic alcohol abuse is typically not sufficient to result in substantial cognitive impairment in young men, the addition of this second disease state (HIV) may con-tribute to cognitive deficits. A possible mechanism for this effect may be an irreversible neuropathologic change brought about by alcohol abuse that can persist even after alcohol intake is reduced. In general, authors examining alcohol and HIV have suggested that alcohol abuse can contribute to the onset of NP impairments, with one study revealing that the relative risk of dementia was nearly six times higher in HIV-seropositive persons having a history of alcohol abuse/dependence [39]. Not all investigators have obtained results that support the additive effects of alcohol use on NP impairment in HIV-seropositive samples [40]; these studies, however, often employed more stringent inclusion criteria (e.g. including only persons with mild histories of current recreational drug or alcohol use).

Variously the results of such studies suggest both independent and interactive effects of HIV and alcohol on NP functioning. These effects may represent the influence of independent mechanisms on CNS structure and function or may represent a heightened vulner-ability engendered by one neurotoxic agent (e.g. alcohol—particularly if predating infection) which creates a greater vulnerability to NP dysfunction in the face of the second neurotoxic agent. As such, possibly heavy alcohol use or diagnostic alcohol abuse/ dependence can decrease cognitive reserve, resulting in a more rapid deterioration of NP performance with the advent of HIV infection [41]. Fein and DiSclafani [41] examined the contribution of alcohol and drug use to functional brain reserve. The authors highlight that often a hereditary component to substance use disorders is present, and as such, many persons who are alcohol abusers had at least one alcohol abusing parent, which could have a deleterious impact on cerebral reserve via the teratogenic effects of alcohol use, as well as through the environmental effects of drug and alcohol use. Drug and alcohol use are often accompanied by poverty, which is a marker for poor health care, education, and exposure to violence and trauma.

In heavy drinkers, cerebellar degeneration can contribute to difficulties with motor control and coor-dination dysfunction, which can be exacerbated in HIV [21]. Rothlind et al [36] suggest that the confluence of HIV-associated subcortical dysfunction and alcohol associated cerebellar and cerebral dysfunction contribute to decrements in complex attention, working memory, sequencing, timing, and motor control. In addition, both alcohol use and

HIV can render the CNS vulnerable to sensory and motor neuropathies that can also affect performance in such domains.

HIV, Alcohol, HAART Adherence and NP Performance

Adherence to HAART has been a critical issue in the management of HIV and AIDS. Suboptimal adherence to HAART has been found to contribute to treatment failure and to the development of resistant viral strains. A number of factors, including psychiatric disorder, low SES, poor knowledge, and health-related cognitions have been cited as contributors to poor adherence. In addition, NP dysfunction, particularly executive dys-function and drug and alcohol use, have been consistently cited as predictors of HAART adherence [42]. A reciprocal relation may be at play here as adherence may also represent a putative mechanism for alcohol and HIV-associated NP decrements. Both alcohol use and HIV contribute to NP decrements, which can then have an adverse impact on medication adherence and, in turn, result in more rapid disease progression, a greater likelihood of viremia, and subsequently, even poorer NP outcomes [36]. An interruption in HAART adherence due to alcohol use can lead to the discontinuation of HAART, which can contribute to development of viral resistance and more rapid disease progression [43].

Little work has examined the combined NP effects of HIV and alcohol in a systematic way in the post-HAART era. Sassoon et al [37] found interactive effects between alcohol and HIV on NP function in a sample of persons comprising a large proportion of HAART users. The investigators compared NP performance between HIV seropositives using and not using HAART and found no differences. Alcohol use can have a negative impact on HAART through a number of mechanisms as alcohol can directly harm adherence or can negatively impact metabolism and therapeutic levels of HAART. This situation can facilitate disease progression and increase the likelihood of NP impairments [11]. Other reports, however, have suggested that heavy drinking does not change the efficacy of HAART [44].

The progressive nature of HIV-related cognitive decline has been described, with greater disease progression associated with greater NP decrements. Typically, significant cognitive impairment is not observed until the advent of symptomatic illness or diagnosis with AIDS. As such, the impact of alcohol on immunologic parameters and the progression of HIV infection may translate into a greater propensity for the development of NP decline and deficits in HIV-seropositive persons who use alcohol. Alcohol has been associated with greater HIV replication in cell culture [6]. The findings also suggest that alcohol consumption can increase the vulnerability to becoming infected with HIV, and that even a single drinking event can depress the immune responses of white blood cells.

Other immunologic parameters affected by alcohol use include fewer tumor necrosis factor receptors on cytokine release, the immune response, simulated macrophages, oxidative stress, the depletion of lympho-cytes, and changes in host mechanisms and the specific immune response [7]. Animal models suggest that alcohol consumption has a negative impact on periph-eral immune function, with alcohol-exposed animals progressing from initial viral infection to an AIDS-comparable condition or death [11]. Taken together, both animal and human models suggest that alcohol use can increase host susceptibility to infectious disease and subsequent progression to AIDS [7]. Other studies, however, have failed to find evidence that chronic drinking influences the rate and progression of HIV infection [45] or NP functioning in HIV-infected individuals [46]. Penkower et al [47] investigated the patterns of change in alcohol consumption as well as the frequency and amount of alcohol consumption in HIV-seropositive men who were followed for approximately 6 years. The level of drinking at study entry was not associated with CD4+ cell counts and/or the develop-ment of AIDS-related symptoms at the final study visit. The authors suggested that the immunosuppressive effects of alcohol use may be overwhelmed by the immunosuppressive effects of the HIV-initiated cascade.

Neuropsychological Assessment of HIV Associated Cognitive Decline

Given that the cardinal symptoms of HIV-associated cognitive impairment are psychomotor and motor slowing, reaction time deficits, memory impairment, and executive dysfunction, test batteries that include multiple measures of these domains are optimal. To date, no single "test" has emerged that can diagnose dementia, although screening measures, such as the HIV Dementia Rating Scale (HDS), can be used to ascertain the need for further assessment. The HDS consists of four brief subtests and has low sensitivity and modest specificity. The measures of psychomotor speed that assess divided attention (e.g. Trail Making Test Part B) are often the most sensitive to the types of impairments observed in persons with HIV. Computerized reaction time tasks are very sensitive to the types of slowed processing observed in HIV, and may be useful with asymptomatic patients for whom NP deficits are likely to be quite subtle. Memory assessment must include measurement of delayed recall as this subset of memory is most profoundly affected, particularly relative to tests that assess recognition. In addition, the assessment of memory should optimally include both verbal and non-verbal measures. The assessment of executive functioning should incorporate measures of set shifting and hypo-thesis formation (e.g. Wisconsin Card Sorting Test), abstraction (e.g. Wechsler Adult Intelligence Scale (WAIS) Similarities) and inhibition (e.g. Stroop Inter-ference Trial).

A detailed clinical interview assessing demographic information, psychiatric history, medical history (particularly neurologic history, current and past drug and alcohol use, current medications, social and occupational history and any functional impairments or ecological manifestations of NP dysfunction) should also be employed. Records on viral load, CD4+ T cells, history of CNS opportunistic infections, and antiretro-viral regimen is also critical when conducting such assessment and diagnosis.

When working with patients or cohorts in whom comorbid alcohol use is at issue, the supplementation of a battery geared toward HIV should be considered. Although some overlap is found in affected domains (e.g. memory, reaction time), certain areas of NP performance are preferentially affected by alcohol use (e.g. visuospatial functioning, visual memory), and the addition of tests that also assess these domains is important. The NP tests are only as good as the norms against which they are interpreted. Whereas certain tests and batteries have well validated norms based on large cohorts stratified by race, age, and education, this condition is not true with all tests. Incumbent on the researcher or clinician is to ensure that the norms being employed sufficiently represent the patient or sample of interest to avoid the under- or over-diagnosis of cognitive impairment.

The National Institute of Mental Health (NIMH) Workgroup on Neuropsychological Assessment Approaches proposed a battery of tests that not only provides a comprehensive assessment of the types of subtle neurocognitive changes observed secondary to HIV, but also detects any focal CNS disturbances, such as opportunistic infections or neoplasms. The proposed battery includes an assessment of the following domains (a) premorbid intelligence; (b) attention; (c) speed of processing; (d) memory; (e) abstraction; (f) language; (g) visuospatial; (h) construction abilities; (i) motor abilities; (j) psychiatric assessment. In the clinical arena, patient history and presenting complaints will guide the clinician to the types and number of tests to use within each of these domains.

Methodological Issues in the Study of Alcohol, HIV, and NP

Overall, whereas some evidence still exists suggesting an interactive effect of alcohol and HIV on NP functioning, this effect has not been consistently observed. A primary contributor to this inconsistency is the difficulty in accurately measuring alcohol use. Numerous indices of consumption and alcohol use are variously employed (number of standard drinks per week, diagnostic abuse or dependence, breathalyzer measurements, average number of drinks per day). Depending on the index employed, different studies have obtained variable findings.

The measures of consumption (e.g. number of drinks per week, number of drinking events) are often inconsistent because alcohol use can be variable, and recall is often quite poor. In addition, whereas most researchers employ "standard drink" measures, even the use of such metrics does not sufficiently address the variability in drinking habits over time. The use of such diagnostic measures as the SCID-I or the PRISM to capture alcohol abuse or dependence often results in greater reliability, yet, the use of such groupings can often miss the relatively heavy drinkers who do not otherwise meet diagnostic criteria. Lifetime histories of alcohol use also contribute to measurement error. The finding that the duration of alcohol use contributes to the severity of NP deficits resulting from alcohol use has been well-documented. Uneven drinking patterns, periods of abstinence, binge drinking periods, and poor recall for past drinking habits result in tremendous heterogeneity within cohorts. As a result, groups that are often treated as "uniform" (e.g. persons who meet the diagnostic criteria for alcohol dependence) often have varied histories that can introduce significant within group error, diminish power, and delimit the ability to draw meaningful conclusions. In addition, persons who are currently abstinent may have histories punctuated by very heavy alcohol use. Most investigators are limited by methodological issues like sample size when attempting to create subgroups on the basis of current drinking habits, current diagnosis, and past histories.

In addition to diagnostic measures and quantity/ frequency indices, such measures as the CAGE and the MAST examine not only the frequency of drinking but also impairments secondary to drinking. Such instru-ments provide a more efficient means of identifying "problem drinking" but are also vulnerable to errors in recall and differential drinking histories. Breathalyzers provide a far more objective index of recent alcohol use, but shed light only on very recent alcohol use and do not assess past or even relatively recent drinking behavior—both of which are critical parameters in understanding NP performance. Given that alcohol exerts an effect on cognition as a function of long-term consumption, as well as recent exposure, the use of multimodal assessments that index current and lifetime diagnostic history, frequency and quantity of drinking in the short term, and other measurements of impairment are needed to ensure internal validity. Techniques such as the Time Line

Followback methodology [48] allow investigators to examine alcohol at an event level, which permits a better quantification of recent alcohol use (typically within the past 3 months). Such data often provide extremely reliable indices of quantity and frequency.

Comorbid Drug Use

A relatively large proportion of persons with HIV and alcohol-use histories have a significant history of comorbid drug use/abuse, with lifetime rates of substance abuse/dependence in currently infected cohorts ranging from 40% to 75% (49). This situation can make it difficult to (a) definitively disentangle the independent effects of HIV on NP performance in heterogeneous cohorts of HIV infected patients and (b) understand the independent, additive, and/or synergistic effects of HIV and substance use on the CNS and NP functioning. Further complicating this issue is that many drug users are polysubstance users with variable histories of current and past use and abuse. Similar to the work on alcohol and HIV, the research on the NP effects of drug use and HIV has been inconclusive, with studies describing both independent and interactive effects.

The Changing Epidemiology of HIV

The epidemiology of HIV in the United States has been shifting, and rates of infection are increasing most rapidly in ethnic minority group members, and among persons of lower socioeconomic status [3]. As such, other co-factors that may contribute to the NP picture of HIV and alcohol use must be considered. Neither HIV infection nor alcohol/drug abuse occurs in a vacuum. Compared with non-drinkers, persons with histories of alcohol use, and particularly those with limited economic resources, are also more likely to have lower levels of education, a greater exposure to environmental toxicities, histories punctuated by violence and attendant injury, and poorer access to health care. As such, alcohol use and poverty may be markers for variables that weaken the cognitive substrate and decrease cognitive reserve [50]. In the face of such CNS insults as HIV and/or substance use, the threshold for the onset of cognitive impairments in persons with such risk factors drops, and they are more vulnerable to an earlier onset of and to more significant NP impairments. Ongoing work with such cohorts must carefully characterize the subjects based on their ethnicity, socio-economic status, and neurologic and health histories.

The Neuropsychology of HIV: Implications for Developing Nations

The incidence of AIDS in developing nations is increasing at an alarming rate. Of the 40 million persons infected worldwide, nearly two-thirds reside in Sub-Saharan Africa [51]. The lack of access to HAART, as well as adequate nutrition and other basic needs, increases the likelihood of neurologic and neuro-psychiatric complications and may be contributors to increased morbidity and mortality. Much of what we learned from the NP studies of HIV conducted before the advent of HAART can provide insight into the patterns of neurocognitive compromise that will be observed in infected persons from developing nations. The current research questions being tackled in the US and in Western Europe today are addressing subtle impairments, ecologic validity, and the effects of HAART on neurocognition—areas of inquiry that are less relevant in countries that are confronting the more dire questions of survival and basic functioning. Studying NP performance in developing nations can be challenging, given that much of the existing instru-mentation is too heavily culture- and language-based to have any utility in most developing nations. Many such tests are heavily language based, and often appropriate translation has not been undertaken, particularly into the myriad dialects that would be needed to use the tests in a wide variety of settings. Cultural differences compli-cate an appropriate assessment of psychopathology. Western diagnostic categories, such as depression and anxiety, often do not translate well, and the symptom expression via somatic complaints is more likely to be observed.

To date, NP investigations in developing nations are very preliminary, and the need for assessment instruments that can capture the cardinal symptoms of HADC and MCMD in samples diverse with respect to language and education is critical. Infected persons and those most vulnerable to infection are often very poor, with histories characterized by low education, mal-nutrition, poor health care, and a greater likelihood of exposure to violence, to environmental toxins, or to other environmental conditions that contribute to CNS injury. As such, the threshold for the onset of cognitive impairment among HIV-infected persons in developing nations is likely to be quite low, and the functional impairments are likely to have a more rapid onset. This situation has far-reaching clinical and cultural impli-cations, particularly for women in such settings as they often have young children in their care or remain responsible for the care of ailing husbands and other family members. Well-designed studies of neuro-psychiatric and NP functioning, using culturally appro-priate instrumentation, culture-fair test cognitive test materials, and meaningful measures of functional impairment are critical for enhancing the treatment and management of HIV in developing nations.

The Neuropsychology of HIV in the Post-HAART Era

Highly active antiretroviral therapy has changed the face of HIV/AIDS. In 1993, AIDS was the leading cause of death in adults 25-44 years of age but has since shifted to the fifth leading cause of death in that age group [52]. As early as 1987, the effects of nucleoside analogues, particularly zidovudine (AZT), were reported and were followed by reports of declines in the incidence of AIDS-related dementias. Even among those already diagnosed with HADC, improvements in NP and neurologic functioning were reported upon the initiation of AZT treatment [53]. Much of what we have learned about NP performance and HIV has been learned in the era before the advent of HAART. HAART has resulted in a lower incidence of HIV related neurobehavioral disorders.

The prevalence of HADC has increased, although an attendant drop in incidence has occurred, a trend that is likely attributable to a greater life expectancy with the use of HAART. Although the incidence rates are dropping, minor neurologic impairments continue to persist, even in the face of HAART treatment [53]. In general, however, studies examining the impact of HAART on cognitive functioning have reported a positive effect on NP performance. Individuals whose antiviral regimen included greater numbers of blood brain barrier penetrating drugs showed a greater reduction in CSF viral load, which corresponded to greater cognitive improvement. Currently unclear is whether specific classes of HAART afford greater protection, but at least some level of protection of cognitive function is assumed to be mediated by HAART-related improvement in immunologic function.

Traditionally, severe immunosuppression was considered requisite for HADC, yet, after the advent of HAART, a proportional increase in HADC was observed even among those having CD4+ T-cell counts in the 201 to 350 range. This shift, with severe immunosuppression no longer a necessary condition for the onset of HADC, and the manifestation of HAD in relatively healthy patients may be due in part to the poor penetration of antiretroviral agents into the brain, a reservoir for HIV from the outset. As such, some of the biological markers that were once useful red flags for clinicians monitoring HADC (e.g. plasma CD4+ T-cell numbers), have lost some of their utility. In the post-HAART period, HADC is believed to develop in approximately 15% of those with AIDS, and MCMD is nearly 40% [54].

The adherence demands of HAART result in a bidirectional relation between neurocognition and adherence. On the one hand, neurocognitive deficits, particularly memory impairment and executive dys-function, have been linked to poor adherence, whereas poor adherence can result in more rapid disease progression, which can result in greater NP impairment. HIV-seropositive drug and alcohol abusers may be at a particularly high risk for suboptimal adherence. Drug and alcohol use can have a deleterious impact on the efficacy of HAART, which can result in a more rapid disease progression and a greater likelihood of NP deficits. Furthermore, the identification of NP compli-cations may help in managing HIV positive patients and enhance their ability to adhere to complex medical regimens. The confluence of studies that raise issues, including the negative impact of HIV-related cognitive decline and alcohol use on adherence, as well as the suggestion that alcohol may facilitate immuno-suppression—thus potentially rendering HAART less effective—indicate that even with the attendant improvements in NP function in the post-HAART era, the subset of patients with a history of both HIV and alcohol use remain vulnerable, perhaps more vulnerable, to HIV related cognitive decline.

Hepatitis C Virus Coinfection

Approximately one third of all individuals with HIV are coinfected with the Hepatitis C virus (HCV), and alcohol use contributes to the progression of HCV [55]. In persons with HIV, the increasing rate of HCV coinfection has been associated with an increased risk of NP impairment. A possible synergistic effect of HIV/HCV coinfection has been suggested, with coinfected individuals demonstrating significantly slower reaction times than those infected with either HIV or HCV alone. Von Giesen et al [56] observed that a greater proportion of HIV/HCV coinfected persons met the criteria for AIDS dementia than did those with advanced HIV only. Some dissociation between the two disease processes has been observed with the HCV-infected-only persons showing slowed information processing, whereas the HIV-infected-only persons evidenced more executive impairment on a Stroop reaction time task. Disentangling the myriad factors that can contribute to greater NP compromise in coinfected persons—immune processes, liver function, CNS changes, and drug use history—

is a complex enterprise. Nevertheless, clinicians working with coinfected clients must remain aware of the heightened likelihood.

FUTURE DIRECTIONS

The literature on the neuropsychological (NP) effects of HIV and alcohol use still lags behind what is known about other drug use and HIV. The issue is complicated on both sides, however, because many HIV-seropositive patients have a history characterized by polysubstance use. The work to date suggests that alcohol and HIV clearly have deleterious effects on the CNS, which are manifested via NP deterioration. Although some studies have observed a multiplicative effect, others have not, and this difference may be due in part to the different methodologies used for quantifying alcohol use. Alcohol use and HIV do not occur in a vacuum, persons with these histories often carry other cofactors including poor health histories, substance use, histories of other neurologic conditions or injuries, low education, or insufficient economic resources—all of which can contribute to augmenting the NP effects of both HIV and alcohol use.

Neuroimaging studies of persons with both HIV infection and alcohol use point to a convergent and divergent involvement of various subcortical and cortical substrates, and future studies should endeavor to continue to describe the CNS changes that accompany alcohol use in persons with HIV. A clear need exists for more studies that examine alcohol use and HIV longitudinally.

The deleterious effects of both HIV and alcohol are best observed over time and given that alcohol is believed to hasten the HIV disease progress, longitudinal studies are necessary to capture this pattern. In addition, a suggestion has been made that during periods of abstinence from alcohol use, some recovery of function can be observed, and that longitudinal models will permit a better examination of whether such recovery is observed in persons with concurrent HIV infection.

Of the many health complications engendered by HIV and AIDS, the NP decline and conditions like dementia may be among the most clinically and personally challenging. The loss of control that accompanies such disorders and the attendant distress for both the patient and caregivers can be psycho-logically taxing and traumatic. Although the advent of HAART has helped to mitigate more severe cognitive symptomatology, subtle deficits still proliferate. In face of ongoing alcohol abuse or dependence, such deficits are likely to be magnified, and the concurrent use of alcohol may expedite mortality and morbidity.

Our understanding of the CNS changes observed in HIV and AIDS are well-developed, though we still are attempting to understand the wide variance in the severity, onset, and progression of NP symptomatology across patients.

As the epidemic rages in the developing world, however, new challenges abound as we attempt to capture the picture of cognitive decline and the difficulties accompanying such decline in infected persons around the world.

ACKNOWLEDGMENTS

This work was supported in part by NIGMS S06 GM08101 (Durvasula – PI). The author also wishes to acknowledge the administrative support of Alvina Rosales, Hitomi Uchishiba, Leslie Lauten, and Tina Watford in the preparation of this manuscript.

REFERENCES

[1]   Bryant KJ. Expanding research on the role of alcohol consumption and related risks in the prevention and treatment of HIV/AIDS. *Subst Use Misuse* 2006;41:1465-1507.

[2]   Justice A, McGinnis K, Atkinson J, Heaton R, Young C, Sadek J, et al. Psychiatric and neuro-cognitive disorders among HIV-positive and negative veterans in care: Veterans Aging Cohort Five-Site Study. *AIDS* 2004;18:S49-S59.

[3]   Centers for Disease Control and Prevention (CDC). Diagnoses of HIV/AIDS--32 States, 2000-2003.*MMWR Morb Mortal Wkly Rep.* 2004; 53(47):1106-10.

[4]   Petry N. Alcohol use in HIV patients: What we don't know may hurt us. *Int. J. STD AIDS* 1999; 10(9):561-70.

[5]   Durvasula RS. Rates of major psychopathology and personality disorders in an HIV infected cohort. Unpublished.

[6]   Bagasra O, Whittle P, Kajdacsy-Balla A, Lischner HW. Effects of alcohol ingestion on in vitro susceptibility of peripheral blood mononuclear cells to infection with HIV-1 and on CD4 and CD8 lymphocytes. *Prog. Clin. Biol. Res.* 1990; 325: 351-8.

[7]   Wang Y, Watson RR. Is alcohol consumption a cofactor in the development of acquired immuno-deficiency syndrome? *Alcohol* 1995;12(2):105-9.

[8]   Samet JH, Horton NJ, Meli S, Freedberg KA. Alcohol consumption and antiretroviral adherence among HIV infected persons with alcohol problems. *Alcohol Clin. Exp. Res.* 2004;28(4):572-7.

[9]   Brew BJ, Rosenbloom MJ, Price RW. Pathogenic implications of neuropathological findings in the AIDS dementia complex. *Psychopharmacology* 1998;24(3):307-10.

[10]   Ho DD, Rota TR, Schooley RT, Kaplan JC, Allan JD, Groopman JE, et al. Isolation of HTLV-III from cerebrospinal fluid and neural tissues of patients with neurological syndromes related to the acquired immunodeficiency syndrome. *N. Engl. J. Med.* 1985;313:1493-7.

[11]   Meyerhoff DJ. Effects of alcohol and HIV infection on the central nervous system. *Alcohol. Res. Health* 2001;25(4):288-98.

[12]   Wood S, Grant I. The Neurology of HIV. In: Gendelman HE, Grant I, Everall IP, Lipton SA, Swindells S, eds. *The neurology of AIDS*. New York: Oxford Univ Press, 2005:606-16.

[13]   Grant I. Neurocognitive complications of HIV infection. In: *Encyclopedia of the human brain*. New York: Elsevier, 2002:475-89.

[14]   American Psychiatric Association. Diagnostic and statistical manual of mental disorders, fourth edition (DSM IV Text revision). Washington, DC: American Psychiatric Press, 2004.

[15]   Harper C. The neurotoxicity of alcohol. *Hum. Exp. Toxicol.* 2007;26:251-7.

[16] Pfefferbaum A, Adalsteinsson E, Sullivan EV. Alcoholism and AIDS: Magnetic resonance imaging approaches for detecting interactive neuropathology. *Alcohol Clin. Exp. Res.* 2002; 26(7):1031-46.

[17] Shear PK, Jernigan TL, Butters N. Volumetric magnetic resonance imaging quantification of longitudinal brain changes in abstinent alcoholics. *Alcohol Clin. Exp. Res.* 1994;18(1):172-6.

[18] Meyerhoff D, MacKay S, Sappey-Marinier D, Deicken R. Effects of chronic alcohol abuse and HIV infection on brain phosphorus metabolites. *Alcohol Clin. Exp. Res.* 1995;19(3):685-92.

[19] Martin P, Gibbs S, Nimmerrichter A, Riddle W. Brain proton magnetic resonance spectroscopy studies in recently abstinent alcoholics. *Alcohol Clin. Exp. Res.* 1995;19(4):1078-82.

[20] Pfefferbaum A, Adalsteinsson E, Sullivan EV. Cortical NAA deficits in HIV infection without dementia: Influence of alcoholism comorbidity. *Neuropsychopharmacology* 2005;30:1392-9.

[21] Sullivan EV, Rosenbloom MJ, Pfefferbaum A. Pattern of motor and cognitive deficits in detoxified alcoholic men. *Alcohol Clin. Exp. Res.* 2000;24(5):611-21.

[22] Rourke S, Loberg T. *Neurobehavioral correlates of alcoholism.* New York: Oxford Univ Press, 1996.

[23] Beatty W, Hames K, Blanco C, Nixon S. Visuo-spatial perception, construction, and memory in alcoholism. *J. Stud. Alcohol* 1996; 57(2):136-43.

[24] Tapert SF, Brown CG, Kinderman SS, Cheung E, Frank LR, Brown SA. fMRI measurement of brain dysfunction in alcohol-dependent young women. *Alcohol Clin. Exp. Res.* 2001;25:236-45.

[25] Schulte T, Mueller-Oehring EM, Rosenbloom MJ, Pfefferbaum A, Sullivan EV. Differential effect of HIV infection and alcoholism on conflict pro-cessing, attentional allocation, and perceptual load: Evidence from a Stroop match-to-sample task. *Biol. Psychiatry* 2005;57:67-75.

[26] Wilkinson DA, Poulos CX. The chronic effects of alcohol on memory. A contrast between a unitary and dual system approach. *Recent Dev. Alcohol* 1987;5:5-26.

[27] Pitel A, Witkowski T, Vabret F, Guillery-Girard B, Desgranges B, Eustache F, et al. Effect of episodic and working memory impairments on semantic and cognitive procedural learning at alcohol treatment entry. *Alcohol Clin. Exp. Res.* 2007; 31(2):238-48.

[28] Zhang X, Begleiter H, Porjesz B, Litke A. Electrophysiological evidence of memory impair-ment in alcoholic patients. *Biol. Psychiatry* 1997; 42(12):1157-71.

[29] Beatty W, Blanco C, Hames K, Nixon S. Spatial cognition in alcoholics: influence of concurrent abuse of other drugs. *Drug Alcohol Depend.* 1997; 44(2):167-74.

[30] Durvasula R, Myers H, Satz P, Miller E, Morgen-stern H, Richardson M, et al. HIV-1, cocaine, and neuropsychological performance in African American men. *J. Int. Neuropsychol. Soc.* 2000; 6(3):322-35.

[31] Basso M, Bornstein R. Effects of past non-injection drug abuse upon executive function and working memory in HIV infection. *J. Clin. Exp. Neuropsychol.* 2003;25(7):893-903.

[32] Fein G, Biggins C, MacKay S. Delayed latency of the event-related brain potential P3A component of HIV disease: Progressive effects with increasing cognitive impairment. *Arch. Neurol.* 1995;52(11): 1109-18.

[33] Fein G, Fletcher D, Sclafani VD. Effect of chronic alcohol abuse on the CNS morbidity of HIV disease. *Alcohol Clin. Exp. Res.* 1998;22(5):196s-200s.

[34] Winsauer P, Moerschbaecher J, Brauner I, Purcell J, Lancaster J, Bagby G, et al. Alcohol unmasks simian immunodeficiency virus-induced cognitive impairments in rhesus monkeys. *Alcohol Clin. Exp. Res.* 2002;26(12):1846-57.

[35] Durvasula R, Myers H, Mason KI, Hinkin C. Relationship between alcohol use/abuse, HIV infection and neuropsychological performance in African American men. *J. Clin. Exp. Neuropsychol.* 2006;28(3):383-404.

[36] Rothlind JC, Greenfield TM, Bruce AV, Meyer-hoff DJ, Flenniken DL, Lindgren JA, et al. Heavy alcohol consumption in individuals with HIV infection: Effects on neuropsychological perfor-mance. *J. Int. Neuropsychol. Soc.* 2005;11:70-83.

[37] Sassoon SA, Fama R, Rosenbloom MJ, O'Reilly A, Pfefferbaum A, Sullivan EV. Component cognitive and motor processes of the digit symbol test: Differential effects in alcoholism, HIV infection, and their comorbidity. *Alcohol Clin. Exp. Res.* 2007;31(8):1351-4.

[38] Green JE, Saveanu RV, Bornstein RA. The effect of previous alcohol abuse on cognitive function in HIV infection. *Am. J. Psychiatry* 2004;161:249-54.

[39] Becker JT, Lopez OL, Dew MA, Ajzenstein HJ. Prevalence of cognitive disorders differs as a function of age in HIV virus infection. *AIDS* 2004;18(1):11-8.

[40] Heaton RK, Grant I, Butters N, White DA, Kirson D, Atkinson JH, et al. The HNRC 500-Neuro-psychology of HIV infection at different disease stages. *J. Int. Neuropsychol. Soc.* 1995;1:231-51.

[41] Fein G, Di Sclafani VD. Cerebral reserve capacity: Implications for alcohol and drug abuse. *Alcohol* 2004;32(1):63-7.

[42] Cook RL, Sereika SM, Hunt SC, Woodward WC, Erien JA, Conigliaro J. Problem drinking and medication adherence among persons with HIV infection. *J. Gen. Intern. Med.* 2001;16(2):83-8.

[43] Samet JH, Horton NJ, Meli S, Dukes K, Tripps T, Sullivan L, et al. A randomized controlled trial to enhance antiretroviral therapy adherence in patients with a history of alcohol problems. *Antivir Ther* 2005;10(1):83-93.

[44] Fabris P, Tositti G, Manfrin V, Giordani MT, Vaglia A, Cattelan AM, et al. Does alcohol intake affect highly active antiretroviral therapy (HAART) response in HIV-positive patients? *J. Acquir. Immune Defic. Syndr.* 2000;25(1):92-3.

[45] Dingle G, Oei T. Is alcohol a cofactor of HIV and AIDS? Evidence from immunological and behav-ioral studies. *Psychol. Bull* 1997;122(1):56-71.

[46] Bornstein RA, Fama R, Rosenberger P. Drug and alcohol use and neuropsychological performance in asymptomatic HIV infection. *J. Neuropsychiatry Clin. Neurosci.* 1993;5(3):254-9.

[47] Penkower L, Dew MA, Kingsley L, Zhou SY, Lyketsos CG, Wesch J, et al. Alcohol consump-tion as a cofactor in the progression of HIV infection and AIDS. *Alcohol* 1995;12(6):547-52.

[48] Sobell L, Sobell M. Timeline follow-back: A technique for assessing self-reported alcohol consumption. Totowa: Humana Press, 1992.

[49] Bing E, Burman M, Longshore D, Fleishman J, Sherbourne C, London A, et al. Psychiatric disorders and drug use among human immuno-deficiency virus-infected adults in the United States. *Arch. Gen. Psychiatry* 2001;58(8):721-8.

[50] Satz P, Morgenstern H, Miller EN, Selnes OA, McArthur JC, Cohen BA, et al. Low education as a possible risk factor for cognitive abnormalities in HIV-1 findings from the multicenter AIDS Cohorts Study (MACS). *J. Acquir. Immune Defic. Syndr* 1993;6(5):503-11.

[51] Joint United Nations Programme on HIV/AIDS (UNAIDS) and the World Health Organization (WHO). AIDS Epidemic Update. December 2006. Report. Geneva, Switzerland: UNAIDS/WHO. Available at: http://data.unaids.org/pub/EpiReport /2006/01-Front_Matter_2006_EpiUpdate_eng.pdf

[52] Minimo AM, Smith BL. Deaths: Preliminary data for 2000. *Natl. Vital. Stat. Rep.* 2001;49(12):25-6.

[53] Dore GJ, Correl PK, Li Y, Kaldor JM, Cooper DA, Brew BJ. Changes to AIDS dementia complex in the area of highly active antiretroviral therapy. *AIDS* 1999;13:1249-53.

[54] Sacktor N, McDermott M, Marder K, Schifitto G, Selnes O, et al. HIV-associated cognitive impairment before and after the advent of combination therapy. *J. Neurovirol.* 2002;8(2):136-42.

[55] Sherman KE. New paradigms in the management of hepatitis C virus co-infections. *Nat. Clin. Pract. Gastroenterol Hepatol.* 2007;4:10-6.

[56] von Giesen HJ, Heintges T, Abbasi-Boroudjeni N, Kucukkoylu S, Koller H, Haslinger BA, et al. Psychomotor slowing in hepatitis C and HIV infection. *J. Acquir. Immune Defic. Syndr.* 2004; 35(2):131-7.

In: Alcohol-Related Cognitive Disorders   ISBN: 978-1-60741-730-9
Editors: L. Sher, I. Kandel, J. Merrick pp. 319-329   © 2009 Nova Science Publishers, Inc.

Chapter 22

FETAL ALCOHOL SYNDROME AND ITS LONG-TERM EFFECTS

Joav Merrick, Efrat Merrick-Kenig, Isack Kandel, Gideon Vardi and Mohammed Morad

ABSTRACT

Ancient scripture and paintings together with several medical reports on the effect of alcohol on the newborn over the past three hundred years finally led to the description of the fetal alcohol syndrome in the 1970s by French and American research groups. Maternal alcohol abuse during pregnancy can result in the specific pattern of malformations and neurocognitive deficits characteric of this syndrome. Diagnostic criteria and classifications have been developed and in the 1990s reports showed the long term consequences for these children. In recent years several studies from different countries have shown that prenatal alcohol exposure will lead to life long consequences on physical development, intellectual development, behavior, social development, occupation, independence, sexuality or sexual behavior and increased risk of suicidality. In this review of long-term observation studies we found that the prenatal exposure to alcohol have permanent and life long damage, which impair both the social and occupational future of the person exposed with a need for life long assistance in order for that person to function at an optimal level. Primary prevention and early intervention with general public health educational efforts seems to be the best way forward.

INTRODUCTION

"The children of Israel continued to do what was evil in the eyes of Hashem, and Hashem delivered them into the hand of the Philistines for forty years. There was a certain man of Zorah, of the family of the Danite, whose name was Manoah; his wife was barren and had not given birth. An angel of God appeared to the women and said to her, "Behold now – you are barren and have not given birth, but you shall conceive and give birth to a son. And now be careful not to drink wine or aged wine, and not to eat anything contaminated......." (Judges

13, 1-4) [1] is most likely one of the first places, where the issue of fetal damage from alcohol is mentioned. Not only in the written media, but also in the art we find early mention of the adverse effects of alcohol. William Hogarth (London, 1697 - 1764) in his famous graving from 1751 called "Gin Lane" showed the dangerous effects of gin. His satire with this engraving had an immediate impact and during the same year parliament passed the Gin act, which regulated the sale of alcohol [1,2].

Health professionals and especially midwives have for the past two hundred years observed the effects on babies [1] and tried to discourage alcohol consumption. Evidence for the earliest suspicion of the teratogenic effects of alcohol started to accumulate with work by two medical officers working in Liverpool prisons in 1899, who found infant mortality and stillborn rates for children born to alcoholic mothers more than two times that for nonalcoholic mothers [3].

In modern times the clinical effects of alcohol on the children were first reported in 1967-68 in France [4,5], but not noticed until published in English in 1973 [6] as case histories of eight unrelated children born to mothers who were chronic alcoholics. These children showed a similar pattern of craniofacial, limb and cardiovascular defects associated with prenatal-onset growth deficiency and developmental delay. Developmental delay, prenatal and postnatal growth deficiency and short palbebral fissures were observed in all eight children.

FETAL ALCOHOL SYNDROME (FAS)

Alcohol is a teratogen, that can cause birth defects or functional impairment in a developing fetus. Some signs may be present at birth, like low birth weight, prematurity and microcephaly. Characteristic facial features may be present at birth, or may become more obvious over time. Signs of brain damage can be delay in development, behavioral abnormalities and mental retardation or intellectual disability, but affected individuals exhibit a wide range of abilities and disabilities.

The adverse effects of alcohol on human development represent a spectrum of structural anomalies and behavioral and neurocognitive disabilities, which today is most accurately termed fetal alcohol spectrum disorders (FASD). Since the first reports in 1967-1973, a lot of work has gone into developing specific criteria for defining and diagnosing this condition. Two sets of diagnostic criteria have been used for evaluation of children with potential diagnoses in the FASD continuum, the 1996 Institute of Medicine (IOM) criteria [7] and the Washington criteria [8], but recently a practical clinical approach to diagnosis has been put forward [9]. This revised classification was validated through the evaluation of 1,500 children, who were prenatally exposed to alcohol from six Native American communities in the United States and one community in the Western Cape Province of South Africa. The children and their families underwent standardized multidisciplinary evaluations, which included a dysmorphology examination, developmental and neuropsychologic testing, with a structured maternal interview, which gathered data about prenatal drinking practices demographic and family information [9]. 164 children with potential FASD were found and data analyzed resulting in revisions and clarifications of the existing IOM FASD diagnostic categories. These revised criteria are listed in Table 1 and currently used in a multicenter study [10] in order to facilitate an easier practical pediatric clinical approach.

Table 1. Revised Institute of Medicine (IOM) criteria for diagnosis of the fetal alcohol spectrum disorders (FASD) (9,10) (FAS=fetal alcohol syndrome; PFAS= partial FAS; ARBD=alcohol related birth defects; ARND=alcohol related neurodevelopmental disorder)

DIAGNOSTIC CRITERIA FOR FAS OR PFAS
(with or without confirmed maternal alcohol exposure)

A. Evidence of a characteristic pattern of minor facial anomalies, including at least two of the following:
   - Short palpebral fissures (less than or equel to the 10th percentile)
   - Thin vermillion border of the upper lip (score 4 or 5 on the
   - lip/philtrum guide (9,10))
   - Smooth philtrum (score 4 or 5 on the lip/philtrum guide (9,10))
B. Evidence of prenatal and/or postnatal growth retardation: height or weight less or equal to the 10th percentile
C. Evidence of deficient brain growth or abnormal morphogenesis, including one or more of the following:
   - Structural brain abnormalities
   - Head circumference less than or equal to the 10th percentile

FAS requires all the above features (A-C); PFAS requires A and B or C or evidence of a complex pattern of behavior or cognitive abnormalities inconsistent with developmental level and that cannot be explained by genetic predisposition, family background or environment alone

DIAGNOSTIC CRITERIA FOR ALCOHOL RELATED EFFECTS (ARBD AND ARND)
(a diagnosis in these categories requires a confirmed history of prenatal alcohol exposure)

   - ARBD requires the characteristic facies plus specific congenital structural defects (including malformations and dysplasias) in at least one organ system (if the patient displays minor anomalies only, at least two must be present). This category assumes the subject to have normal growth and intellectual/behavioral characteristics
   - ARND assumes the subject to have normal growth and structure and at least one of the following (A or B):
A. Evidence of deficient brain growth or abnormal morphogenesis, including one or more of the following:
   - Structural brain abnormalities
   - Head circumference less than or equal to the 10th percentile
B. Evidence of a complex pattern of behavior or cognitive abnormalities inconsistent with developmental level and that cannot be explained by genetic predisposition, family background or environment alone
   - This pattern includes: marked impairment in the performance of complex tasks (complex problem solving, planning, judgement, abstraction, metacognition and arithmetic tasks); higher level receptive and expressive language deficits; and disordered behavior (difficulties in personal manner, emotional lability, motor dysfunction, poor academic performance and deficient social interaction)

The true epidemiology of FASD is not known, since cases can go undetected at birth and even later in life [9], but various studies have reported the occurence in the range of 0.5-3 per 1,000 births in most populations [7]. The less severe types of FASD may even effect as much as one percent of children born in United States and the burden to society estimated at billions of dollars each year [9,11].

LONG TERM EFFECTS OF PRENATAL ALCOHOL EXPOSURE

In 1991 the first report on the long term effects was published from Seattle [12]. 61 adolescents and adults with prenatal alcohol exposure were presented. After puberty, the faces of patients with fetal alcohol syndrome or fetal alcohol effects were not as distinctive, but they tended to remain short and microcephalic, although their weight was somewhat closer to the mean. The average IQ was 68, however the range of IQ was quite large, as low as 20 (severely impaired) to as high as 105 (normal). The average achievement levels for reading, spelling, and arithmetic were fourth grade, third grade and second grade, respectively. The Vineland Adaptive Behavior Scale was used to measure adaptive functioning in these individuals. The composite score for this group showed functioning at the level of a seven-year-old. Daily living skills were at a level of nine years, and social skills were at the level of a six-year-old. Maladaptive behaviors such as poor judgment, distractibility, and difficulty perceiving social cues were common with unstable family environments.

This group has published further data regarding the disabilities in children, adolescents and adults with FASD [13] finding major problems with adaptive behavior. They used five operationally defined adverse outcomes and 18 associated risk/protective factors. Their study used a life history interview with knowledgeable informants of 415 patients with FASD (median age 14 years, range 6-51; median IQ 86, range 29-126). Most of the study participants (80%) were not raised by their biological mothers, but the study also found some other disturbing facts. The life span prevalence was 61% for disrupted school experiences, 60% for trouble with the law, 50% for confinement (in detention, jail, prison, or a psychiatric or alcohol/drug inpatient setting), 49% for inappropriate sexual behaviors on repeated occasions and 35% for alcohol/drug problems. These and other adverse effects will be described in more details below.

Physical Development

One study from Munster in Germany followed 52 persons with FASD over a number of years with a mean age of 21.6 years (range 18-32 years) and found that growth disorder persisted in some of the patients, while others had some catch-up in length, weight and head cirsumference. At birth 42% were of small stature (below 3rd percentile), 53% underweight and 45% microcephalic. Before reaching puberty 17% had caught up to the normal percentile level in weight. After puberty the absolute weight and the weight/length ratio had further increased in 16% of the children with their stature remaining small, but they were overweight. As adults 26% were below normal in weight, 30% below normal in height and microcephaly persisted into adulthood (46%). The typical dysmorphic features of FAS in childhood seemed less marked or malformed in adulthood [14].

From another study of 21 persons with heavy prenatal alcohol exposure (8-22 years, mean 12.6 years) with 21 normal controls it was found that the brain growth continues to be adversely affected long after the prenatal insult with the frontal and inferior parietal/perisylvian area most implicated consistant with the behavioral imparments [15].

Intellectual Development

In children with fetal alcohol syndrome disorders (FASD) the IQ (intelligence quotient) can range from 50 to 115 [16]. In studies of six years old with FASD a mean decrease of seven IQ points was found and in studies of adolescents and adults the intellectual functioning was found in the mild to moderate range of impairment with 46% having an IQ of less than 69[16]. Mean verbal IQ was 65 while performance IQ was 79 with significant specific deficits in academic and adaptive functioning [16].

Even in the case of a normal IQ these children tend to have compromised learning with poor short term memory (but intact long term memory), difficulty in establishing routines, decreased academic performance, problems with verbal memory and defects in spatial memory and poor retention of learned tasks [16]. Speech and language impairment (difficulties in word comprehension, naming ability, articulation, expression and receptive language skills) is a typical finding in these children [16].

In the study from Germany [14] the school age years were characterized by late entry into school, frequent school change, failure to advance to higher classes and premature ending of the formal school. 56% were in special school and none graduated from secondary school. Deficits were measured in regard to learning, which pointed to complex cerebral abnormalies and cognitive disorders. Slow thought process, abstraction and difficulty on concentration were found together with poor memory (61%).

Behavior

Already in the first follow-up study from the Seattle Longitudinal Study on Alcohol and Pregnancy maladaptive behaviors were found [12]. Poor judgment with an inability to appreciate the consequences of an action, distractibility and difficulty perceiving social cues, which combined with frustration can lead to impulsive behavior and conflict with society. Friendliness towards strangers and lack of inhibitions can also lead to exploitation.

At age 14 years a significant association was found between prenatal alcohol exposure and increased behavior or learning difficulties during adolescence resultingin anti-social behavior, school problems and self perceived learning difficulties [12]. Another study from the same research group found major problems with adaptive behavior [13]. Disrupted school experience was found in 14% of school children and 61% in adolescents and adults. 53% of adolescents had been suspended from school and 29% expelled. 70% reported attention problems, 58% had problems with peers and 55% made repeated disruptions in class [13].

A number of children (14%), adolescents and adults (60%) had trouble with the law [13] in the form of law violations against persons (45%), such as shoplifting, theft, assault, burglary or domestic violence. 13% of the children, 67% of the adolescents and 87% of the adults were actually charged, arrested and convicted. The mean age for onset of trouble with the law was 12.8 years.

8% of the children were confined (psychiatric hospitalization), while among the adolescents and adults 35% were reported ever incarcerated for a crime, 23% ever hospitalized for psychiatric problems and 15% ever hospitalized for alcohol and drug treatment [13].

Concerning alcohol and drug problems it was found for 29% of adolescents and 46% for adults with overall more alcohol (33% than drug problems (23%). The mean age for onset for alcohol and rug problems was 13.4 years [13].

At 21 years [18] a further follow-up study showed that prenatal alcohol exposure was significantly associated with current alcohol problems. This relationship was independent of the family history, nicotine exposure, other prenatal exposure or postnatal environmental factors. Of the 433 offspring 82.9% reported themselves as current drinkers and 17.1% as life-long or current alcohol abstainers. 35 or 8.1% scored at or above 10 on the ADA (Alcohol Dependence Scale), which is an indication of mild alcohol dependence.

A smaller study from San Diego with 27 adolescents (10-18 years) exposed prenatally to alcohol and 29 controls showed that the exposed group performed at a lower level of moral maturity and with a significantly higher rate of delinquent behaviors (19).

Others disagree with the above findings around the connection between prenatal alcohol exposure and later adolescent delinquency [20]. A study from Atlanta, Georgia with 250 adolescents (mean age 15.1 years) and their mothers or primary care givers had 48 controls not exposed to prenatal alcohol, 39 exposed with dysmorphy, 77 exposed without dysmorphy and 84 students in special education classes, a total of 248 cases. The assessment and analysis of the findings revealed that the exposure groups did not differ from the controls on measures of variety and frequency of delinquent behavior, but males engaged in a wider range of delinquent acts than girls. The regression analysis found that higher adolescent life stress, higher self reported drug use and lower parental supervision were significantly related to delinquent acts than alcohol exposure prenatally [20]. This study had the limitation of being conducted with only low income, black families and the average age of only 15.1 years.

The study from Germany [14] found that eight out of 52 adults exposed prenatally to alcohol showed some kind of physical aggressiveness, but marked anti-social behavior or conflict with the law was rare. One was pyromanic, two sexual offences, two store thefts and three cases of stealing handbags or cars.

Social Development, Occupation and Independence

Every person has to achieve social development in order to function optimally in a diverse society, which with the above problems can be seen as a hard task for persons exposed to alcohol in uterine life and due to the effects on brain development. So far there are few long term follow-up studies into adulthood, but the study from Germany showed that 52 adults had a limited spectrum of occupational qualifications and types of job [14]. 15 had achieved an occupation with apprenticeship (like mining technician, cook, mechanic, nurse, kindergarten teacher, physician assistant, carpenter), 19 an occupation without apprenticeship (building worker, weaver, waiter, painter, gardener, door-keeper, labourer), 15 had a simple occupation (agricultural labourer, household helper, workshop for the disabled), while three we unemployed and kept by their carers. None had achieved a higher education [14].

Sexuality or Sexual Behavior

Inappropriate sexual behaviors on repeated occasions was the most frequent adverse life outcome over the life span (median age 14 years, range 6-51) found in the follow-up study from Seattle [13]. This behavior increased over age (39% in children, 48% in adolescents and 52% in adults) with the most repeated inappropriate sexual behavior for children was exposing (20%) and inappropriate sexual touching (19%), for adolescents and adults promiscuity (26%) and inappropriate sexual advances (18%). The mean age for onset of inappropriate sexual behavior was 9.6 years [13].

While these people could be likely to present to offender treatment programs, it would be doubtful that these programs would recognize these persons as victims of prenatal alcohol exposure [21]. It is therefore recommended that professionals working with sexual offenders consider FASD as a cause for the sexual behavior and use this knowledge in the treatment program [21].

Suicidality

Suicide is a leading cause of death in Western society. Several case studies and also a pilot study from the Seattle Longitudinal Study on Alcohol and Pregnancy found increased suicide attempts. 18% had a severe suicide attempt, 27% had a moderate risk attempt, 9% a low risk attempt and 46% had no lifetime attempts. Compared to the general population rate of 4.6% these rates are much higher for persons exposed to prenatal alcohol [22].

PREVENTION

It is obvious that primary prevention is the solution [7]. Universal prevention intervention in the form of explanation to society and potential parents that drinking and pregnancy does not go together should be done through public education at all levels. Health professionals (family physicians, health visitors, obstetricians and gynecologists) and teachers would be the natural partners in such education programs.

Selective prevention intervention [7] would target persons with greater risk, such as women who drink alcohol in their reproductive age range, but also their partners. Health professionals should seek out the population of women at high risk in order to find ways to intervene.

Home visitation or the nurse visitor has its origin in United Kingdom and Denmark from the beginning of the 1900 [23] as an effective and general preventive intervention in pregnancy and early childhood. In the United States it has not been an universal program, but rather intervention in high risk populations and now taken the form of Nurse Family Partnership (NFP) [24]. This is an intervention where mothers receive home visitation by registered nurses pre- and postnatally in order to reduce mothers' vulnerability to the effects of stressful life events. A recent study of mothers (N = 324), who were generally low-income, young and unmarried at the time of the birth of their first child with structured interviews done with mothers about 15 years after the program began showed that experiencing uncontrollable stressful life events, such as the death of a loved one, led to fewer negative outcomes (fewer mental health problems, less binge drinking, and better parenting practices) among nurse-visited mothers than among mothers receiving no visitation [24].

INTERVENTION

Home visitation has been effective in prevention of child abuse and neglect, but has also recently been used as an intervention program for young women with fetal alcohol spectrum disorders (FASD) [25], but using para-professional advocate case managers instead of nurses. This pilot program was implemented in 2001 through the University of Washington, Seattle and a standard existing program (Parent Child Assistance Program-PCAP) adapted for the target population. PCAP usually work with one case manager per 15 families for a three year period beginning during pregnancy or shortly after birth of the child. The purpose of the case manager/advocate is to develop a positve and empathic relationship with the cliet, help address a wide range of environmental issues, connect the client and family with existing services and teach how to access these services. Further to coordinate services, help the client to follow recommendations, assure a safe home environment for the child and ensure health care.

This pilot study [25] with 19 women (mean age 22.3, range 14-36 years) were characterized as mainly white (63%), unmarried (84%), poorly educated (47% with 9th grade or less), earlier incarceration (68%) and prior childhood physical or sexual abuse (94%). Physical and mental health was characterized as serious, chronic medical conditions (47%) and 71% reported earlier psychiatric evaluation.

The intervention with a case manager/advocate for women with FASD showed (over an observed 12 month period within a three year program) improved outcomes, which included decreased alcohol and drug abuse, increased use of contarceptives, increased medical and mental health care service utilization and more stable housing. The advocates found this population far more complex and demanding than their usual target population, because of the lack of comprehension, poor memory and difficulty in executing a plan, most likely due to the brain damage from prenatal alcohol exposure in these clients. This study showed that it was possible to move forward and also protect the children, but these women will need coordinated assistance across the lifespan [25].

CONCLUSIONS

This population of children born after prenatal alcohol exposure is a population at risk in many ways. These children are at risk for abuse and neglect, not only because the families in which they are born are with a troubled life history, but also because these children with developmental and cognitive problems lack a sense of consequence of their actions, usually with a very friendly behavior towards other people and therefore prone to maltreatment [16,25]. Follow-up studies [25] have found a high level of childhood exploitation (94%), when interviwed in adulthood, so intervention early on is an important factor in prevention.

In this review of long-term observation studies [12-14] we found that the prenatal exposure to alcohol have permanent and life long damage, which impair both the social and occupational future of the person exposed with a need for life long assistance in order for that person to function at an optimal level. This is indeed a burden to the person, the family but also to society.

There seems to be universal agreement among professionals, professional societies and committees about the way forward [7,16,25]:

- Primary prevention of FASD should involve educational programs (school based or even starting earlier), early recognition and treatment of women at risk
- Health care providers should ask and consult women on the issue of drinking and pregnancy
- Health care providers should identify newborn and babies in order for early intervention
- Intervention programs should involve family and community
- Assessment and intervention is a multidisciplinary approach
- This service should be funded by the public
- Interventions should be evaluated and investigated for effectiveness
- Interagency collaboration is a must
- Long-term intervention
- Cultural based holistic approach

REFERENCES

[1]   Merrick J. [Alcohol and the fetus]. In: Merrick J, ed. [Children in alcohol and drug-abusing families. Copenhagen: *Hans Reitzel*, 1985:49-56. [Danish]
[2]   Website: http://www.artoftheprint.com/artistpages/hogarth_william_ginlane.htm
[3]   Sullivan WC, Scholar S. A note on the influence of maternal inebriety on the offspring. *J. Mental Sci.* 1899;45:489-503.
[4]   Lamarche AM. [Reflexions sur la descendance des alcoholiques]. *Bull Acad. Natl. Med.* 1967;151:517-21. [French]
[5]   Lemoine P, Harousseau H, Borteyro JP, Menuet KJC. [Les enfants de parents alcoholiques. Anomalies observees. A propos de 125 cas]. *Quest Medical* 1968;25:476-82. [French]
[6]   Jones KL, Smith DW, Ulleland CN, Streissguth AP. Pattern of malformation in offspring of chronic alcoholic mothers. *Lancet* 1973;1(7815):1267-71.
[7]   Stratton KR, Howe CJ, Battaglia FC, eds. *Fetal alcohol syndrome: Diagnosis, epidemiology, prevention and treatment.* Washington, DC: Nat Acad Press, 1996.
[8]   Astley SJ, Clarren SK. Diagnosing the full spectrum of fetal alcohol-exposed individuals: Introducing a 4-digit diagnostic code. *Alcohol Alcohol* 2000;35:400-10.

[9]   Hoyme HE, May PA, Kalberg WO, Kodituwakku P, Gossage JP, Trujillo PM, Buckley DG, Miller JH, Aragon AS, Khaole N, Viljoen DL, Jones KL, Robinson LK. A practical clinical approach to diagnosis of fetal alcohol spectrum disorders: Clarification of the 1966 Institute of Medicine criteria. *Pediatrics* 2005;115:39-47.

[10] Autti-Ramo I, Fagerlund A, Ervalahti N, Loimu L, Korkman M, Hoyme HE. Fetal alcohol spectrum disaorders in Finland: Clinical delineation of 77 older children and adolescents. *Am. J. Med. genetics* 2006;140A:137-43.

[11] Sampson PD, Streissguth AP, Bookstein FL, Little RE, Clarren SK, Dehaene P, Hanson JW, Graham JM. Incidence of fetal alcohol syndrome and prevalence of alcohol-related neurodevelopmental disorder. *Teratology* 1997;56:317-26.

[12] Streissguth AP, Aase JM, Clarren SK, Randels SP, LaDue RA, Smith DF. Fetal alcohol syndrome in adolescents and adults. *JAMA* 1991;265:1961-7.

[13] Streissguth AP, Bookstein FL, Barr HM, Sampson PD, O'Malley K, Young JK. Risk factors for adverse life outcomes in fetal alcohol syndrome and fetal alcohol effects. *J. Dev. Behav. Pediatr* 2004;25(4):228-38.

[14] Loser H, Bierstedt T, Blum A. Fetal alcohol syndrome in adults: Long-term observations on 52 patients. *Dtsch Med. Wschr* 1999;124:412-8.

[15] Sowell ER, Thompson PM, Mattson SN, Tessner KD, Jernigan TL, Riley EP, Toga AW. Regional brain shape abnormalities persist into adolescence after heavy prenatal alcohol exposure. *Cerebral Cortex* 2002;12:856-65.

[16] Godel J, Bay H. Fetal alcohol syndrome. *Paediatr. Child Helth* 2002;7(3):161-74.

[17] Olson HC, Streissguth AP, Sampson PD, Barr HM, Bookstein FL, Thiede K. Association of prenatal alcohol exposure with behavioral and learning problems in early adolescence. *J. Am. Acad Child Adolesc. Psychiatry* 1997;36(9):1187-94.

[18] Baer JS, Sampson PD, Barr HM, Connor PD, Streissguth AP. A 21-year longitudinal analysis of the effects of prenatal alcohol exposure on young adult drinking. *Arch. Gen. Psychiatry* 2003;60:377-85.

[19] Schonfeld AM, Mattson SN, Riley EP. Moral maturity and elinquency after prenatal alcohol exposure. *J. Stud. Alcohol* 2005;66:545-54.

[20] Lynch ME, Colews CD, Corley T, Falek A. Examining delinquency in adolescents differentially prenatally exposed to alcohol: The role of proximal and distal risk factors. *J. Stud. Alcohol* 2003;64:678-86.

[21] Baumbach J. Some implications of prenatal alcohol exposure for the treatment of adolescents with sexual offending behaviors. *Sex Abuse* 2002;14(4):313-27.

[22] O'Malley K, Huggins J. Suicidality in adolescents and adults with fetal alcohol spectrum disorders. *Can. J. Psychiatry* 2005;50(2):125.

[23] Merrick J, Hjorth PS, Garden L, eds. [Childhood. A book about child health and development during the last 300 years]. Copenhagen: Danish Nursing Publ, 1988. [Danish]

[24] Izzo CV, Eckenrode JJ, Smith EG, Henderson CR, Cole R, Kitzman H, Olds DL. Reducing the impact of uncontrollable stressful life events through a program of nurse home visitation for new parents. *Prev. Sci.* 2005;6(4):269-74.

[25] Grant T, Huggins J, Connor P, Pedersen JY, Whitney N, Streissguth A. A pilot community intervention for young women with fetal alcohol spectrum disorders. *Community Ment. Health J.* 2004;40(6):499-511.

PART FOUR: REFLECTIONS

In: Alcohol-Related Cognitive Disorders   ISBN: 978-1-60741-730-9
Editors: L. Sher, I. Kandel, J. Merrick pp. 333-336   © 2009 Nova Science Publishers, Inc.

Chapter 23

ALCOHOL, IMPULSIVITY AND SUICIDE: PLENTY OF ROOM FOR NEW RESEARCH

Leo Sher and Joav Merrick

Although alcohol is used by many in a safe and enjoyable manner, there are individuals who develop difficulties with alcohol. These problems include intoxication, abuse, and dependence. Alcohol use disorders are a major medical and social problem facing many countries [1-2]. In the United States today, more than 15 million Americans are estimated to suffer from alcoholism [1]. In the United Kingdom, the number of 'dependent drinkers' was calculated at over 2.8 million in 2001 [2].

The consumption of alcoholic beverages has risen steadily since World War II, and drinking begins at an earlier age [3]. The steady increase in alcohol production and consumption is related to the broader growth of commodity production in industrialized societies in which alcoholic beverages are consumed in tandem with other new forms of commodities and foods [4]. In the business world, misleading and confusing information is often used to win consumers without considering the effects of the product on the health of the user [5]. Alcohol advertising is countered by warnings from the health professions, but the individual is expected to sort out the contradictory information and make a rational decision. Seeking the causes of alcohol abuse within the person diverts attention from the invisible economic, political, and social parameters that promote the lucrative industry of alcohol production and consumption.

Alcohol use is a major contributing factor for head injuries, motor vehicle accidents, violence, and assaults [6]. Estimates are that alcohol is involved in 45% of violent crimes, 45% of episodes of marital violence, 20% of non-fatal industrial accidents, and 15% of non-fatal traffic accidents [6]. The cost of alcohol-related mortality and morbidity in the United States is estimated at $136 billion per year [6]. Beyond the money also lies the pain and suffering of all individuals, not only the alcoholic affected.

In the United States, over 30,000 people commit suicide each year [7]. The rate of attempted suicide can be as much as ten times higher than the rate of completed suicide [8]. Of community-residing persons, 4.6% admit to attempting suicide at least once in their lifetime [9]. Alcohol use is associated with suicide risk [6,7]. Alcohol plays two different roles. Ongoing alcohol use disorders can contribute to suicide risk by effects on mood and impulsive-aggressive traits. Acute alcohol consumption at the time of a suicide attempt can have a disinhibiting effect. Alcohol is involved in 40% of suicide attempts [6]. Some reports have found that lifetime mortality due to suicide in alcohol dependence is as high as 18% [10]. Murphy and Wetzel [11] reviewed the epidemiologic literature and found that the lifetime risk of suicide among individuals with alcohol dependence treated in outpatient and inpatient settings was 2.2% and 3.4%, respectively. Nonetheless, the suicide risk in individuals with alcohol dependence is 60 to 120 times greater than in the non-psychiatrically ill population.

In European countries, studies report that a positive and significant relation between per capita alcohol consumption and gender- and age-specific suicide rates was revealed most often in northern Europe and was found least often in southern Europe, thus concluding that the population-level association between alcohol and suicide is conditioned by cultural factors [12]. Also, a variation across country groups (traditional wine countries of southern Europe, beer countries of central Europe and the British Isles, spirits countries of northern Europe) in alcohol effects was observed, particularly those on violent deaths [13].

Based on a comprehensive review of the literature, Conner and Duberstein [14] proposed a model to explain the elevated risk of suicide among alcohol-dependent individuals. This model includes aggression/ impulsivity, severe alcoholism, negative affect, and hopelessness as key predisposing factors; and major depressive episodes and stressful life events, particularly interpersonal difficulties, as key precipitating factors for suicide. This model suggests that effective treatment of comorbid alcoholism and depression may prevent attempted and completed suicides. Alcohol diminishes impulse control and increases aggressive-ness and if combined with life dissatisfaction, may result in depression and suicidal behavior.

Impulsivity is a complex construct for which a variety of criterion measures are noted [15]. The various impulsivity measures may be conceptualized as repre-senting three broad categories of techniques: (1) self- or observer-reports; (2) physiological/biological measure-ments, and (3) laboratory behavioral measures [16]. Moeller et al [16] have provided a number of conclusions that support the relation between alcohol/substance abuse and impulsivity—alcohol/substance abusers are more impulsive on self-report and laboratory behavioral measures; impulsive groups have higher incidence of alcohol/substance abuse; impulsivity is both a risk factor for the development of alcohol/substance abuse and a resulting consequence of alcohol/substance abuse; impulsivity is a significant predictor of quitting alcohol/ drug treatment; and treatments for impulsivity improve outcome in alcohol/substance abuse. Dysfunction of the serotonin neurotransmitter system has been cited most consistently as a possible mechanism for impulsive and suicidal behaviours [17-19], as well as impulsive behavior and alcohol/substance abuse [20-21]. Serum cholesterol is another emerging factor that could be related both to impulsive and to suicidal behaviors [22-23], although this aspect may not be relevant to the interaction of these behaviors with alcohol and substance abuse [24].

The large population of individuals with alcoholism, the relative frequency of suicides and suicide-related behaviors in this population, and the devastating effects of attempted and completed suicides on individuals, families, and society make this a topic that requires our attention. Further research studies are needed to better define risk factors for suicidal behavior in individuals with alcohol use disorders and to devise prevention programs for this high-risk group.

REFERENCES

[1]   Gabbard GO (editor). Treatments of psychiatric disorders, 3rd ed. Arlington, VA: *Am. Psychiatr. Publ*, 2001.

[2]   UK Cabinet Office Strategy Unit. Alcohol misuse: How much does it cost? September 2003.

[3]   Walsh DC. Social responses to substance abuse. In: *Freeman HE, Levine S, eds. Handbook of medical sociology,* 4th ed. Englewood Cliffs, NJ: Prentice-Hall, 1989:128-43.

[4]   SingleE, Morgan P, Lint J. *Alcohol, society, and the state*. Vol. 2. Toronto: Addiction Research Foundation, 1981.

[5]   Nikelly AG. Alcoholism: social as well as psycho-medical problem. The missing "big picture. *J. Alcohol Drug. Educ*. 1994: 1-12.

[6]   Winokur G, Clayton PJ, eds. *Medical basis of psychiatry*, 2nd ed. Philadelphia: WB Saunders, 1994.

[7]   Sher L. Alcoholism and suicidal behavior: a clinical overview. *Acta Psychiatr. Scand* 2006;113:13-22.

[8]   Hawton K, Arensman E, Wasserman D. Relation between attempted suicide and suicide rates among young people in Europe. *J. Epidemiol. Community Health* 1998;52:191-4.

[9]   Kessler RC Borges G Walters EE. Prevalence of and risk factors for lifetime suicide attempts in the National Comorbidity Survey. *Arch. Gen. Psychiatry* 1999;56:617-26.

[10]   Roy A, Linnoila M. Alcoholism and suicide. Suicide Life Threat Behav 1986;16:244-73.

[11]   Murphy GE, Wetzel RD. The lifetime risk of suicide in alcoholism. *Arch. Gen. Psychiatry* 1990;47:383-92.

[12]   Ramstedt, M. Alcohol and suicide in 14 European countries. *Addiction* 2001;96(Suppl 1): S59-75.

[13]   Norstrom, T, Skog, OJ. Alcohol and mortality: methodological and analytical issues in aggregate analyses. *Addiction* 2001;96(Suppl 1): S5-17.

[14]   Conner KR, Duberstein PR. Predisposing and precipitating factors for suicide among alcoholics: empirical review and conceptual integration. *Alcohol Clin. Exp. Res.* 2004;28:6S-17S.

[15]   Dougherty DM, Mathias CW, Marsh DM, Moeller FG, Swann AC. Suicidal behaviors and drug abuse: impulsivity and its assessment. *Drug Alcohol Depend* 2004;76(Suppl):S93-S105.

[16]   Moeller FG, Barratt ES, Dougherty DM, Schmitz JM, Swann AC. Psychiatric aspects of impulsivity. *Am. J. Psychiatry* 2001;158:1783-93.

[17]   Cremniter D, Jamain S, Kollenbach K, Alvarez JC, Lecrubier Y, Gilton A, Jullien P, Lesieur P, Bonnet F, Spreux-Varoquaux O. CSF 5-HIAA levels are lower in impulsive as compared to nonimpulsive violent suicide attempters and control subjects. *Biol. Psychiatry* 1999;45:1572–9.

[18]   Oquendo MA, Mann JJ. The biology of impulsivity and suicide. *Psychiatr. Clin. N Am.* 2000;1:11–25.

[19] Sher L, Oquendo MA, Grunebaum MF, Burke AK, Huang Y, Mann JJ. CSF monoamine metabolites and lethality of suicide attempts in depressed patients with alcohol dependence. *Eur. Neuropsychopharmacol.* 2007;17:12-15.

[20] Moeller FG, Steinberg JL, Petty F, Fulton M, Cherek DR, Kramer G, Garver DL. Serotonin and impulsive/aggressive behavior in cocaine dependent subjects. Prog. Neuropsychopharmacol. *Biol. Psychiatry* 1994;18:1027–35.

[21] Soloff PH, Lynch KG, Moss HB. Serotonin, impulsivity, and alcohol use disorders in the older adolescent: a psychobiological study. *Alcohol Clin. Exp. Res.* 2000;24:1609–19.

[22] Apter A, Laufer N, Bar-Sever M, Har-Even D, Ofek H, Weizman A. Serum cholesterol, suicidal tendencies, impulsivity, aggression, and depression in adolescent psychiatric inpatients. *Biol. Psychiatry* 1999;46:532–41.

[23] Kaplan JR, Muldoon MF, Manuck SB, Mann JJ. Assessing the observed relationship between low cholesterol and violence-related mortality: implications for suicide risk. In: Stoff DM, Mann JJ, eds. The neurobiology of suicide: From the bench to the clinic. *Ann. NY Acad. Sci.* 1997;836:57–80.

[24] Roy A, Gonzalez B, Marcus A., Berman J. Serum cholesterol, suicidal behavior and impulsivity in cocaine-dependent patients. *Psychiatry Res.* 2001;101:243–7.

PART FIVE: ACKNOWLEDGMENTS

In: Alcohol-Related Cognitive Disorders   ISBN: 978-1-60741-730-9
Editors: L. Sher, I. Kandel, J. Merrick pp. 339-341   © 2009 Nova Science Publishers, Inc.

Chapter 24

ABOUT THE AUTHORS

Taylor W Acee, MA, Educational Psychology, University of Texas at Austin Austin, Texas, 78701 USA. E-mail: aceet@mail.utexas.edu

Marsha E Bates, PhD, Cognitive Neuroscience Laboratory, Center of Alcohol Studies. Rutgers - The State University of New Jersey, 607 Allison Road, Piscataway, New Jersey, 08854 USA. E-mail: mebates@rutgers.edu

Heather Becker, PhD, University of Texas at Austin School of Nursing, 1700 Red River, Austin, Texas, 78701 USA. E-mail: hbecker@mail.nur.utexas.edu

Matthias Brand, PhD, Physiological Psychology, University of Bielefeld, POBox 10 01 31, D-33501 Bielefeld, Germany. E-mail: m.brand@uni-bielefeld.de

Larry Burd, PhD, North Dakota Fetal Alcohol Syndrome Center, Department of Pediatrics, University of North Dakota School of Medicine and Health Sciences, 501 N Columbia Road Stop 9037, Grand Forks, North Dakota, 58202-9037 USA. E-mail: laburd@medicine.nodak.edu

Christine Carlson, BS, MS-1, Department of Pediatrics, University of North Dakota School of Medicine and Health Sciences, 501 N Columbia Road Stop 9037, Grand Forks, North Dakota, 58202-9037 USA. E-mail: treykenneth@yahoo.com

Christine Cronk, ScD, Department of Pediatrics, Medical College of Wisconsin, Translational and Biomedical Research Center Office 2490, Children's Research Institute, PO Box 26509, 8701 Watertown Plank Road, Milwaukee, Wisconsin, 53226-4801 USA. E-mail: ccronk@mcw.edu

Irene Daum, PhD, Institute of Cognitive Neuroscience, Dept Neuropsychology, GAFO 05/616, Ruhr-University of Bochum, 44780 Bochum, Germany. E-mail: irene.daum@ruhr-uni-bochum.de

Carol L Delville, MSN, University of Texas at Austin School of Nursing, 1700 Red River, Austin, Texas, 78701 USA. E-mail: cdelville@mail.utexas.edu

Ramani Durvasula, PhD, California State University, King Hall – Psychology, 5151 State University Drive, Los Angeles, Clifornia, 90032, USA. E-mail: rdurvas@calstatela.edu

Mark T Fillmore, PhD, Department of Psychology, University of Kentucky, Lexington, Kentucky, 40506-0044 USA. E-mail: fillmore@uky.edu

Frances Finnigan, PhD, Department of Psychology, Glasgow Caledonian University, Cowcaddens Road, Glasgow, G4 0BA, United Kingdom. E-mail: f.finnigan@gcal.ac.uk

Karen E. Grattan-Miscio, PhD, Department of Social Science, Canadore College, 100 College Dr., North Bay, ON P1B 8L7 Canada. E-mail: kegm@sympatico.ca

Peter G Hepper, BSc, PhD, FBPsS, CPsychol, School of Psychology, Queen's University Belfast, Belfast BT7 1NN United Kingdom. E-mail: p.hepper@ qub.ac.uk

Isack Kandel, MA, PhD, Faculty of Social Sciences, Department of Behavioral Sciences, Academic College of Judea and Samaria, Ariel, Israel. E-mail: kandelii@zahav.net.il

Elisabeth Kapaki, MD, Department of Neurology, Eginition Hospital, 74 Vas Sophias Ave, 11528 Athens, Greece. E-mail: ekapaki@med.uoa.gr

Jacob Kerbeshian, MD, Department of Neuroscience, University of North Dakota School of Medicine and Health Sciences, 501 N Columbia Road Stop 9037, Grand Forks, ND 58202-9037 USA and Department of Pediatrics, Altru Health System, 1200 S. Columbia Road, Grand Forks, North Dakota, 58206-6002 USA. E-mail: jkerbeshian@altru.org

Gideon Koren, MD, FRCPC, Motherisk Program, The Hospital for Sick Children, 555 University Ave, Toronto M5G 1X8 Canada. E-mail: gidiup_2000@yahoo.com

Ioannis Liappas, MD, Department of Psychiatry, Eginition Hospital, 74 Vas Sophias Ave, 11528 Athens, Greece. E-mail: iliappas@eginitio.uoa.gr

Krisztina L Malisza, PhD, Institute for Biodiagnostics, MR Research and Development, 435 Ellice Avenue, Winnipeg, MB, R3B 1Y6 Canada. E-mail: kris.malisza@nrc-cnrc.gc.ca

Josef Marksteiner, MD, Department of Psychiatry and Psychotherapy, Landeskrankenhaus Klagenfurt, St. Veiterstrasse 47, A-9020 Klagenfurt, Austria. E-mail: josef.marksteiner@kabeg.at

Graham J McDougall Jr, RN, PhD, FAAn, University of Texas at Austin School of Nursing, 1700 Red River, Austin, Texas, 78701, USA. E-mail: gmcdougall@mail.nur.utexas.edu

Christie L McGee, MS, San Diego State University/University of California-San Diego Joint Doctoral Program in Clinical Psychology, 6363 Alvarado Ct. #200, San Diego, California, 92120 USA. E-mail: cmcgee@projects.sdsu.edu

Joav Merrick, MD, MMedSci, DMSci, Division for Mental Retardation, Ministry of Social Affairs, POBox 1260, IL-91012 Jerusalem, Israel. E-mail: jmerrick@zahav.net.il

Efrat Merrick-Kenig, MD, National Institute of Child Health and Human Development, Office of the Medical Director, Division for Mental Retardation, Ministry of Social Affairs, POBox 1260, IL-91012 Jerusalem, Israel. E-mail: efratmerrick@gmail.com

Miriam Z Mintzer, Department of Psychiatry and Behavioral Sciences, Behavioral Biology Research Center, Johns Hopkins University School of Medicine, 5510 Nathan Shock Drive, Baltimore, Maryland, 21224 USA. E-mail: mmintzer@jhmi.edu

Mohammed Morad, MD, Clalit Health Services Shatal Clinic, Rehov Similanski 79, IL-84223 Beer Sheva, Israel. E-mail: moradmo@clalit.org.il

Kelly Nash, The Hospital for Sick Children, 555 University Ave, Toronto, ON, M5G 1X8 Canada. E-mail: knash@oise.utoronto.ca

Mary J O'Connor, PhD, ABPP, Semel Institute for Neuroscience and Human Behavior, 760 Westwood Plaza, Rm. 58-239A, Los Angeles, Califiornia, 90024, USA. E-mail: BPaley@mednet.ucla.edu

Blair Paley, PhD, UCLA Semel Institute for Neuroscience and Human Behavior, 760 Westwood Plaza, Rm. 58-239A, Los Angeles, California, 90024 USA. E-mail: BPaley@mednet.ucla.edu

George P Paraskevas, MD, Department of Neurology, Eginition Hospital, 74 Vas. Sophias Ave, 11528 Athens, Greece. E-mail: ekapaki@med.uoa.gr

Carmen Rasmussen, PhD, Department of Pediatrics, University of Alberta, 137 Glenrose Rehabilitation Hospital, 10230-111 Avenue, Edmonton, Alberta, T5G 0B7 Canada. E-mail: carmen@ualberta.ca

Suchismita Ray, PhD, Center of Alcohol Studies. Rutgers, The State University of New Jersey, 607 Allison Road, Piscataway, New Jersey , 08854 USA. E-mail: shmita@rci.rutgers.edu

Edward Riley, PhD, Center for Behavioral Teratology, 6363 Alvarado Ct, #209, San Diego, California, 92120, USA. E-mail: eriley@mail.sdsu.edu

Joanne Rovet, PhD, Department of Psychology, The Hospital for Sick Children, 555 University Ave, Toronto, ON, M5G 1X8 Canada. E-mail: joan.rovet@sickkids.ca

Daniela Schulze, PhD, Trainee Clinical Psychologist, NHS Tayside Drug Problem Service, Constitution House, 55 Constitution Road, Dundee, DD1 1LB United Kingdom. E-mail. daniela.schulze@nhs.net

Erin Sheard, PhD, Department of Psychology, The Hospital for Sick Children, 555 University Ave, Toronto, M5G 1X8 Canada. E-mail: erin.sheard@sickkids.ca

Leo Sher, MD, Division of Molecular Imaging and Neuropathology, Department of Psychiatry, Columbia University, 1051 Riverside Drive, Suite 2917, Box 42, New York, NY 10032 USA. E-mail: LS2003@columbia.edu

Jonathan Smallwood, BA Hons, PhD, Department of Psychology, University of Aberdeen, William Guild Building Room F10, Aberdeen, Scotland, United Kingdom. E-mail: j.smallwood@abdn.co.uk

Ilia Theotoka, PhD, Department of Psychiatry, Eginition Hospital, 74,Vas Sophias Ave, 11528 Athens, Greece. E-mail: iliatheotoka@mail.gr

Jennifer Uekermann, PhD, Institute of Cognitive Neuroscience, Dept Neuropsychology, GAFO 05/607, Ruhr-University of Bochum, 44780 Bochum, Germany. E-mail: Jennifer.Uekermann@ruhr-uni-bochum.de

Gideon Vardi, MD, MPH, Zussman Child Development Center, Soroka University Medical Center , Ben Gurion University of the Negev, POB 151, IL-84101 Beer-Sheva, Israel. E-mail: gideonva@gmail.com

Philip W Vaughan, MA, University of Texas at Austin School of Nursing, 1700 Red River, Austin, Texas, 78701 USA. E-mail: p_v@mail.utexas.edu

Joris C Verster, PhD, University of Utrecht, Utrecht Institute for Pharmaceutical Sciences, Department of Psychopharmacology, PO Box 80082, 3508 TB Utrecht, the Netherlands. E-mail: j.c.verster@uu.nl

Elisabeth M Weiss, MD, PhD, Department of General Psychiatry, Anichstrasse 35, A-6020 Innsbruck, Austria. E-mail: elisabeth.weiss@i-med.ac.at

Marianne Weiss, DNSc, RN, University College of Nursing PO Box 1881 Milwaukee, Wisconsin, 53201-1881 USA. E-mail: marianne.weiss@marquette.edu

Katy Wyper, BSc, Department of Educational Psychology, University of Alberta, Edmonton, Alberta, T5G 0B7 Canada. E-mail: kwyper@ualberta.ca

In: Alcohol-Related Cognitive Disorders
Editors: L. Sher, I. Kandel, J. Merrick pp. 343

ISBN: 978-1-60741-730-9
© 2009 Nova Science Publishers, Inc.

Chapter 25

ABOUT THE EDITORS

Leo Sher, MD is a psychiatrist with a background in internal medicine. His areas of research and clinical expertise include neurobiology, diagnosis, and treatment of mood, anxiety, and personality disorders, alcoholism, and suicidal behavior. He is Associate Clinical Professor of Psychiatry at Columbia University and Research Psychiatrist in the Division of Molecular Imaging and Neuropathology at the New York State Psychiatric Institute in New York City. He has authored more than 250 scientific publications, is a reviewer for numerous medical journals, the recipient of several awards and the first researcher in North America who introduced the use of the combined dexamethasone suppression/corticotropin-releasing hormone stimulation test for psychiatric purposes. E-mail: LS2003@columbia.edu Website: http://asp.cumc.columbia.edu/facdb/profile_list.asp?uni=ls2003andDepAffil=Psychiatry

Isack Kandel, MA, PhD, is senior lecturer (assistant professor) at the Faculty of Social Sciences, Department of Behavioral Sciences, Ariel University Center of Samaria, Ariel. During the period 1985-93 he served as the director of the Division for Mental Retardation, Ministry of Social Affairs, Jerusalem, Israel. Several books and numerous other publications in the areas of rehabilitation, disability, health and intellectual disability. E-mail: kandelii@zahav.net.il

Joav Merrick, MD, MMedSci, DMSc, is professor of pediatrics, child health and human development affiliated with Kentucky Children's Hospital, University of Kentucky, Lexington, United States and the Zusman Child Development Center, Division of Pediatrics, Soroka University Medical Center, Ben Gurion University, Beer-Sheva, Israel, the medical director of the Division for Mental Retardation, Ministry of Social Affairs, Jerusalem, the founder and director of the National Institute of Child Health and Human Development in Israel. Numerous publications in the field of pediatrics, child health and human development, rehabilitation, intellectual disability, disability, health, welfare, abuse, advocacy, quality of life and prevention. Received the Peter Sabroe Child Award for outstanding work on behalf of Danish Children in 1985 and the International LEGO-Prize ("The Children's Nobel Prize") for an extraordinary contribution towards improvement in child welfare and well-being in 1987. E-Mail: jmerrick@internet-zahav.net; Website: www.nichd-israel.com; Home-page: http://jmerrick50.googlepages.com/home

In: Alcohol-Related Cognitive Disorders   ISBN: 978-1-60741-730-9
Editors: L. Sher, I. Kandel, J. Merrick pp. 345-347   © 2009 Nova Science Publishers, Inc.

Chapter 26

ABOUT THE NATIONAL INSTITUTE OF CHILD HEALTH AND HUMAN DEVELOPMENT IN ISRAEL

The National Institute of Child Health and Human Development (NICHD) in Israel was established in 1998 as a virtual institute under the auspicies of the Medical Director, Ministry of Social Affairs and Social Services in order to function as the research arm for the Office of the Medical Director, but also as a national research and policy institute on child health and human development.

In 1998 the National Council for Child Health and Pediatrics, Ministry of Health and in 1999 the Director General and Deputy Director General of the Ministry of Health endorsed the establishment of the NICHD.

MISSION

The mission of a National Institute for Child Health and Human Development in Israel is to provide an academic focal point for the scholarly interdisciplinary study of child life, health, public health, welfare, disability, rehabilitation, intellectual disability and related aspects of human development. This mission includes research, teaching, clinical work, information and public service activities in the field of child health and human development. The Institute should eventually be the obvious resource to turn to for professionals, politicians, the general public and the media concerned with the care of children, the disabled and the intellectually disabled in our society.

SERVICE AND ACADEMIC ACTIVITIES

Over the years many activities became focused in the south of Israel due to collaboration with various professionals at the Faculty of Health Sciences (FOHS) at the Ben Gurion University of the Negev (BGU). Since 2000 an affiliation with the Zusman Child Development Center at the Pediatric Division of Soroka University Medical Center has resulted in collaboration around the establishment of the Down Syndrome Clinic at that center. From 2002 a full course on "Disability" was established at the Recanati School for

Allied Professions in the Community, FOHS, BGU and seminars for specialists in family medicine. From 2005 collaboration was started with the Primary Care Unit of the faculty and disability became part of the master of public health course on "children and society". From the academic year 2005-2006 a one semester course on "aging with disability" was started as part of the master of science program in gerontology in collaboration with the Center for Multidisciplinary Research in Aging. In 2006 we also started the annual World Down Syndrome Day as a seminar day with both academic and social components in collaboration with international organizations.

Academic activity has also taken place within the Ministry of Social Affairs for medical and allied health professionals in collaborations with most universities in Israel and relevant academic colleges.

RESEARCH ACTIVITIES

The affiliated (volunteer) staff has over the years published work from projects and research activities in this national and international collaboration (about 1,000 publications since 1998). In the year 2000 the International Journal of Adolescent Medicine and Health and in 2005 the International Journal on Disability and Human development of Freund Publishing House (London and Tel Aviv), in the year 2003 the TSW-Child Health and Human Development, in 2006 the TSW-Holistic Health and Medicine of the Scientific World Journal (New York and Kirkkonummi, Finland) and in 2008 the International Journal of Child Health and Human Development, International Journal of Child and Adolescent Health and the Journal of Pain Management all published by Nova Science, New York), all peer-reviewed international journals have been affiliated with the National Institute of Child Health and Human Development.

This collaboration with seven international journals has resulted in further projects worldwide and the possibility to publish the research in special peer-reviewed issues or other publications.

NATIONAL COLLABORATIONS

Nationally the NICHD works in collaboration with the Faculty of Health Sciences, Ben Gurion University of the Negev; Department of Physical Therapy, Sackler School of Medicine, Tel Aviv University; Autism Center, Assaf HaRofeh Medical Center; National Rett and PKU Centers at Chaim Sheba Medical Center, Tel HaShomer; Department of Physiotherapy, Haifa University; Department of Education, Bar Ilan University, Ramat Gan, Faculty of Social Sciences and Health Sciences; College of Judea and Samaria in Ariel and recently also collaborations has been established with the Division of Pediatrics at Hadassah, Center for Pediatric Chronic Illness, Har HaZofim in Jerusalem.

INTERNATIONAL COLLABORATIONS

Internationally with the Department of Disability and Human Development, College of Applied Health Sciences, University of Illinois at Chicago; Strong Center for Developmental Disabilities, Golisano Children's Hospital at Strong, University of Rochester School of Medicine and Dentistry, New York; Centre on Intellectual Disabilities, University of Albany, New York; Centre for Chronic Disease Prevention and Control, Health Canada, Ottawa; Chandler Medical Center and Children's Hospital, Kentucky Children's Hospital, Section of Adolescent Medicine, University of Kentucky, Lexington; Chronic Disease Prevention and Control Research Center, Baylor College of Medicine, Houston, Texas; Division of Neuroscience, Department of Psychiatry, Columbia University, New York; Institute for the Study of Disadvantage and Disability, Atlanta; Center for Autism and Related Disorders, Department Psychiatry, Children's Hospital Boston, Boston; Department of Paediatrics, Child Health and Adolescent Medicine, Children's Hospital at Westmead, Westmead, Australia; International Centre for the Study of Occupational and Mental Health, Dusseldorf, Germany; Centre for Advanced Studies in Nursing, Department of General Practice and Primary Care, University of Aberdeen, Aberdeen,United Kingdom; Quality of Life Research Center, Copenhagen, Denmark; Nordic School of Public Health, Gottenburg, Sweden, Scandinavian Institute of Quality of Working Life, Oslo, Norway; Centre for Quality of Life of the Hong Kong Institue of Asia-Pacific Studies and School of Social Work, Chinese University, Hong Kong.

CONTACT PERSON

Joav Merrick, MD, MMedSci, DMSc
Office of the Medical Director, Division for Mental Retardation, Ministry of Social Affairs and Social Services, POB 1260, IL-91012 Jerusalem, Israel
E-mail: jmerrick@zahav.net.il
Website: www.nichd-israel.com

INDEX

D

G

H

I

M

O

P

Q

R

service provider, 104
services, iv, 10, 11, 30, 83, 84, 88, 89, 102, 104, 126, 326
SES, 74, 95, 127, 128, 307
severity, 31, 47, 60, 72, 99, 103, 113, 116, 117, 118, 119, 144, 147, 148, 225, 227, 236, 238, 257, 293, 300, 301, 309, 313
sex, 40, 41, 47, 73, 79, 81, 102, 129, 132, 140, 207, 230, 267, 269, 270, 293, 294, 298, 300
sex differences, 207, 230, 293, 294
sex offenders, 132
sexual abuse, 126, 326
sexual activity, 136
sexual behavior, xi, xvi, 11, 31, 79, 101, 125, 126, 129, 132, 137, 319, 322, 325
sexual intercourse, 134
sexual offences, 324
sexual offending, 328
sexual risk behavior, 299
sexuality, xvi, 46, 319, 325
SGA, x, 67
shape, 7, 55, 133, 141, 328
sheep, 86
Sher, Leo, 341
short period, 212
short term memory, 323
short-term, 23, 159, 253, 261, 302, 303
short-term memory, 23, 159, 261, 302, 303
sibling, 121, 129
siblings, 112, 122
side effects, 104
sign, 301
signal transduction, 31
signaling, 192, 272
signals, 32, 165, 229
signs, 1, 71, 87, 112, 117, 237, 250, 254, 257, 258, 266, 294, 320
simulation, 52, 226
single photon emission computed tomography (SPECT), ix, 29, 32, 36, 37, 39, 40, 46, 48, 53, 54, 237, 241
sites, 75, 279
skills, xi, xiii, 9, 10, 11, 14, 15, 24, 26, 30, 71, 74, 81, 91, 92, 95, 100, 103, 104, 107, 109, 115, 130, 131, 135, 143, 149, 150, 155, 171, 172, 200, 209, 221, 223, 226, 227, 228, 230, 238, 242, 288, 302, 322, 323
sleep, 38, 58, 99, 117, 150, 215, 220, 224, 225, 226
sleep disorders, 117
sleeping problems, 99
small palpebral fissures, 91, 144
smoking, 80, 106, 108, 112, 113, 134
smooth philtrum, 6, 91, 144

sobriety, ix, 200, 293
social behavior, ix, 65, 106, 107, 139, 155, 208, 323, 324
social behaviour, 150
social cognition, xiv, 96, 148, 150, 235, 236, 238, 239, 240
social competence, 97, 240
social context, 9, 133, 151
social costs, 1
social cues, 9, 14, 130, 150, 322, 323
Social deficits, 105, 130
social development, xvi, 319, 324
social drinkers, xii, xiii, 169, 174, 188, 191, 192, 195, 199, 200, 207, 211, 212, 218, 244, 289, 296, 303
social drinking, 93, 171, 180, 208
social impairment, 12, 95, 130
social information processing, 105
social isolation, 289
social learning, 92
social network, 103
social norms, 151
social perception, 71
social phobia, 274
social problems, 58, 96, 98, 102, 105, 239
social responsibility, 95
social rules, 104
social services, 30, 102, 104
Social Services, 343, 345
social situations, 92, 105
social skills, xi, 9, 24, 26, 30, 91, 95, 103, 107, 109, 115, 130, 135, 155, 322
social skills training, 26, 109
social stress, 118
social withdrawal, 98, 150
socialization, 9, 95, 130, 150
socioeconomic, xvi, 74, 79, 83, 97, 101, 127, 299, 310
socioeconomic background, 101
socioeconomic status, xvi, 74, 79, 83, 97, 101, 127, 299, 310
socioemotional, xi, 143, 144, 145, 148, 150, 153, 156
Socioemotional functioning, 150, 154
sociology, 333
soft drinks, 226
software, 70, 76, 202
solutions, 205
somatic complaints, 311
somatosensory, 50
sorption, 112
South Africa, 22, 70, 72, 78, 85, 88, 112, 320

T

vascular disease, 270
ventral striatum, 96, 240
ventral tegmentum, 240
ventricles, 36, 264
ventromedial prefrontal cortex, 132
verbal and nonverbal fluency, 8
verbal fluency, 130, 219, 248, 254, 255, 257
verbal reasoning, 8, 306
Vermont, 26, 107
veterans, 274, 314
victimization, 10
victims, 126, 138, 325
Victoria, 2, 139, 245
Vineland Adaptive Behavior Scales, 9, 17, 26, 95
violence, 1, 102, 126, 136, 306, 310, 311, 324, 331, 334
violent, 131, 136, 140, 331, 332, 333
violent behavior, 136
violent crime, 331
violent crimes, 331
violent offences, 131
viral infection, 307
virus, xvi, 299, 301, 304, 316, 317
virus infection, 316
vision, 115, 202
visual acuity, 85
visual attention, 168, 173, 305
visual environment, 167
visual memory, 284, 308
visual motor integration, 9, 27
visual perception, 9, 32, 46
visual processing, 48
visual stimuli, 59
visualization, 294, 298
visual-motor deficits, 10
Visual-spatial, 9
Visual-spatial problems, 9
visuospatial, 131, 155, 213, 292, 293, 294, 302, 303, 308, 309
visuospatial function, 131, 292, 302, 308
visuo-spatial memory deficits, 149
vitamin B1, 250
vitamin B1 (thiamine) deficiency, 250
vitamins, 291
vodka, 61, 180, 227
voice, 241
voiding, 127
vulnerability, xiv, 102, 137, 142, 149, 169, 235, 236, 238, 250, 251, 256, 292, 300, 306, 307, 326

W

Wales, 180

walking, 15
war, 222
warrants, 303
water, 61, 149, 155, 180, 203, 264
water maze, 149
WCST, 41, 130, 131
wealth, xii, 159, 170
weapons, 134
Wechsler Adult Intelligence Scale (WAIS), 308
Wechsler Individual Achievement Test, 17, 26
Wechsler Intelligence Scale, 17, 18, 26
Wechsler Intelligence Scale for Children, 17, 18, 26
Wechsler Memory Scale, 18
weight management, 279
Weinberg, 141, 154
welfare, 341, 343
well-being, 57, 341
Wernicke-Korsakoff syndrome, 1, 259, 264, 294, 298, 302
Western Cape Province, 88, 320
Western Europe, 311
white blood cells, 307
white matter, 1, 7, 36, 237, 291, 293, 295, 300, 302, 303, 304
William Hogarth (London, 1697 - 1764), 320
Williams syndrome, 6
wine, 61, 62, 63, 281, 319, 332
winning, 254
Wisconsin, x, 18, 27, 41, 67, 68, 76, 79, 80, 81, 85, 88, 130, 149, 163, 244, 247, 254, 255, 308, 337, 339
Wisconsin Card Sorting Test, 18, 27, 130, 163, 244, 247, 254, 255, 308
Wisconsin Fetal Alcohol Syndrome Screening Project, 79, 81, 88
withdrawal, 1, 10, 98, 150, 263, 291
withdrawal from school, 10
withdrawal syndromes, 1
women, 57, 62, 63, 68, 73, 74, 77, 79, 85, 93, 103, 104, 111, 117, 121, 133, 173, 193, 197, 207, 227, 230, 238, 241, 244, 246, 247, 278, 282, 286, 289, 293, 294, 297, 298, 300, 311, 319, 325, 326, 327
word comprehension, 9, 323
word frequency, 194, 195
word naming, 149
word recognition, 197, 218
workers, 228
working memory, x, xiii, xv, 8, 20, 22, 29, 30, 31, 36, 37, 40, 41, 46, 47, 48, 51, 52, 54, 131, 137, 145, 148, 152, 154, 162, 174, 196, 211, 212, 213, 216, 218, 223, 224, 239, 246, 253, 254, 256, 260, 261, 262, 266, 291, 292, 296, 302, 303, 305, 306, 315